Physiotherapy: A Psychosocial Approach

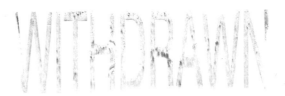

For Butterworth-Heinemann:

Senior Commissioning Editor: Heidi Allen
Development Editor: Robert Edwards
Project Manager: Gail Wright
Senior Designer: George Ajayi

Physiotherapy: A Psychosocial Approach

Edited by

Sally French BSc MSc(Psych) MSc(Soc) PhD MCSP DipTP

Senior Lecturer, Department of Allied Health Professions, University of Hertfordshire, Hatfield, UK

Julius Sim BA MSc(Soc) MSc(Stat) PhD FSS

Professor, Department of Physiotherapy Studies and Primary Care Sciences Research Centre, Keele University, Keele, UK

THIRD EDITION

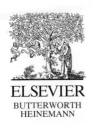

ELSEVIER
BUTTERWORTH
HEINEMANN

EDINBURGH LONDON NEW YORK OXFORD PHILADELPHIA ST LOUIS SYDNEY TORONTO 2004

BUTTERWORTH-HEINEMANN
An imprint of Elsevier Limited

First edition 1992
Second edition 1997
Third edition 2004
  Reprinted 2005

ISBN 0 7506 5329 9

British Library Cataloguing in Publication Data
A catalogue record for this book is available from the British Library

Library of Congress Cataloging in Publication Data
A catalog record for this book is available from the Library of Congress

Note
Medical knowledge is constantly changing. Standard safety precautions must be
followed, but as new research and clinical experience broaden our knowledge,
changes in treatment and drug therapy may become necessary or appropriate.
Readers are advised to check the most current product information provided by
the manufacturer of each drug to be administered to verify the recommended
dose, the method and duration of administration, and contraindications. It is the
responsibility of the practitioner, relying on experience and knowledge of the
patient, to determine dosages and the best treatment for each individual patient.
Neither the Publisher nor the editors or contributors will be liable for any loss
or damage of any nature occasioned to or suffered by any person acting or
refraining from acting as a result of reliance on the material contained in this
publication.

The Publisher

ELSEVIER your source for books,
journals and multimedia
in the health sciences
www.elsevierhealth.com

Working together to grow
libraries in developing countries
www.elsevier.com | www.bookaid.org | www.sabre.org
ELSEVIER   BOOK AID International   Sabre Foundation

The
publisher's
policy is to use
paper manufactured
from sustainable forests

Printed in China

Contents

Contributors

Nicola Adams BSc(Hons) PhD MCSP CPsychol
Reader in Health and Social Care, Centre for Research in Health Care, Faculty of Health and Applied Social Sciences, Liverpool John Moores University, Liverpool, UK

Karl Atkin BA(Hons) DPhil
Director for the Centre for Research in Primary Care, and Senior Lecturer in Primary Care and Ethnicity, Centre for Research in Primary Care, University of Leeds, Leeds, UK

Sally French BSc MSc(Psych) MSc(Soc) PhD MCSP DipTP
Senior Lecturer, Department of Allied Health Professions, University of Hertfordshire, Hatfield, UK

Paul Kingston MA PhD CertEd RNMH RMN RNT
Professor of Primary Healthcare, School of Health, University of Wolverhampton, Wolverhampton, UK

Mary F. McAteer MEd PhD MCSP MICSP DipTP
Senior Lecturer, School of Physiotherapy, University College Dublin, Dublin, Ireland

Jane S. Owen Hutchinson BA MA MA(Ed) CertEd CertHlthEd DipRehabCouns MCSP
Manager, Physiotherapy Support Services, Royal National Institute for the Blind, London, UK

Tamar Pincus BSc MSc MPhil PhD
Senior Lecturer, Department of Psychology, Royal Holloway, University of London, London, UK

Frances Reynolds BSc DipPsychCouns PhD
Senior Lecturer in Psychology, Department of Health and Social Care, Brunel University, London, UK

Helen Roberts BA(Hons) Maîtrise DPhil
Professor of Child Health, Child Health Research and Policy Unit, City University, London, UK

Julius Sim BA MSc(Soc) MSc(Stat) PhD FSS
Professor, Department of Physiotherapy Studies and Primary Care Sciences Research Centre, Keele University, Keele, UK

Marion V. Smith BA(Hons) MPhil PhD
Lecturer, School of Social Relations, Keele University, Keele, UK

John Swain BSc PGCE MSc PhD
Professor of Disability and Inclusion, School of Health, Community and Education Studies, University of Northumbria, Newcastle-upon-Tyne, UK

Janine Talley BSc PhD PGCE
Staff Tutor, School of Health and Social Welfare, Open University, Milton Keynes, UK

Ayesha Vernon BA PhD
Freelance Disability Trainer, Leicester, UK

Jackie Waterfield MSc PGCert GradDipPhys MCSP ILTM
Senior Lecturer, Department of Physiotherapy Studies, Keele University, Keele, UK

Christopher A. Whittaker MEd DAES ACP TCert
Honorary Fellow, School of Education, University of Durham, Durham, UK

Chapter 1

Introduction

Sally French and Julius Sim

1.1 THE NEED FOR A PSYCHOSOCIAL PERSPECTIVE

In recent years there has been an increasing interest in, and concern for, the psychological, sociological, cultural and ethical aspects of health, illness, impairment and disability. It is arguable that since the first edition of this book, in 1992, these concerns have increased across all health care professions, including physiotherapy. This is owing, at least in part, to the changing ways in which health and social care are practised and delivered. Policy initiatives in the UK – such as the NHS and Community Care Act (1990), the Direct Payment Act (1996), the Carers (Recognition and Services) Act (1996) and the Human Rights Act (1998) – have brought about profound changes both in the way health and social care are delivered and in the relationship between professionals and their patients and clients. Users of health and social care have greater voice and influence than they had in the past, and physiotherapists are no longer trusted on the basis of their professional standing alone. With growth in information technology, such as the internet, many more people now have access to medical information, and legislation, such as the Disability Discrimination Act 1995, has translated many 'needs' – for example accessible health care facilities – into 'rights' (Brothers et al 2002). Increasingly, the development of physiotherapy knowledge and the practice of physiotherapy can be seen to be subject to, and often constrained by, a variety of professional, policy and regulatory structures (Sim & Richardson 2004). All of these changes have added to the importance of physiotherapists becoming fully aware of the social, psychological, ethical, philosophical and cultural issues that underpin and influence their work.

Whereas, in the past, the focus of physiotherapy education was on bio-medical issues and on learning practical skills and techniques, it is now recognized that these aspects, however important they may be in them-selves, are insufficient for the effective practice of physiotherapy. Illness, for example, also has psychological, social and cultural aspects, and whether or not someone adheres to physiotherapy advice will depend on a range of factors including the person's lifestyle and social and material resources. The origin, severity and chronicity of pain have been shown to relate strongly to psychosocial factors, and may have little relationship to the 'objective' biological features of a condition (Waddell & Waddell 2000, Pincus et al 2002). It can no longer be assumed that disabled people want to be 'cured' or made 'normal', and differences of culture and eth-nicity influence the ways in which illness is perceived, experienced and managed. In the UK, these issues are reflected in the *Curriculum Frame-work of the Chartered Society of Physiotherapy*, where it is stated that phys-iotherapy 'uses physical approaches to promote, maintain and restore physical, psychological and social well-being, taking account of variations in health status' (Chartered Society of Physiotherapy 2002a: 19), and where it is argued that graduating physiotherapists need to be competent in:

- Optimizing health and well-being
- Promoting equality
- Seeking evidence and applying new knowledge
- Responding to changing demands
- Working in partnership with patients and clients
- Understanding social theory
- Understanding relevant social policy and legislation
- Making paramount patient/client experience.

With changes in social policy, such as the closure of long-stay institu-tions for people with learning disabilities and mental health problems, the work of physiotherapists has increasingly become based in the com-munity where therapists are likely to be more involved with the every-day lives of their patients and clients and those who assist them. Talking of physiotherapy with people with learning difficulties, Standing (1999: 259) states:

> Traditional techniques and skills are not always appropriate … Working in partnership with people with learning disabilities demands of therap-ists far more than learning new techniques and treatment, it involves a willingness and capacity to respond imaginatively to every person as a unique individual and to help and support each person in the achieve-ment of his or her own aspirations and desired lifestyle.

Psychosocial issues thus form the context in which physiotherapy is practised but, more than that, these issues have a profound impact on physiotherapy practice itself by, for example, explaining differences in physical sensations such as pain, and exploring the dynamics of the client–professional relationship. These and other issues are examined in this new edition with reference to particular theoretical models and understandings from psychology, sociology and philosophy, related to health and illness. The emerging discipline of disability studies is also explored, as well as insights from the social policy literature.

1.2 STRUCTURE OF THE BOOK

The remainder of this book is divided into four sections. The first section, 'The Nature of Health and Illness', investigates the broad social influences on health and illness in society today. This section explores the ways in which broad societal factors impact on health and illness to produce inequalities in health status throughout life. The very meaning of health and illness is examined, as well as the ways in which people behave when unwell and how this is influenced by their beliefs and past experiences.

The second section, 'The Psychosocial Context of Health and Illness', examines the impact of social and psychological factors on health, illness and development. Psychological and sociological factors influencing pain are explored, as well as the influence of ethnicity, sex and gender on health status and experience. Aspects of the subjective experience of illness, and the specific experience of loss, are explored. The psychosocial development of the child is also examined to provide physiotherapists with a detailed understanding of typical child development, and the factors that influence it, when working with children and their carers.

Section 3, 'Patients and Practitioners', explores the relationship and interaction between physiotherapists and their patients and clients. This section examines the ways in which professionals and clients communicate with each other and how their communication is enmeshed within wider social processes. Broad issues of professionalism and power are also explored, as well as the process of ethical decision-making in physiotherapy.

Section 4, 'Psychosocial Aspects of Physiotherapy Care', explores the impact of psychosocial issues on the work of physiotherapists. The challenges posed to physiotherapists by the social model of disability are explored. Particular psychosocial interventions that may be used by physiotherapists, such as counselling skills and behaviour modification, are also covered.

This edition of *Physiotherapy: A Psychosocial Approach* completely updates the second edition and, as with previous editions, aims to provide physiotherapists and physiotherapy students with a comprehensive exploration of psychological and sociological factors as they apply to health, illness, impairment and disability. Such topics range from the minutiae of interpersonal communication to the broad impact of political factors on health status. This third edition introduces new topics of relevance to physiotherapists, and includes many new authors who have knowledge and experience of physiotherapy and physiotherapy education and who are experts in their particular fields. The book is particularly intended for undergraduate physiotherapy students but qualified physiotherapists may also find it useful, as well as other health care professionals. Each chapter is self-contained, though links are made to other chapters where appropriate, and fully referenced. Although the authors are from the UK, and UK terminology has been adopted (e.g. 'physiotherapy' rather than 'physical therapy'), the issues covered in this volume will be of relevance to readers from all countries.

The issues and arguments presented in this volume are not always easy to confront. Health, illness and disability are contested areas, which can be viewed in different ways and which bring to the fore issues of power, suffering, inequality and morality. It is our belief, however, that physiotherapists who are willing to explore and confront these issues will be in a better position to practise in the twenty-first century.

SECTION 1

The nature of health and illness

Chapter **2**

Change, diversity and influences on patterns of health and ill health

Janine Talley

2.1 INTRODUCTION

While death is one of the few certainties of life, when we are going to die, what we will die of, and the health and ill health we will experience during our lifetime are less certain. In exploring patterns of health and ill health we seek answers to fundamental questions. What is the health experience of people today? How does the experience of people living in one place compare with those in another? How does our experience today compare with that of people in the past? How can we improve health both for ourselves and for people in the future? To answer these questions presents many challenges. Most importantly it requires obtaining and analysing contemporary and historical data on patterns of health and ill health and their determinants. Physiotherapists' concern with people's health and well-being makes it necessary for them to understand these broad and complex issues.

2.1.1 SOURCES OF DATA ON PATTERNS OF HEALTH AND ILL HEALTH

The relatively recent development of epidemiology and the introduction of systematic mechanisms for the collection of health-related data on a national scale in many countries has enabled us to gain a much clearer picture of the experience of health and disease than has been available in previous centuries. In Britain, the introduction of the 10-yearly census in 1801 was a major step in the collection of mortality and other health-related data (Gray 2001a). Other important developments arose as a result of social and public health reformers of the Victorian era recognizing the value of data on mortality and morbidity as a basis for action to improve health. The setting up of the General Register Office in 1837 and the appointment of a superintendent of statistics was a key landmark (Department of Health 1998a). This was followed by the medical certification of death in 1838 (compulsory from 1874) and notification of certain infectious diseases in 1889 (Pelling et al 1993, Gray 2001a). In the UK today, death registration, censuses, hospital records, disease notification systems, surveys and other tools generate valuable data on health, mortality and morbidity (Katz 2000).

Due to the difficulty of defining and measuring a concept as subjective as health, proxy measures are more commonly used. These include crude death rates, age-standardized death rates (such as standardized mortality ratios), life expectancy, years of life lost, infant mortality rates (IMRs), deaths from specific causes, physical and physiological measurements (e.g. blood pressure, obesity) and morbidity data. The disability adjusted life year (DALY), developed in the 1990s as a single measure to describe both mortality and morbidity (Gray 2001b, Jelsma et al 2002), combines years of life lost due to premature death with loss of healthy life resulting from disability. A large amount of data for some of these indicators is available for some countries.

While the available data are valuable and relatively reliable, their limitations need to be recognized. Data are only as good as the methods by which they are obtained. If, for example, incorrect data are inserted on to a death certificate, or a mistake in coding made when these data are transferred to the records, inaccuracies will result. Similarly, changes in diagnostic categories and medical nomenclature can cause problems when interpreting data. Terminology causes particular problems (Gray 2001c); for example, what do we mean by 'disability' or 'illness'? How do we define and use concepts such as ethnicity?

Despite the fact that all systems have some limitations, they do nevertheless give us some insight into many aspects of health and disease in the recent past and present. What is more difficult is to build up a picture for those periods and for those parts of the world for which such data are not available. In some countries of the developing world, there are still no official systems of death registration. In situations where relatively comprehensive and reliable data are unavailable, we are dependent on other, more patchy or unreliable sources such as oral history, informal documentary evidence (e.g. family records), artefacts and archaeological remains. In recent years, new technologies have enabled us to extend our understanding of health and ill health in the past. Ground-breaking work has been done on archaeological remains. At the University of Manchester

in England, for example, Egyptian mummies have been investigated using modern techniques such as endoscopy, radiology, fluoroscopy, tomography, stereoscopy, microscopy and immunochemistry.

Since mortality rates do not give an accurate picture of morbidity rates (because many conditions do not lead to an early death), separate assessments of morbidity are sometimes attempted. However, this is fraught with difficulties. Whether someone is dead or alive is clear, but whether someone is ill or well is much less clear. Much ill health goes unreported and unrecorded by official systems, and diagnosing and defining ill health can be problematic. Ill health is a subjective concept. For example, what is perceived as stress by one person may be unproblematic for another.

Nevertheless, despite these limitations we can look back in time and across the world and get some idea of how our contemporary experiences compare to the experiences of others, past and present, and how we can explain the patterns that we find.

2.2 WE'VE NEVER HAD IT SO GOOD … OR HAVE WE?

Looking at available data shows that patterns of health and ill health vary with time and place. One of the most fundamental human concerns is how long we live. For this reason, expectation of life at birth (the average lifespan of a newborn) is often used in comparisons of health experience, and provides a useful measure of health intervention outcomes (Department of Health 2001c). We know that in the UK today most people stand a good chance of living at least 'three score years and ten'. In the year 2000, the expectation of life at birth in the UK was nearly 78 years (Rosenberg 2000). In this respect, it could be argued, we have never had it so good. Since the beginning of the last century death rates have been falling and life expectancy increasing (Department of Health 1998a). For example, the crude death rate in England had fallen from 18 per 1000 in 1896 to 11 per 1000 in 1996 (Department of Health 1998a). Current average life expectancy in the UK is higher than that experienced by many of our ancestors and contemporaries. It has been estimated that in Roman times average life expectancy was 22–24 years (Rosenberg 2000). Even in 1900, world life expectancy at birth was still only 30 years. Life expectancy in low-income countries such as Malawi, Mozambique and Zambia is still currently much lower than that in the UK at just over 37 years in 2000 (Rosenberg 2000).

Rapidly rising life expectancy has also been a trend worldwide. Since the middle of the twentieth century, some parts of the world have seen average life expectancy increase by more than 65% (Gray 2001d). By 1985, world life expectancy had increased to 62 years (Rosenberg 2000). Figures for England over a period of just 14 years between 1984 and 1998 provide a striking illustration of the rate of change, with life expectancy at birth increasing by over 2 years for women and 3 years for men (Department of Health 2001d). Indeed, between 1998 and 2000, life expectancy had increased by 2 years or more in 23 countries (Rosenberg 2000).

It should be noted, though, that one limitation of using life expectancy at birth as a measure is the fact that it is heavily influenced by childhood mortality (Gray 2001d). The negative relationship between expectation of life at birth and infant mortality (so that where childhood mortality is high the expectation of life at birth will be low) conceals the fact that life expectancy for individuals surviving the first few years of life may actually be quite high, and differences narrow when life expectancy at later ages is compared. The IMR provides a better measure than life expectancy of health outcomes in childhood (Department of Health 2001c). It is often used as a general measure of health because the data are more readily available in some countries, and it is strongly correlated with adult mortality (Gray 2001d). But, even if we look separately at IMR, we still find that the UK experience has improved with time and is better than that of many other countries. In the last half of the twentieth century, the UK IMR decreased steadily from 24 per 1000 (Gray 2001d) to fewer than six per 1000 in 1999 (Department of Health 2001c). This compares with 149 per 1000 in Mali and 96 per 1000 in the Central African Republic (1998 figures; Gray 2001d). In general, infant and child mortality has decreased dramatically in developing countries over recent decades (Leon & Walt 2001).

When we do die, in the UK we are most likely to die in old age from degenerative diseases such as ischaemic heart disease, cerebrovascular disease, cancers and respiratory disease (Gray 2001a, 2001d). The first two of these alone account for over a third of all deaths and together they account for almost three-quarters of deaths in the developed world (Gray 2001d). Worldwide, coronary heart disease (CHD) is the leading cause of death (BBC 1998, Gray 2001b) and has been described as a modern epidemic (Le Fanu 1999, Taubes 2001). Most cancer deaths result from cancers of the trachea, bronchus and lung (Gray 2001b). Other important causes of death in developed countries include diabetes, road traffic accidents and liver cirrhosis (Gray 2001d).

Although ischaemic heart disease, cerebrovascular disease, and respiratory infections also feature among the major causes of death for the developing world, other causes of death are a significant problem. Of particular note here are infectious and parasitic diseases, maternal and perinatal conditions, and nutritional deficiencies, which alone caused almost two-thirds of deaths in Africa in 1998 (Gray 2001d). HIV/AIDS, diarrhoeal diseases, childhood diseases (such as measles), tuberculosis and malaria are more important as causes of death in the developing world than in the developed world (Gray 2001b). In the developing world malaria causes 1.1 million deaths a year and is second to tuberculosis as the most serious communicable disease (Gray 2001b).

Using years of life lost as a measure of mortality places greater emphasis on causes affecting younger age groups. In this case, the most important causes of years of potential life lost are road traffic accidents in the developed world and communicable diseases in the developing world (Gray 2001b).

We know that patterns of mortality we see today differ from those in the past. For several million years, our early hunting and gathering ancestors are likely to have had a short life expectancy. For them, death will have occurred most commonly as a result of starvation, accidents during the course of hunting, violence, childbirth and environmental stressors such as exposure (Kiple 1996, Gray 2001e). However, in the 12 000 years or so preceding the twentieth century this pattern appears to have changed. A settled agricultural mode of existence became dominant and infectious disease became the main limiting factor on human survival (Kiple 1996, Gray 2001e). This period saw the emergence of viral and bacterial diseases such as smallpox, tuberculosis, plague, cholera, typhoid and influenza as major threats to survival. Parasites also became an increasing problem (Ortner & Theobald 1993).

Mortality crises have been a common feature of the historical disease pattern. Famines, epidemics and pandemics of diseases such as plague, cholera, smallpox, typhus, dysentery and influenza have swept through past populations claiming millions of lives. Plague has caused many of the most devastating crises (Gray 2001a). Of the infectious diseases, however, it has been argued that tuberculosis has been responsible for the most destruction of life and debilitation overall, due to its large impact over a prolonged period (Webster 1994). The disease has been estimated to have caused millions of deaths in the nineteenth century (Kiple 1996), including at least a quarter of all deaths in Europe in the early nineteenth century (Webster 1994).

In both the developed and developing world, there has been a shift in time from communicable to non-communicable diseases (Leon & Walt 2001). CHD is now the major cause of death worldwide (BBC 1998), though acute infectious diseases have only disappeared as the major killers in countries with high life expectancy, such as the UK, over the last century (Gray 2001b). Three-quarters of the reduction in mortality seen in the period from the mid nineteenth century to 1971 has been attributed to the decline in infectious disease (Gray 2001a). Over a period of just 60 years between 1931 and 1991 the pattern of disease in England changed dramatically with an increase in the proportion of deaths caused by circulatory disease and cancers and a decrease in the proportion caused by respiratory diseases (Jones 2000a). These changes are reflected in the work of physiotherapists.

Up to 17.5% of reduced mortality is suggested to be due to a decline in tuberculosis (Gray 2001a). None the less, in some parts of the world where life expectancy is low, infectious diseases including tuberculosis still remain a serious threat to survival. Tuberculosis alone accounts for approximately 3.2% of deaths in the developing world (Gray 2001b). In the last quarter of the twentieth century, death rates in England also fell for other important causes such as lung cancer (in men), CHD and stroke (Department of Health 1998a). There is debate over the trajectory of progress of CHD deaths, but available evidence on the US pattern shows a steady rise in deaths over the first half of the twentieth century with a steady fall from the 1950s (Le Fanu 1999, Taubes 2001).

The fact that many important diseases have declined should not, however, obscure the fact that old diseases can resurface and new diseases emerge as threats to health. AIDS has emerged as an important cause of death in recent decades, causing 2.6 million deaths in 1999 alone (Gray 2001b). The problem has been particularly acute for the developing world where the majority of those with HIV/AIDS are found (Gray 2001b). Malaria has increased around the world since the 1970s (Gray 2001b) and tuberculosis has notably returned as a threat to health in the developed world over the last few decades.

Overall, though, it might be argued that we have something to celebrate in that we have generally rising life expectancy. But do we? While life may be longer, the problem is that these extra years are not necessarily years of good health (Department of Health 1998a). In the UK, 'healthy life expectancy' has not actually been increasing. We have not added years of life free from ill health, but years with chronic disease and disability. A rise in the proportion of people reporting a limiting long-standing illness (from 15% to 22% since 1975), and a doubling in the proportion reporting illness in the 2 years previous to a recent study (from 9% to 16%), have been reported (Department of Health 1998a).

Morbidity is an enduring fact of life. Data on our ancestors continue to accumulate and show that they too experienced many health problems, including skeletal and dental problems. We know that people today continue to suffer a range of health problems. At the end of the last century, there was little evidence of any reduction in morbidity and disability compared to the previous 10 or 20 years (Department of Health 1998a). The most commonly documented conditions today in the UK are mental health problems, skin disorders, circulatory problems, problems of the digestive system, cancers, musculoskeletal disorders, injuries and respiratory conditions (Gray 2001c). Other conditions such as malaria and HIV/AIDS also cause considerable ill health in the developing world (Gray 2001b).

If we look at the DALY as a combined measure of mortality and morbidity (Gray 2001b) we find that, worldwide, communicable diseases in particular, but also maternal, perinatal and nutritional problems, are the most significant health problems. Lower respiratory infections and diarrhoeal diseases are the top communicable diseases (Gray 2001b).

What data on patterns of health and ill health also reveal is striking variation and inequality in health experience. Although expectation of life in many countries is relatively high and has increased in recent years, this is not universally the case. The UK, for example, does not have the highest life expectancy in the world. In 2000, Andorra, San Marino and Japan had the world's highest life expectancies – respectively 83.5, 81.1 and 80.7 years (Rosenberg 2000). Although in England IMRs have improved over recent years, the rate (5.7 deaths per 1000 births) remains above the European average (Department of Health 2000a, 2001c) at about 2 per 1000 more than best European Union rates of 3.5 per 1000 in Luxembourg and 3.8 per 1000 in Sweden (Department of Health 2001c).

Many countries have low life expectancies, and life expectancies have even decreased in some countries in recent years (BBC 1998, Rosenberg 2000). Between 1998 and 2000, life expectancy fell in 21 countries, for example Mozambique, where it fell from 45.4 to 37.5 years (Rosenberg 2000). AIDS has been identified as the major contributor to falling life

expectancies in African countries (Leon & Walt 2001) and it has been estimated that in some African countries AIDS will reduce life expectancy
from 61 years to 39 years by 2010 (BBC 1998).

2.3 CLASS, GENDER AND ETHNICITY

Reports of generally increasing life expectancy conceal differing rates of
increase. Globally, the gap between the health experiences of the best and
the worst is increasing rather than decreasing. If we look at the associations between patterns of health and a range of variables we find that
health experience varies with factors such as socioeconomic position,
gender, age, ethnicity, place, year of birth, marital status and a range of
other social and physical variables.

Socioeconomic position has been shown to have a particularly strong
association with health status. A range of measures have been used to
determine socioeconomic position, including occupation, education, ownership of assets and measures based on characteristics of residential area
(Department of Health 1998a). International comparisons commonly use
income in the form of gross national product (GNP) per capita (per head)
and development indicators such as literacy, education and calorie supply (Gray 2001f). Worldwide comparisons show a significant health
divide between rich and poor countries. Low-income countries generally
experience lower life expectancy and higher mortality and morbidity
than middle- and high-income countries (Gray 2001d). While all health
indicators may be improving generally for both rich and poor countries,
the slower rate of change in poorer countries means that there is a widening rather than diminishing gap (Gray 2001d).

In UK studies, occupational social class is commonly used to measure
socioeconomic position. The relationship between class and health in
England has been described in some detail by the Department of Health
and Social Security (1980), Whitehead (1988), the Department of Health
(1998a), and others. Again, the general pattern emerges of a positive relationship between health indicators and socioeconomic status. Those at
the top of the scale generally have the best health in terms of mortality
and morbidity. People who are less well off tend to be ill more often and
die sooner (Department of Health 1999). This pattern of inequality has
been shown for mortality in general and for a range of specific causes of
death. These include CHD, stroke, lung cancer and suicides among men
and respiratory disease and lung cancer among women (Department of
Health 1998a). Social class gradients are evident for accidents, which are
an important cause of mortality and morbidity, especially in the young
and old (Department of Health and Social Security 1980, Green 2001).
In the early 1970s death rates from accidents in the 1–14 age range
were between three (females) and five (males) times greater for social
class 5 (the lowest social class) than social class 1 (the highest social class;
Green 2001).

In the early 1970s, the lowest social class had an overall death rate twice
as high as the highest social class. By the early 1990s, this had jumped to

a threefold difference (Department of Health 1998a). Those in higher social classes can expect to live up to 5 years longer than those in lower social classes (Department of Health 1998a). The life expectancy of a boy born into the poorest social class is over 9 years less than a boy born into the most affluent social class (Department of Health 2000a). Infants born to fathers in unskilled or semi-skilled occupations have a mortality rate 1.6 times higher than those in professional or managerial occupations (Department of Health 2000a). In common with the situation between countries, there continues to be a widening gap between those at the top of the social scale and those at the bottom (Department of Health 1998a, 2001c). In the last three decades, the UK has become wealthier and healthier, but income inequalities and health inequalities have increased (Graham 2001).

Looking at health indicators by gender also shows a marked divide. Worldwide, life expectancy is generally higher for women (Rosenberg 2000). The world life expectancy of 63 years conceals the fact that life expectancy is only 61 for males compared to 65 years for females. In England in 1998, the expectation of life at birth for a woman was likely to be 5 years longer than for a man, with expectancies respectively 80 and 75 years (Department of Health 2001a). However, when we look at healthy life expectancy the gap is smaller (Department of Health 1998a). Moreover, the gap in life expectancy between the genders is decreasing in England (Department of Health 2001a) as rates of mortality from conditions such as lung cancer and accidents increase for women (Jacobson et al 1991). Death rates in general are higher for men than for women at all ages. Deaths from accidents account for much of the gender difference in mortality for children in England (Department of Health 1998a). In developing countries, the gender divide is less marked due to higher female mortality (Gray 2001b). This has been attributed to greater risks in childbirth, poorer nutrition and social factors resulting in poorer health (Gray 2001b).

The gender divide is not as polarized in the UK if we look at morbidity. While rates are higher in males for accidents and some conditions such as CHD, for many others there is no difference or female rates are higher (e.g. rheumatoid arthritis) (Gray 2001c). Reported rates of long-standing illnesses are higher for females (Gray 2001c).

Data on health indicators show that in England minority ethnic groups generally experience poorer heath than the majority (Department of Health 1998a). Children of women born in Pakistan are twice as likely to die in their first year than children of women born in the UK (Department of Health 2000a). West African and South African immigrants have high rates of cerebrovascular disease (stroke), while people from the Indian subcontinent have high rates of ischaemic heart disease, stroke and diabetes (Gray 2001c). Irish and Scottish immigrants have high mortality from accidents and violence (Gray 2001c). Black (Caribbean, African and other) groups have more long-standing illness (Department of Health 1998a).

Geographical variations are also evident. In England, there is a difference in IMR of three-and-a-half times between the health authorities with the highest and the lowest IMRs (Department of Health 2000a). Health differences exist between urban and rural areas and between north and south. For example, the death rate from CHD in people under 65 is almost three times higher in Manchester than in Oxfordshire (Department of Health 1999). Variation in environmental conditions leads to geographical variations in the incidence of diseases such as malaria.

Variations in health are evident throughout the lifespan. Mortality rates generally increase with age after early childhood in the developed world (Gray 2001c), but exceptions exist. Mortality from accidents is higher in the young and elderly and suicide is more common in younger age groups (Gray 2001c). Similar patterns emerge for morbidity. Most cancers increase with age, for example.

2.4 EXPLAINING PATTERNS OF HEALTH AND ILL HEALTH

There is clearly much change and diversity in patterns of health, but how can this be explained? As with any data, apparent patterns or associations may be artifacts of the methodology used. Taubes (2001) describes some of those for the post-war CHD 'epidemic'. These include the use of new terminology, changed wording on death certificates, and the suggestion that rising numbers may be due to more people living long enough to die from CHD rather than any real increase in risk (since the decline in infectious disease has caused a shift to degenerative diseases of old age). It has been argued that differences in numbers of individuals in the different social classes, and use of categories which exclude individuals such as people not in employment, could lead to a distorted picture of contemporary inequalities in health between social classes (Alcock et al 2000). In the case of England, however, even if adjustments are made to minimize this distortion, significant differences appear to remain (Jones 2000b).

Where there are associations between variables, interpretation can be problematic. Several factors may be involved, links may not be direct, and there may be time lags between cause and effect (Hennekens & Buring 1987). The direction of causality may be an issue so, for example, with social class inequalities in health, does poor health cause people to drop down the social scale or is being lower down the social scale the cause of poor health? The evidence would not support the former explanation in this instance (Jones 2000b).

Despite these arguments, in many cases it seems reasonable to accept that the observed patterns reflect the real situation. If we do this, then what we do know is that there are no simple explanations. Patterns of health and ill health seem to result from complex interactions between biological, psychological, social, political, economic, cultural, and environmental factors, and other determinants. The final biological event leading to death or ill health (the proximal cause) will be the result of many, more distant, contributory causes (distal causes) – the end of a chain or web of events (McConway 1994). Health and ill health result from the interaction between an individual and his or her social and material environment.

The Lalonde Report (1974) was influential in widening perceptions of the influences on health, describing four main fields of influence as environment, biology, health services and lifestyle. Dahlgren & Whitehead's (1991) model is conceptually useful in presenting health determinants as layers of influence. Fixed factors such as age, sex and genetic constitution are at the centre, while those which have potential to be modified radiate out from these and include lifestyle factors, social and community factors and general socioeconomic, cultural and environmental conditions. The complexity of influences underpins contemporary multicausal theories of disease (Jones 2000b), such as those accepted for CHD and cancers.

We know that biological factors can contribute to patterns of health and disease in various ways. Age, sex and constitutional factors are at the centre of the spheres of influence on health. A number of disorders and diseases, for example cystic fibrosis and haemophilia, are genetic in origin. Genetic factors also contribute to a number of other conditions, including CHD (Payne 2001). Historically, biological changes such as a reduction in the virulence of causal organisms seem to have played an important role in the decline of certain diseases, such as scarlet fever and plague (Gray 2001a). Co-evolution can occur between humans and microbial pathogens to reach an acclimatization, whereby diseases become mild and endemic rather than major threats to life. Examples include measles in the UK. Cases of people with AIDS who do not manifest symptoms have been reported, suggesting accommodation of the virus.

However, it is argued that most significant differences in health are not due to genetics, nor are they biologically inevitable (Leon & Walt 2001). Biological explanations alone cannot account for many of today's most important causes of mortality and morbidity, including CHD (Gray 2001a). Other determinants have been implicated. They include individual psychology, health beliefs, behaviour and lifestyle. Risk factors which have been linked to CHD include smoking, excessive alcohol consumption, high levels of free radicals, low exercise levels, being overweight, high blood pressure, psychological stress and being born small (Payne 2001). Smoking is accepted as the most significant of these (Payne 2001). A number of these risk factors have also been linked to other diseases such as stroke and diabetes.

Health-damaging behaviours such as smoking have been used to explain health inequalities. There is, for example, evidence of relationships between social class and health-damaging behaviour in England (Department of Health 1998a). Social class gradients in CHD are mirrored by social class gradients in smoking and poor diet (low in fruit, vegetables and dietary fibre) (Department of Health 1998a). Data for 1996 show 12% of professional men and 41% of unskilled manual working men smoked, while the figures for women in these respective classes were 11 and 36% respectively (Department of Health 1998a).

The reasons why individuals engage in health-damaging behaviours have been debated. Are people making a free choice or are choices constrained and influenced by other factors? There is strong evidence from research to support the latter view. A number of studies show that the smoking behaviour of young working-class mothers of under-5s is linked to their social circumstances (Jones 2000b). Smoking provides time out and respite in the midst of stressful demands. Studies on accidents and other causes of mortality and morbidity have similarly shown behaviour to be dependent on context (Jones 2000b). This has implications for the advice that physiotherapists may give to their patients. However, we do know that some individuals, for whatever reason, have a greater psychological capacity to adapt to adverse conditions in less health-damaging ways than others. Explanatory mechanisms include Antonovsky's (1993) sense of coherence theory.

Materialist explanations of health and disease patterns emphasize the influence of social and material factors. From this perspective, health and health inequalities are ultimately determined by factors such as wealth, environmental conditions, living and working conditions and social networks (Jones 2000b, Graham 2001). The Acheson Report (Department of Health 1998a) argues that 'the weight of scientific evidence points to a socieconomic explanation of health inequalities. This traces the roots of ill-health to determinants such as income, education and employment as well as to the material environment and lifestyle'.

But what are the mechanisms by which socioeconomic factors are linked to health? Certainly, poverty and health can be obviously linked through higher exposure and susceptibility to communicable disease as a result of poor sanitation, hygiene, housing, and malnutrition (Leon & Walt 2001). However, this does not explain non-communicable diseases and patterns whereby ill health is greater in advantaged groups or persists in the absence of deprivation. Psychosocial hypotheses have been suggested which link circumstances with stress, the physiological results of which raise risks of ill health (Leon & Walt 2001). Factors such as income equity, social capital and cohesion have been implicated. Theories such as the programming hypothesis link early life circumstances to later experience of health and ill health (Davey 2001).

If we look historically, some important turning points in patterns of disease have been associated with social and economic revolutions and interventions (Kiple 1996). One of the most significant changes in patterns of health in human history was the rise of infectious disease as a major cause of mortality. When we examine the circumstances surrounding this change it can be seen that the start of the period in history dominated by infectious disease is marked by a major transition in human social organization – the change from nomadic hunter–gatherer societies to settled agricultural lifestyles. This 'agricultural revolution' has been linked to the rise of infectious diseases as the main cause of illness and death (Gray 2001e).

Kiple (1996) describes how, for the 4.5 million years during which our ancestors lived as hunter–gatherers, the small, low-density communities (50–100 individuals) provided conditions that were not favourable to the spread and survival of contagious diseases. In order to flourish, airborne and contact diseases such as measles and smallpox need large populations, living in close proximity. Similarly, waterborne diseases such as cholera and typhoid will only be favoured where populations live sufficiently long in an area to contaminate water supplies.

The shift to a settled agricultural lifestyle created the conditions for a rise both in population and in infectious disease (Gray 2001e). Greater availability of food allowed increased population size and consequently the conditions for increased transmission of disease and epidemic outbreaks. A settled lifestyle meant closer proximity to other humans, animals and accumulated waste with consequent increased exposure to, and opportunity for transmission of, communicable diseases (Ortner & Theobald 1993). Close contact with domesticated animals has been linked to measles, smallpox and influenza, for example (Kiple 1996).

Insufficient food was a major contributory cause of death and disease in the past and is a significant problem in the developing world today (Gray 2001f). Settled agriculture is likely to have resulted in reduced diversity of foodstuffs and increased malnutrition, leading to greater susceptibility to infectious disease (Kiple 1996). A vicious circle can be set up where weakened individuals become unable to procure food or absorb nutrients due to illness (Kiple 1996, Gray 2001b).

In the same way, diarrhoeal disease and malnutrition are linked today in low-income countries, and affect the growth and development of millions of children (Gray 2001b). Malnutrition, ill health and poverty are thus inextricably associated. The concept of entitlement relations makes an important contribution to understanding this link (Gray 2001f). If people do not have the means to produce their own food, or the resources (e.g. money) to procure food, then they have no direct or indirect entitlement to it and may not receive it. Famines and malnutrition can, therefore, occur amid plenty. This has been argued to be the case for many important famines of the past and present, including the Irish potato famine of 1845–9.

In the last few centuries, other major socioeconomic changes have influenced patterns of health, including the industrial revolution, industrialization, urbanization and the growth of cities. Major changes during the industrial revolution in England in the eighteenth and nineteenth centuries included the removal of common land into private ownership and dislocation of peasant farmers, alongside urbanization and industrialization. Again, these changes initially brought conditions conducive to communicable diseases, such as overcrowding, poverty, poor living conditions and loss of direct entitlement to food (Ortner & Theobald 1993, Leon & Walt 2001). Extended trade and commerce have also provided routes for transmission of disease (Ortner & Theobald 1993), and the health experience of many developing countries has been significantly influenced in various ways by colonization and relationships with industrialized countries.

2.4.1 THE ROLE OF MEDICINE

The relative contributions of biological, environmental, social and medical factors to the pattern of declining mortality since the nineteenth century have been the subject of debate in recent years (Gray 2001a). For much of the twentieth century, medical science was commonly perceived as the key to improved health. Developments in the latter half of the last century have been described as a medical revolution (Porter 1996). The

introduction of vaccinations, therapeutic drugs and other medical interventions and discoveries have certainly been successful in significantly
reducing, eliminating or ameliorating some of the causes of mortality
and ill health. Notable examples in the developed world include vaccinations for polio and diphtheria (McKeown 1984). Le Fanu (1999) lists
some definitive medical 'moments', among which he includes developments such as penicillin, cortisone, chlorpromazine for the treatment
of schizophrenia, open heart surgery, hip replacement and kidney
transplants.

However, critics have provided persuasive arguments in support of
the view that overall, medicine has made a limited or even negative contribution to health. Thomas McKeown (1984) provided evidence that
over the twentieth century many important diseases were in decline
before medical intervention or that interventions were directed at conditions that were not the most significant threats to health. His argument is
exemplified by data showing there had already been a 92% decline in
mortality from tuberculosis in England and Wales before the introduction of drug therapies (Le Fanu 1999). According to the 'McKeown
hypothesis', improved diet and social conditions have been more important than medical interventions. While the relative importance of these
factors has been disputed by other authors, explanations for the modern
decline in mortality generally emphasize the establishment of public
health administration and legislation and improvements in nutrition and
standards of living (Gray 2001a).

The fact that many medical interventions have not been evaluated or
have been proven to be ineffective has recently led to the evidence-based
medicine movement and a range of other activities such as clinical governance in health care. Critics have highlighted the fact that medical
intervention may also be positively harmful. One of the best-known critics of medicine, Ivan Illich (1976), explored the concept of iatrogenesis:
medically created ill health, and the disempowering effects of medicine
in society. Illich argues that medical intervention has not just been ineffective against many significant causes of morbidity and mortality, but
has actually contributed to the burden of ill health through the direct and
indirect side-effects of treatments (clinical iatrogenesis). More widely, he
argues that medicine encourages sickness through medicalization (social
iatrogenesis), and disempowers people by destroying the ability to cope
with and address their own morbidity and mortality (cultural iatrogenesis). Even if effective medical interventions are available, we also need to
recognize that they may not be used, owing to economic, social, political
or other factors – treatment for infertility or cosmetic surgery may, for
example, be limited in the UK National Health Service (NHS).

Disillusionment with medical approaches and recognition of the limits
of biomedicine and formal health care have led to the re-emergence of
public health agendas and an emphasis on social policy as a means of
improving health and reducing inequality. Social constructionist perspectives have emerged to challenge the view of ill health and disability
as biologically determined rather than socially constructed (Gerhardt
1989, Saraga 1998a; see also Chs 3 and 17).

2.5 APPROACHES TO PROMOTING HEALTH AND REDUCING INEQUALITY

There is a long history of action to improve health and reduce inequalities. In Britain, the public health reformers of the nineteenth century instigated landmark social and environmental reforms aimed at reducing ill health, particularly among the urban poor (Pelling et al 1993). These encompassed clean water, good sanitation, clean air, adequate housing and a range of other structural changes. In the twentieth century, health improvement and the reduction of inequalities were driving forces behind the setting up of the welfare state and the NHS in 1948.

A number of key strategic developments in health policy took place in the latter years of the twentieth century. The Lalonde Report (1974) was particularly powerful in broadening agendas and shifting the emphasis from a focus on treatment, health care and medical interventions to prevention and promotion with recognition of social and environmental determinants of health as well as lifestyle factors. On an international level, many subsequent strategies and policies showed a similar shift. These included the influential World Health Organization's *Health for All by the Year 2000* strategy (World Health Organization 1977), and the *Health for All in Europe* targets that followed (World Health Organization 1985). The World Health Organization Alma Ata declaration (World Health Organization 1978) focused particularly on the developing world with an emphasis on primary care, agriculture, education, housing and other social and economic factors. In all of the World Health Organization strategies, recognition was given to building healthy public policy, working to create supportive environments, and to the importance of different sectors working together. They also raised the issue of equity and health and the need to reduce inequalities between rich and poor (Jones & Douglas 2000). The Rio Earth Summit, organized by the United Nations Conference on Environment and Development in 1993, brought environmental issues to the fore.

These international developments gave shape to national policies around the world in the 1980s and 1990s. However, successive government reports in the UK between 1976 and 1999 still emphasized targeting people's personal behaviour and lifestyles (Jones 2000b). The English *Health of the Nation* strategy document published in 1992 was criticized particularly for a failure to address the effects of poverty on health. With a change in government in 1997, new strategies were launched between 1997 and 1999 by the nations of the UK: *Saving Lives: Our Healthier Nation* (England), *Towards a Healthier Scotland*, *Better Health Better Wales*, *Well into 2000* (Northern Ireland) (Jones & Douglas 2000). *Saving Lives* was more direct than previous English policies in addressing the structural determinants of health, including poverty, and in considering inequality.

Although both nationally and internationally the emphasis is currently on public policy as a route to improving health and reducing inequalities, it has been observed that the focus in the UK and other European countries is on socioeconomic inequalities and primary prevention, whereas in low- to middle-income countries the emphasis is on equitable access to health care and socioeconomic inequalities are largely ignored (Leon & Walt 2001). The reason suggested for this is that health care is more readily available in developed than in developing countries. The past modelling of health services on the developed world has proved to be inappropriate for developing countries and the importance of community development and bottom-up initiatives such as barefoot doctors has now been acknowledged (Walt 2001).

2.5.1 ACTIONS TO REDUCE INEQUALITIES IN HEALTH

The issue of inequalities in health has been a particular focus of attention worldwide in recent years. It was recognized in the mid-1970s that the UK was slipping behind other countries in health improvement and that there were significant inequalities in health. This led to the establishment of the Government Working Group on Inequalities in Health, chaired by Sir Douglas Black, in 1977, and publication of the Black Report in 1980 (Department of Health and Social Security 1980). This report has been described as 'a rare example, perhaps the first anywhere in the world, of an attempt authorized by Government to explain trends in inequalities in health and relate these to policies intended to promote as well as restore health' (Department of Health 1998a). The report influenced public health debates both nationally and internationally.

Despite the Black Report and other reports on inequalities in health, such as the reports *Health Divide* (Whitehead 1988) and *Variations in Health* (Department of Health 1995), inequality did not appear to be given any official priority in the UK through the 1980s (Department of Health 1998a). While it was given some consideration in the *Health of the Nation* strategy (Department of Health 1991), the diminution of its significance is embodied in the use of the more neutral term 'variations' in health. However, with the election of a new (Labour) government in 1997, health inequalities became a more central issue (Graham 2001). An independent inquiry on inequalities in health was conducted to review the data and to identify a range of areas for future policy development. The Acheson Report (Department of Health 1998a) which emerged from this recommended actions to improve structural factors such as poverty, income tax and benefits, education, housing and environment, employment, mobility, transport and pollution and nutrition. Subsequently, the main government strategy for health, *Saving Lives: Our Healthier Nation* (Department of Health 1999), required the setting of local targets for reducing health inequalities and introduced strategies for action. These included local partnerships, health improvement programmes, health action zones and healthy living centres. The *New NHS: Modern – Dependable* White Paper (Department of Health 1997) also outlined changes relevant to inequalities and the NHS plan published in 2000 (Department of Health 2000a) for the first time reinforced local targets by the creation of national health inequalities targets, to narrow the health gap in childhood and throughout life between socioeconomic groups and between the most deprived areas and the rest of the country (Department of Health 2001c). These policies acknowledged that the roots of inequalities lay in poverty, lack of educational attainment, unemployment and social exclusion (Graham 2001). The Department of Health's *Cross-Cutting Review* on health inequalities (Department of Health 2002) reinforced the practical commitment to reducing inequalities through reviewing targets and setting in place long-term strategies to achieve this.

Health strategies are also being developed to reduce health inequalities outside Europe (Graham 2001). Action at a range of levels is required (Leon & Walt 2001), including the reduction of poverty and provision of aid to the poorest countries and poorest groups. Consideration of the wider determinants of health feature large, with value placed on the strengthening of individuals and communities. Building up the evidence base of data on health experience will be essential to global progress.

2.6 CONCLUSION

What, then, are the implications for the physiotherapist? What relevance does this chapter have for the practitioner who, for example, is rehabilitating a patient following a stroke or a fall? As well as using all their medical knowledge and all the techniques at their disposal, physiotherapists also need to consider some broad social questions. Could something have been done to prevent the situation arising? Why this person and not another? Perhaps the patient who has fallen and fractured a hip is elderly, living in circumstances that have contributed to the situation and which will influence recovery. Perhaps poverty, malnutrition and confusion have contributed to the fall and isolation and depression will prevent the use of follow-up services.

It is well known that health and ill health do not 'just happen'. Some inequalities in health, such as genetic differences, are unavoidable but many others are not and are the result of differences in opportunity, access to services, material resources, lifestyle choices and other factors (Department of Health 2002). Making a contribution to promoting health and preventing ill health is something everyone can do in a personal capacity, but for professions such as physiotherapy there are additional opportunities. Every individual interaction with a patient provides the chance to influence physical, mental and social well-being, but looking beyond the immediate context offers the chance to have a more far-reaching impact. The UK Department of Health review on tackling health inequalities (Department of Health 2002) provides some useful starting points in thinking about ways in which health professionals can influence patterns of health and contribute to reducing health inequalities:

• Ensure services respond to local needs and that local people are involved in the needs assessment process

• Form links, partnerships and alliances with others to promote the health of the individuals and communities you work with

• Ensure services are user-centred and joined up at the point of delivery

• Ensure that activities are relevant, flexible and acceptable (i.e. culturally and educationally appropriate), and that settings are accessible and appropriate

- Show commitment and take action to achieve greater investment in community-based programmes

- Ensure that community initiatives include appropriate training and support for volunteers, peer educators and local networks

- Engage with national and local policies and visibly show political support and commitment.

Chapter 3

Health, health education and physiotherapy practice

Jane S. Owen Hutchinson

3.1 INTRODUCTION

Because of their centrality within practice, most physiotherapists will, during the course of their work, have considered the concepts of health and health education. Opportunities to reflect upon these subjects are amply provided within the literature of the human sciences, including that of physiotherapy, where various definitions and models of health and health education have been documented (see, for example, Warren 1985, 1986, Burkitt 1986, Twomey 1986, Ritchie 1989, Sim 1990b, 2002, Condie 1991, Parry 1991, Roberts 1994, Higgs & Titchen 1995, Hills 1995). Personal experience supported by written evidence, however, suggests that while many physiotherapists may be acquainted with a wide range of health models on an abstract, theoretical level, their practice is nevertheless predominantly characterized by the biomedical model (see, for example, McIntosh 1989, Ritchie 1989, Sluijs 1991, Balfour 1993, Sluijs et al 1993, Adamson & Nordholm 1994, Marshall & Walsh 1994, Stachura 1994, Jaggi & Bithell 1995, Jorgensen 2000). Most therapists continue to regard members of the public to whom they give a service as 'patients'. These patients are perceived as individuals presenting with a physical diagnosis: the patient is not infrequently classified as 'a back', 'a fractured shaft of femur' or 'a ruptured tendo Achilles'. The diagnosis may refer to an acute or a chronic condition: the former demands immediate 'cure', the latter requires long-term management by the 'expert'.

Research conducted by Hills (1995) indicates that physiotherapists also seem to favour a model of health education (as described by Coutts & Hardy 1985, Burkitt 1986, Webb 1994a, 1994b, Ewles & Simnett 1999) whose principal focus is on the individual. The aim is prophylaxis or prevention (at primary, secondary and tertiary levels) of that individual's problem through the dissemination of factual information delivered by traditional teaching approaches and methods. Thus physiotherapists attending a workshop on health education organized by the Chartered Society of Physiotherapy (CSP) and the former Health Education Council (HEC) in 1985 reported that they perceived their role 'mainly in terms of tertiary prevention on a one-to-one basis, but increasingly moving towards secondary prevention, in the form of, for example, back schools and contributing to radio programmes' with 'initiatives … towards primary prevention, for example, working with sports coaches and keep-fit teachers' (CSP 1988: 602). It is noted in the same document that physiotherapists work with individuals and groups and give specific and general 'information and advice' about selected conditions and their management and emphasize the importance of health education (associated with the 'treatment' and 'prevention' of particular conditions) for carers and other professional personnel. Other surveys confirm these findings. Leathley (1988) reported that 85% of her sample of physiotherapists considered 'back care education' to be 'the most important health education activity', while 47% ranked 'ante- or post-natal work' as most important. The respondents identified 'hospital staff' and 'carers, particularly those in the community' as the primary target groups for health education (see also Lilley 1983, Lyne 1985, 1986, Leathley & Stone 1986, Shore 1986, Twomey 1986, Hayne 1988, Glazer-Waldman et al 1989, McIntosh 1989, Sluijs 1991, Sluijs et al 1993, Hills 1995).

Furthermore, it appears that many physiotherapists tend to equate the role of health educator with high status and power. According to the report from the CSP's workshop, physiotherapists perceive themselves as experts capable of influencing '"the system" at a policy/decision-making level' by educating employers, hospitals/social service managers and education authorities in the importance of appropriate staff training and good ergonomic design of the workplace (CSP 1988). Physiotherapists describe how, through their involvement with ergonomic issues, they are able to influence company policy. One physiotherapist comments that her 'skills as a physiotherapist and knowledge of the body is a real help when looking at such matters as designing footwear'. Physiotherapists also influence the behaviour of employees. One practitioner 'encourages staff to think of other ways of maintaining a healthy life-style; liaises with the catering department to run events on healthy eating; and runs courses on subjects like Alexander Technique and self-defence'. Another interviewee states that: 'We can identify the problems and work on rehabilitation to get the person back to full fitness. It helps keep people at work and prevents their well-being from deteriorating'.

Unfortunately, however, this zealous (and characteristically biomedical) approach to health education has not met with unqualified success. Edmonds (1988) identifies the problem:

> The current debate within the National Health Service (NHS) on the approach to treatment based on the whole needs of the patient, and treating the patient as a person, is nowhere more pertinent than in the physiotherapy profession. It is unfortunate that the motivation of those who are deeply caring tends to emerge as judgmental and directive. Anecdotal evidence is embarrassingly abundant of instances where consideration of the person rather than the patient would have led to a more satisfactory outcome of consumer/practitioner interaction. Actual practice has too often resulted in the effect of 'institutionalising' and 'taking over' patients rather than seeking to care for them as people (Edmonds 1988: 27).

Given this situation, an attempt to refocus attention on the limitations of the biomedical model of health and health education seems to be particularly appropriate. Clearly, within the confines of a short chapter it would be impossible to do more than to introduce a selection of what many writers consider to be the crucial issues in this area. It is hoped, however, that the following discussion will stimulate further analytical and critical reflection upon the concept of health and its education which will lead, subsequently, to a reappraisal of the underlying philosophy of physiotherapy, together with a re-evaluation of some of the techniques employed in its practice.

3.2 THE BIOMEDICAL MODEL OF HEALTH

Let us remind ourselves that the biomedical model of health evolved as a consequence of the scientific revolution, which commenced in Europe in the seventeenth century. Doyal (1991: 28–29) describes how 'the natural science which developed during the Renaissance transformed the Aristotelian view of the world which had dominated Western thought for 1500 years'. Doyal continues:

> Increasingly, science was no longer concerned with understanding the essence or teleological purpose of the natural/supernatural world. Rather, the scientist (or natural philosopher as he was called) attempted to discover and explain those regular and recurring sequences of events which could be described and codified in a quantitative and generalisable way. It was believed that this would make possible the utilisation of nature through the making of accurate predictions based on these codified generalisations. In other words, the new science increasingly equated an understanding of the natural world with a capacity to control it (Doyal 1991: 29).

Within the medical context, the Renaissance scientist was preoccupied with the exploration and documentation of the body's structure and function. It is important to emphasize Doyal's (1991: 29) point that: 'These early investigations were largely founded upon a mechanistic view of the nature of men, and of human sickness and health. That is to say, they followed the more general pattern of Renaissance science in analysing living things as sets of mechanical parts – as machines rather than organically integrated wholes.' The Aristotelian emphasis on 'the organic unity of living things' was effectively challenged by such philosophers as Thomas Hobbes and René Descartes, whose mechanistic conception of human beings is generally reflected in contemporary orthodox medical practice which sanctions the biomedical model of health. Undoubtedly, the ideological roots of this model lie in Cartesianism. Descartes believed in a particular variety of dualism with which his name has hitherto been associated. This theory holds that the (immaterial) 'mind' and the (material) 'body' of a given individual, although they somehow interact, are essentially distinct entities (Descartes 1989, Doyal 1991, Jones 1994, Roberts 1994). In common with many other Renaissance thinkers, Descartes was preoccupied with the concept of knowledge, its origins and criteria. He was committed to scientific reductionism, as defined by Popper (1972), Flew (1983), Pratt (1989) and Roberts (1994), an allegiance which influenced his mechanistic approach to physiological analysis (see below). Descartes considered a body to be 'healthy' if, like a properly functioning machine, that body was in good working order; conversely, a body was classified as 'diseased' if an impairment of its function could be detected (Descartes 1989).

Doyal (1991) points out that modern orthodox medicine is generally regarded as being primarily concerned with the body at the expense of attending to the mind and thus continues to espouse a mechanistic concept of health. This approach is consistent with 'The scientific paradigm or empiricist model of knowledge … [which] provides the basis for the medical model' (Higgs & Titchen 1995: 522–523). Empiricism is a perspective that sets 'first-hand observation and other forms of sensory experience' as the only valid source of knowledge (Sim & Wright 2000: 8). Fundamentally, therefore, the scientific paradigm:

> relies on observation and experiment in the empirical world, resulting in generalizations about the content and events of the world which can be used to predict future experience. Knowledge is discovered (i.e. universal and external truths are grasped) and justified on the basis of empirical processes which are reductionist, value-neutral, quantifiable, objective, and operationalisable. Only statements publicly verifiable by sense data are valid (Higgs & Titchen 1995: 522–523).

Beattie (1993: 261) juxtaposes the life sciences against the human sciences and provides further valuable insight into the characteristics of the biomedical perspective: 'Within the professions and institutions of medicine, "mechanistic" approaches to analysis are still dominant: they are seen as "hard", and in keeping with the canons of the natural science tradition. In contrast, "humanistic" approaches are given a place at the margins, but are seen as "soft", and associated with the less prestigious traditions of sociological or literary inquiry.' In the biomedical tradition, health is 'determined secondarily to disease; if a definition of disease can be formulated, health can then be thought of as its polar opposite' (Sim

1990b: 423). Health is thus perceived in negative terms: as the absence, or antithesis of disease. Sim (1990b: 423) suggests that 'because the two concepts are seen to lie on a single dimension' the 'variety of sophisticated means of detecting and quantifying disease processes in the patient ... are equally measures of [biological] health'. Diagnosis of a disease is contingent upon the identification of a particular collection of signs and symptoms presented by the individual 'sufferer' or 'victim'. The objective is, unquestionably, to 'cure' the disease or impairment by means of medical intervention (see, for example, Oliver 1983, 1990, Galler 1993, Swain et al 1993, Keith 1994, Morris 1995).

The central focus of attention within biomedical ideology is upon individuals (Beattie 1993, Fatchett 1994). Emphasis is, however, on a certain kind of 'individualism' that, as Hyland (1988) suggests, finds fullest expression in the writings of Descartes. Jewson's tripartite analysis of the modes of production of scientific knowledge (Jewson 1993) is helpful in providing a historical background to the development of the biomedical model of health. Jewson suggests that scientific medicine passed through three stages: 'bedside medicine', 'hospital medicine' and 'laboratory medicine', and that this last stage consolidated medicine as an experimental science, firmly committed to 'biological reductionism' which reinforced the tendency to view the patient as an object to be manipulated – a trend which has reached its apotheosis in post-war scientific medicine (Doyal 1991).

Other significant characteristics of the biomedical model deserve mention. Jones (1994) states that priority is given to the provision of specialist medical services, in mainly institutional settings, and Beattie notes that the biomedical model adopts a paternalistic, or top-down approach to health and policy-making (Beattie 1993). As Jones (1994) suggests, the objective is to return patients to 'normality' within the shortest possible time-span in order that they may resume productive labour. Such an approach requires the patient to submit to the authority of an omniscient and omnipotent clinical 'expert' whose dominance within the relationship is legitimized by the privileged possession of scientific knowledge, which is closely guarded (Collier 1989). This empowers the clinician to restore the patient's physical health by making an accurate diagnosis of the disease whose process can subsequently be reversed or retarded by the administration of appropriate 'treatment'.

In this latter context, the clinician's role is often to educate the patient in the management of a particular disorder by imparting carefully selected, relevant factual information and prescriptive instruction concerning that individual's body. Risk factors are emphasized and strategies designed to minimize future problems are presented (Jones 1994). The premise seems to be that, if facts are presented in such a way as to promote understanding, patient 'compliance' can be anticipated (see, for example, Glossop et al 1982, Sluijs et al 1993). Having received this knowledge and 'advice', patients are expected to take ultimate responsibility for their subsequent actions. The biomedical approach believes that since each person has the capacity for choice in all matters, people can choose to be more or less healthy. Incontrovertibly, a rational individual would choose to be healthy, particularly when that choice is facilitated by the possession of 'correct' factual information. To ignore such information is irrational according to authoritarian clinicians, who regard their patients' lapses from obedience to the prescribed 'rules' as a serious offence. Clinicians are often irritated and affronted by what they consider to be the patient's flagrant breach of the tacitly agreed medical contract. Clinicians frequently express their 'disappointment' in the patient's conduct and blame the patient for what is perceived as a failure in compliance due either to an inability to understand and learn information and instructions or to a rejection of established – and therefore incontrovertible – 'scientific facts' (Coutts & Hardy 1985, Currer & Stacey 1986, Hyland 1987, 1988, Morgan et al 1988, Turner 1988, Sim 1990b, Doyal 1991, Beattie et al 1993, Armstrong 1994, Jones 1994, Davey et al 1995, Ewles & Simnett 1999).

3.3 DIFFICULTIES WITH THE BIOMEDICAL DEFINITION

Having outlined the characteristics of the biomedical model of health, we shall begin our discussion by considering some of its theoretical difficulties as related to metaphysical, ethical and sociological issues, and show how these have implications for health education. Inevitably, this investigation will reveal some theoretical problems associated with alternative models of health and health education. Turning next to an example from contemporary practice, we shall identify the biomedical model's salient features as exemplified by the practitioner's approach and choice of language. Undertaking this analysis will enable us to appreciate the importance of theoretical consistency in the context of health care practice. Finally, we shall propose an alternative concept of health to that offered by the biomedical model. While it is acknowledged that this paradigm is not without its disadvantages, we shall suggest that it provides a more rational theoretical framework upon which to base physiotherapy practice.

3.3.1 METAPHYSICAL CONSIDERATIONS

Our first criticism of the biomedical model of health may be levelled at its Cartesian foundations (see Section 9.3). Cartesian dualism has received serious challenges from exponents of metaphysical doctrines such as alternative versions of (non-Cartesian) dualism and monism (comprising idealism and various forms of materialism including behaviourism, functionalism and physicalism) (see, for example, Campbell 1970, Ryle 1973, Teichmann 1974, McGinn 1982, Strawson 1984, Williams 1985, Smith & Jones 1987). Of particular significance to physiotherapy practice is that Cartesian dualism fails to provide a satisfactory account of how interaction between two separate, contrasting entities (mind and matter) can occur, given that, according to this theory, each possesses a different (but equal) ontological status. If the body is conceived of as a mere machine, how is it connected to the mind (Teichman 1974)? Indeed, problems of intelligibility arise when it comes to understanding what, in fact, mind is, since it tends to be described negatively: it is not, for example, the brain. If mind is not located in space, a logical difficulty arises as to how mind–body interaction can occur. How can a causal relationship exist between a non-physical substance and a physical entity? For Descartes to locate the mind in the pineal gland and then to suggest that it can cause a physical response rests upon the contradiction that immaterial substances can be 'located' anywhere in space (McGinn 1982).

Exponents of this 'official doctrine' are guilty of making a 'category mistake' (Ryle 1973). Cartesian dualism 'represents the facts of mental life as if they belonged to one logical type or category ... when they actually belong to another'. The upshot of this is the representation of a person as a 'ghost mysteriously ensconced in a machine'. Citing Rudolf Klein, Fatchett (1994: 67) notes 'that people have likened the NHS to "a garage for putting faulty human bodies back on the road again"'. Thus a health educator, having made this initial 'category mistake', predictably conceives of health education as providing the 'ghost' with relevant facts about 'machine' maintenance and then supervising the repair job! It is not surprising, therefore, that many 'ghosts' find these facts meaningless, become disenchanted with the tedium of this work and frequently abandon their 'machine' when the supervisor is not watching! As Whitehead (1989: 5) revealingly comments: 'In schools ... there is evidence that single lesson lectures are still commonly employed with the aim of influencing social problems like illegal drug use, sexual activity in relation to AIDS, smoking and drinking habits and so on, even though any long-term behaviour change is highly unlikely with such a method.'

Let us assume, then, that one of a health educator's aims is to change a person's behaviour; Ryle's objections to Cartesianism lead us to conclude that the biomedical approach to practice seems unlikely to produce these permanent alterations. Ryle's behaviourist perspective prompts him to argue that the Cartesian concept of the 'ghost' in the 'machine' has no appropriate practical application in terms of its ability to describe intelligent performance since it necessarily relies upon an infinite regress. He states that:

> The crucial objection to the intellectualist legend is this. The consideration of propositions is itself an operation the execution of which can be more or less intelligent, less or more stupid. But if, for any operation to be intelligently executed, a prior theoretical operation had first to be performed and performed intelligently, it would be a logical impossibility for anyone ever to break into the circle (Ryle 1973: 31).

Thus, for Ryle, the question 'how' mental activity causes physical activity is irrelevant. He claims that 'my performance has a special procedure or manner, not special antecedents'. Thus on this account, it would seem to be necessary for a therapist to establish certain behavioural criteria of 'health' and 'disease' against which a person's physical state could be judged following an assessment of behavioural patterns. Once the problem had been identified, 'health education' would consist of various forms of behaviour modification until the individual displayed appropriate 'healthy' behaviour (Ewles & Simnett 1999).

As we might expect, however, behaviourism, in common with other branches of materialism, is not without its problems. In contrast to Cartesianism, behaviourism classifies persons as merely physical bodies: mental processes are reduced to brain processes. It is a serious objection to behaviourism that because 'mind' is identified with 'brain', the theory fails to provide a satisfactory explanation of the subjectivity of human experiences, for example, those of pain, or 'feeling unwell'. Thus, in the context of general health care management, behaviourism may fail to acknowledge such subjective feelings because its primary focus would be on the person's observable behaviour. In view of this inadequacy, therefore, behaviourism seems to be only marginally superior to Cartesianism in terms of its ability to provide a satisfactory metaphysical basis for physiotherapy practice.

3.3.2 SOCIOLOGICAL AND ETHICAL CONSIDERATIONS

Turning now from the metaphysical to considerations of a more sociological and ethical nature, Sim (1990b) identifies other limitations of the biomedical model of health. He observes that 'its stamp of objectivity rests upon a "realist" view of diseases – i.e. they have an independent existence, which is unaffected by both the fact and the mode of their perception by the observer' (Sim 1990b: 423). That 'the very identification of disease' is inextricably linked with the making of 'certain value judgments' implies that diseases 'become social constructs': 'they are developed within, and therefore embody, specific social values and processes' (Sim 1990b: 424).

We have noted above that the biomedical model owes much to a certain kind of individualism. Because its orientation is in terms of 'individual physiology, this model tends to seek only biological causes of disease' (Sim 1990b: 424). Clearly, this perspective ignores the undeniable socioeconomic and cultural determinants of disease as identified by numerous writers (see, for example, Frank & Maguire 1988, Morgan et al 1988, Turner 1988, Beattie et al 1993, Armstrong 1994, Bond & Bond 1994, Wilkinson & Kitzinger 1994, Benzeval et al 1995, Davey et al 1995, Ewles & Simnett 1999, Siegrist 2000, Marmot 2001, Wilkinson 2001, Freund et al 2003). In their study of the former HEC's campaign against coronary heart disease, Farrant & Russell (1986) examined the council's publication *Beating Heart Disease*. Their research exposes similar weaknesses of the biomedical model. In contrast to Downie (1988), they remain unimpressed by science and highlight the inadequacy of the 'explanatory power of the conventional risk factors' utilized by the HEC to 'educate' the general public about how to avoid chronic heart disease. Underlying Farrant & Russell's specific criticism of the biomedical approach is the important, general point to which we have earlier alluded: that a practitioner's concept of a person will necessarily determine how he or she conceives 'health'; this in turn will influence his or her ideas about how such persons are to be 'educated' and which methods are most suitable. Given the biomedical model's individualistic conception of persons, and given the HEC's allegiance to this ideology, it is not surprising that Farrant & Russell (1986) discover that the booklet focuses on the personal risk factors of CHD and that the responsibility for reducing risk factors is placed firmly upon the individual. They highlight the HEC's reluctance to view the person as existing within a socioeconomic framework, reflected in the booklet's failure to mention other contributory factors to

CHD prevalence such as: 'the role of the food industry and tobacco industry in maintaining unhealthy consumption patterns, or … the social and economic factors (poverty, stress associated with adverse living and working conditions…) that are related to social inequalities in diet, smoking etc., and that militate against attempts at individual risk factor reduction' (Farrant & Russell 1986: 34).

As these authors emphasize, 'a model of CHD aetiology has been hypothesized that locates the primary cause of CHD (and therefore the appropriate point for intervention) in the wider social and economic environment' which 'utilizes the concept of chronic psychosocial stress as the major linking factor between an individual's environment and his or her cardiovascular system' (Farrant & Russell 1986: 19–20). Thus, exhortations to stop smoking, eat less fat, take more exercise, and so forth, sound hollow and insincere when delivered by the 'expert'. Health education that ignores social influences and whose style is prescriptive and patronizing is thus doomed to failure.

Significantly, however, Farrant & Russell (1986) report that this failure in health education is not solely associated with the HEC's disregard of social issues. The bourgeois attitude often adopted by orthodox health professionals towards their patients is also considered to contribute to communication breakdown. Farrant & Russell identify misconceptions in professionals' beliefs that the prevalence of 'lay ignorance of orthodox medical "facts" about disease aetiology' justifies the corrective role of health education. Their findings suggest that 'it is not ignorance of "the facts" so much as the credibility the individual accords to these facts, as presented in health education literature, vis-à-vis personal "proof" that has been built up over years of observation and experience' (Farrant & Russell 1986: 49). Thus, when confronted with professional perspectives on health, the layperson is likely to engage in sophisticated information processing in an attempt to establish which behaviours are more 'healthy' than others; this evaluation will then determine their subsequent choice of action (see also Beattie et al 1993, Davey et al 1995). Clearly, these findings must be acknowledged by all health professionals and their practice modified accordingly. One of the dangers – particularly with reference to physiotherapy – seems to be that the practitioner's attention is often diverted by the wealth of other research and advice concerning effective methods of communication (see, for example, Glossop et al 1982, Wagstaff 1982, Hasler 1985, Slack 1985, Robinson 1986, Skinner 1986, Griffiths 1987, Hargreaves 1987, Hough 1987, 2001, Jobling 1987, Ley 1988, Payne 1989, Burnard 1992, Webb 1994a). This is not to deny the value of such work to practitioners; rather, it is to suggest that much of it focuses on the efficacy of specific communication techniques and – with the exception of Hough's contributions – rarely questions the professional's (predominantly biomedical) attitudes and assumptions concerning the nature and abilities of those persons designated as 'patients'.

In connection with the above comments, it seems pertinent to examine further the role of the health worker. In this connection Sim (1990b) notes the biomedical model's failure to acknowledge the 'social, cultural and institutional context in which health care occurs'. He contends that this dimension is crucial for physiotherapists who 'require an "action-oriented" theory that will make sense not only of health, but also of health *care* as an activity' (Sim 1990b: 424, original emphasis). Significantly, physiotherapists – together with many other professional groups – often identify themselves as 'health care workers' and as members of 'the caring professions' and Sim's request for the development of a theoretical basis for health care practice is surely legitimate. We might further supplement Sim's analysis by suggesting that therapists additionally require a theory of 'care' and 'caring' upon which to base practice. It is relevant to observe that the concepts of 'care' and 'caring', while they have been hijacked by members of the biomedical fraternity to serve political ends, seem to be associated with a model of health which conceives of the patient as an integrated and unique human being whose overall concerns and needs form the basis of practice. Although these ideas are apparently of little interest to some members of the physiotherapy profession, they have captured the imagination of other professional groups. The positive view of health associated with notions of 'care' and 'caring' has, for example, been well developed within the context of nursing where these ideas seem to have contributed significantly to the practitioner's understanding of the concepts of 'persons', 'health' and 'health education' (see, for example, Griffin 1983, Warren 1988, Watson 1988, Watson & Ray 1988, Barker 1989, MacPherson 1989, Morrison 1989, Ray 1989, Orem 1991, Jolly & Brykczynska 1992, Johns 1994, Andrews & Boyle 1995).

Turning to wider issues, the biomedical influence on government ideology and policy is clear and is reflected in the way in which health issues are addressed in the UK (see, for example, Jacobson et al 1991, Vallance Owen 1992, Harrison & Pollitt 1994). The NHS is increasingly run according to commercial principles: health is a purchasable commodity. Indeed, the gradual shift towards this commercial ethos could be taken as evidence of central government's public sanction of the continued and unrivalled dominance of the biomedical model within health care practice.

The biomedical model's negative view of health colours its interpretation of the related notions of 'protection' and 'education', considered by Tannahill (1985) to fall under the umbrella concept of 'health promotion'. Since concentration is on the elimination of disease within the individual, 'health promotion' becomes a restricted activity, directed solely towards the ' "maintenance" or "restoration" ' of individuals' health (Sim 1990b). Leathley (1988: 218) makes a similar point, although her notion of 'prevention' seems to carry biomedical overtones. She suggests that 'the general orientation of the National Health Service towards sickness rather than health' presents 'obstacles to increasing the preventive and educational aspects' of physiotherapists' work. Not surprisingly, this negative orientation is reflected in central government's general approach to health matters, as revealed in Whitehead's (1989) investigation into health trends in Britain. While she is encouraged by 'the evidence of growing interest in education for health … during the 1980s', Whitehead concludes that 'the total amount of effort and resources put into education for health is still significant in relation to the size of the task and in relation to the resources allocated to other policies of arguably lower priority' (Whitehead 1989: 5).

Whitty & Jones (1995) echo Whitehead's sentiments. They note the tripartite components of the public health function as laid down in the Acheson Report (Department of Health 1998a): to survey the health of the population; to promote and maintain health; and to ensure that the means are available to evaluate existing health services. Whitty & Jones (1995: 385) are concerned, however, about the 'growing misconception that "purchasing for health gain"' is the process by which '"promoting and maintaining health"...will be achieved'. They contend that this confusion has been fed by the government's paper *The Health of the Nation*, which, because it equates health promotion with 'changes in individual life-style as the means of preventing disease', demonstrates a 'misunderstanding of effective health promotion strategies'. That the government requires evidence of 'health service utilization' testifies to its wish to perpetuate the myth that purchasing health services will improve the health of the population, a myth with which members of the medical profession seem all too eager to comply in order to retain their clinical autonomy (see below). Additionally, it is particularly worrying to witness the 'strong political direction' to which the health service is becoming increasingly subjected and to observe the relentless process whereby its financial and human resources are, under the tight control of administrators, being continually pruned.

Within the reactive approach characteristic of the biomedical model, there is little room to embrace the positive idea of health as going beyond the mere absence of disease in collections of isolated, freely choosing individuals. Because it cannot accommodate the concept of 'social health', the model fails to reflect crucial areas of human experience. It rejects the Aristotelian conception of society as comprising interdependent human beings. It ignores the painful truth of social inequality: that people's life-chances, and therefore their opportunities to make choices, are necessarily unequal (Rodmell & Watt 1986, Morgan et al 1988, Townsend et al 1992, Beattie et al 1993, Jones 1994, Benzeval et al 1995, Davey et al 1995). Furthermore, as noted above, the model conceives of health as a commodity rather than as a basic human right. Policy based on this philosophy shows no genuine desire to create a society in which the current disparities in health would be minimized. Acknowledgement of the validity of subjective human experience would prompt central government to adopt more positive health strategies since its principal concern would be the restoration and maintenance of social health. Burkitt (1986), Coutts & Hardy (1985), and Ewles & Simnett (1999) describe sociological models of health education that appear to be based on a recognition of the need to encompass lay perspectives and experiences concerning health and illness (Sim 1990b). Acknowledging the socioeconomic determinants of health, the practitioner 'stresses the need for social planning, e.g. housing estates that allow family generations and social networks to be maintained, challenging the power relationship between the professional and the client' (Burkitt 1986: 3). As Sim (1990b) suggests, this model provides an additional – and distinct – conceptual framework within which a professional may work; its importance lies in its ability to 'show that strictly medical concepts and definitions are insufficient if we are to understand the way in which individuals conceive of health and illness and how this understanding shapes their behaviour' (Sim 1990b: 424). Certainly, the biomedical model is unable to accommodate the concepts of 'disability' and 'handicap' (see, for example, Oliver 1983, 1990, Brechin et al 1988, Swain et al 1993, 2003a, French 1994a, Morris 1995).

Perhaps, however, there is a more sinister reason behind central government's apparent preference for the biomedical above other models of health upon which to base policy. It has already been suggested that the NHS reforms have endorsed this above other models and it would be naive to assume that this was accidental. Sim (1990b: 424) alerts us to what he perceives as the most serious objection to the biomedical approach: 'it makes those who are experts on disease the sole arbiters of health. The layperson's views and experiences related to health are thereby disqualified'. As many sociologists observe, this has led to the 'medicalization' of health, in which the characteristic inequalities within the clinician/patient relationship are systematically preserved by the 'expert' in the interests of medical hegemony (Morgan et al 1988, Collier 1989, Jones 1994, White 2002, Scambler 2003); professional knowledge is a means of maintaining professional power. Following Freidson (1970), Morgan et al (1988: 23) suggest that 'the medical profession's power to control what constitutes health and illness has been used to extend the medical monopoly over areas of life and behaviour which were not traditionally the concern of the medical profession'. Thus, the medical profession effectively 'creates' illness in order to 'extend its professional dominance, with authority deriving from its professional status and claims of competence' (Morgan et al 1988: 23). Morgan et al (1988) cite childbirth as an area that has become increasingly medicalized by professional intervention (see also Coutts & Hardy 1985, Armstrong 1994, Jones 1994). Farrant & Russell (1986) offer further evidence of this 'vested interest' in relation to the former HEC's literature on CHD:

> Furthermore, the 'population' versus 'high risk' preventive strategy debate, within the medical literature, has, in part, to be seen in the context of the medical profession's own interests in keeping coronary prevention within medical control and within a conventional paradigm of medical intervention. One of the arguments that has been advanced in favour of a high-risk strategy of CHD prevention is that it offers for physicians (and patients) a more familiar and comfortable model of medical practice. The WHO notes that 'Doctors often lack the training and hence also the motivation to enlarge their responsibilities beyond the care of the sick'. However, Rose points out that much harder to overcome than this … 'is the enormous difficulty for medical personnel to see health as a population issue and not merely as a problem for individuals'. Thus, whilst epidemiological theory points towards a population approach to CHD prevention, reviews of current practice and initiatives in the medical literature … suggest an emphasis by the medical profession on the role of high-risk screening strategies within a medical setting (Farrant & Russell 1986: 22).

The above issues are linked to the social questions previously considered. For how long can the professionals continue to ignore the socio-economic and environmental determinants of disease and disability as identified by so many writers (for example, Burkitt 1986, Currer & Stacey 1986, Morgan et al 1988, Armstrong 1994, Jones 1994, Siegrist 2000, Marmot 2001, Wilkinson 2001, Freund et al 2003)? The unwillingness to acknowledge this aspect of health, together with the discrediting of people's knowledge and subjective experiences by professionals (Farrant & Russell 1986), seems to be a practice in which central government covertly, but actively, colludes.

3.3.3 OTHER MODELS: SOME FURTHER PROBLEMS

The 'illness' model of health that validates the subjective experience of being unwell has limitations, however, not dissimilar to some of those identified in the biomedical 'disease' model. Firstly, 'health' is a negative concept, derived from the notion of 'illness': its presence implies a corresponding absence of illness. This perspective therefore fails to reflect the potentially complex relationship between health and illness, either at an individual or social level. It cannot, for example, accommodate the possibility of the coexistence of both in a permanently disabled person. This individual may not feel 'ill' but it would not be meaningless or inappropriate for a physiotherapist to discuss strategies directed towards enhancing that individual's 'health'. Conversely, a person who is considered to be in good health might nevertheless testify to 'feeling unwell' and may be unable to identify the reasons for these feelings. Second, the 'illness' model focuses on the importance of restoring and maintaining a person's 'health' rather than on its positive improvement. Thus the sociological and environmental health education strategies described by Burkitt (1986) and by Ewles & Simnett (1999) could be viewed in this light and not necessarily as examples of proactive policy.

This positive aspect is captured in the 1946 definition of the World Health Organization (WHO), which presents health as a multidimensional, all-embracing concept that could apply to almost any aspect of a person's life (World Health Organization 1946). The WHO defines health as 'The complete physical, mental and social well-being and not simply the absence of disease or infirmity' (see also Webb 1994b). The definition, however, raises many problems, not the least of which is related to its terminology. For example, how are we to understand the notion of 'well-being'? Is it identical with that of 'health'? On an Aristotelian analysis, the association between 'well-being' and human flourishing suggests that 'health' is a necessary, but not a sufficient condition for *eudaimonia* – happiness (see Aristotle 1986). The attainment of a happy life is to some extent dependent upon good fortune; thus it would seem possible for a person to be 'healthy' but not to experience 'happiness' or 'well-being'.

Together with these theoretical difficulties, adopting the WHO's (1946) concept of health poses potential practical problems. Insofar as it purports to reflect a generally shared ideal, the WHO's notion of health does not fully acknowledge the view expressed by Ewles & Simnett (1999) that being healthy means different things to different people. A similar allegiance to (liberal) individualism is embodied in exhortations to treat health as a matter of opinion rather than of fact (Coutts & Hardy 1985). In any case, as implied earlier, the WHO's notion of health is utopian and therefore probably unattainable by the majority of individuals. With reference to health education, it proves difficult to implement. Because health is equated with all the positive aspects of life experience, the clear identification and, indeed, achievement, of a person's health goals becomes extremely problematic.

3.4 FROM THEORY TO PRACTICE

In an attempt to crystallize the arguments adduced above concerning the disadvantages of the biomedical model, it now seems appropriate to examine one health educator's account of practice. The account highlights further difficulties associated with this particular health educator's (unsuccessful) struggle to extricate himself from a fundamental conviction in the efficacy of a biomedical approach. To focus on these kinds of ideological problems seems to be particularly relevant to a discussion whose chief aim is to encourage a more analytical and critical approach to physiotherapy practice.

David Muir, promotions officer at the Look After Yourself Project Centre, Christchurch College, Canterbury, outlines a training course which comprised part of the popular Look After Yourself programme in which many UK health authorities have been involved (Muir 1989). That the writer's fundamental allegiance is to the biomedical model of health is evident from the tone of the opening claim: 'Good health is considered by most people to be the single most important thing that they want in their lives, and yet many do little about it' (Muir 1989: 59). In a characteristically Cartesian manner, he then compares bodily health with inanimate objects such as 'cars and household appliances' and criticizes those who 'prefer to wait until something goes wrong' rather than taking preventive action. Although Muir's intention seems to be to discredit the biomedical model, his language betrays an allegiance to its tenets. He asserts that 'Health is sometimes mistaken for fitness' but rejects this limited perspective because it neglects 'other important aspects of a healthy life-style' such as making 'sound' dietary choices, maintaining 'correct' physical weight and the ability to 'cope adequately' with life stress, all of which he sees as playing 'an integral part in helping to achieve the sort of health which makes you feel good' (Muir 1989: 59).

For Muir, then, 'health' is detectable in individuals by the application of prescribed objective criteria (including those of aesthetics, rational ability and emotional resilience). That 'health' is also identified with 'life-style' and 'well-being', however, seems to indicate Muir's recognition of the shortcomings of a biomedical model and, it appears, his wish to convey an indebtedness to other models, for example the model that incorporates the subjective notion of 'illness' (Sim 1990b) against which 'wellness' is judged (see also Armstrong 1994, Scambler 2003). In this context, we may now enquire as to whether Muir believes that the notions of 'health' and 'well-being' refer to synonymous states? Does his concept of 'health' incorporate the Aristotelian idea of *eudaimonia* (Harré 1990)? If Muir equates 'health' with 'flourishing', perhaps he also has in mind a positive conception of 'health' based on the somewhat utopian definitions of the WHO.

However eclectic Muir's conception of health may appear to be, he takes it to be a self-evident truth that health comprises an appropriate subject for education. The premise is characteristic of the biomedical model of health education (Burkitt 1986, Hyland 1988). This premise, which carries the status of a priori truth, is that if teachers equip individuals with skills and knowledge that are appropriate to their health needs, those individuals will be able to take positive steps towards achieving what Muir considers to be this desirable state. Indeed, such tuition will enable class participants to 'make gradual changes' to 'their life-style'. Muir is keen to demonstrate a commitment to a 'progressive' educational philoso-phy: his 'integral' group training scheme is participative. Significantly, however, its objectives are couched in familiar terminology: 'gaining an understanding of relevant health topics', instructing individuals how to exercise 'safely and regularly' and teaching 'understanding and coping with stress and knowing how to practise simple relaxation techniques' (Muir 1989: 59).

Finally, Muir manages to introduce another concept: 'holism' (as described by Flew 1983, Burkitt 1986, Newbeck 1986, Newbeck & Rowe 1986, Pietroni 1987, Seedhouse & Cribb 1989, Barnitt & Pomeroy 1995, Davey et al 1995, Ewles & Simnett 1999). He seeks to link his concepts to 'health' and 'health education' by advertising his training programme as an example of a 'holistic' approach to management. Muir (1989: 59) is confident that: 'The importance of this "holistic" or "total" approach to health and well-being is recognized by an increasing majority of those involved in promoting good health, and many see it as essential to their work...' In common with some physiotherapists (see, for example, Williams 1986, Jackson 1987), Muir perceives it to be a legitimate (and professionally advantageous) strategy to synthesize 'science' and 'art' and 'orthodoxy' and 'alternativism' within practice. Since 'holism' repre-sents a philosophy whose principles stand in direct opposition to those of scientific reductionism, however, further questions arise. Is it empirically likely, and indeed, theoretically consistent, for a health educator to sub-scribe to both these philosophical perspectives? To indicate an indebted-ness to both within the scope of one paper, therefore, would seem to reflect either a genuine, or a contrived, metaphysical inconsistency, neither of which can pass unobserved. Certainly, to base practice on such a philosophical confusion cannot be countenanced, irrespective of other demonstrable weaknesses associated with the biomedical approach.

3.5 TOWARDS A PHILOSOPHY OF HEALTH

That our discussion of some of the problems associated with the biomed-ical approach to health and health education has inevitably exposed other difficulties in some alternative concepts of health should not disconcert us. Disadvantages, as well as advantages, are to be found with any model that can inform practice. There are no simple solutions to this complex problem. Acceptance of these conclusions need not, and indeed, should not, lead us to abandon our search for an attractive theoretical foundation upon which to base physiotherapy.

Our response to such intellectual challenges should be positive and constructive if qualitative improvements in physiotherapy practice are to be effected. Sim (1990b: 426) believes that physiotherapists require a primary, proactive model of health on which to base practice. He contends that 'a more ambitious and wide-ranging definition is necessary' if management is to incorporate 'activities concerned with enhancing health and extending its boundaries'. Sim then cites two theorists, Whitbeck (1981) and Seedhouse (1986), who conceive of health in terms of human aspiration or potential. For Sim, the attractions of such a concept are twofold. First, 'a high degree of health may coexist with illness or disease'; second, 'health as a concept extends beyond the sphere of medical care, and may even be incompatible with certain aspects of medicine'. 'Health', thus 'embraces all spheres of the individual's life in which human aspirations can be realised' (Sim 1990b: 426). Katherine Mansfield's description of health (cited in Coutts & Hardy 1985) and the WHO's (1946) definition (cited in Whitehead 1989) embody this ideal.

Certainly, Seedhouse's philosophy is attractive in many respects, as reflected in his concept of health: 'A person's optimum state of health is equivalent to the state of the set of conditions which fulfil or enable a person to work to fulfil his or her realistic chosen and biological potentials. Some of these conditions are of the highest importance for all people. Others are variably dependent upon individual abilities and circumstances' (Seedhouse 1986: 61).

Because they comprise the foundations of Seedhouse's general philosophy, it is worth expanding on some of the ideas contained within the above definition. The fundamental, ethical premise is that health is 'an undefined yet self-evident "good"' (Seedhouse 1994). Seedhouse's concept of a person (Seedhouse 1988) seems to owe much to the Aristotelian ideology discussed earlier, which conceives of persons as interdependent social human beings whose individual potential for achievement is inextricably linked with that of the flourishing of society in general (see MacIntyre 1985). For Seedhouse, each person possesses certain basic rights, among which is the right to health. Since the attainment of a person's health is necessarily linked with the realization of 'his or her realistic chosen and biological potentials', it is evident that Seedhouse is committed to a fundamental belief that each person has the right to claim personal autonomy, central to which is the notion of 'choice' (Seedhouse & Cribb 1989, Seedhouse & Lovett 1992, Seedhouse 1994; see also Raz (1986) for a full discussion of personal autonomy). Seedhouse's concept of persons is also informed by his stated commitment to other ethical principles: equality, fairness and justice (Seedhouse & Cribb 1989, Seedhouse & Lovett 1992, Seedhouse 1994). Persons are, for Seedhouse, intrinsically valuable: they have the right to be treated according to specific moral precepts.

Given that he adopts this particular concept of a person, it is consistent for Seedhouse to conceive of the health worker as having a duty to guarantee these basic rights. He thus characterizes 'Work for health' as 'essentially *enabling*' (Seedhouse 1986: 64, original emphasis) and associates it with 'providing the appropriate foundations' to facilitate the achievement of personal potentials. The health worker is encouraged to remove obstacles to the attainment of a person's 'biological and chosen goals' and to provide 'the basic means by which [such] goals can be achieved'. Seedhouse openly acknowledges the 'fuzzy' boundaries of the concept of health: 'The world is an interconnected whole: nothing is finally clear-cut'. Using a time-honoured metaphor, Seedhouse makes a crucial point, pertinent to all those engaged in health work: 'Work for health is work on building a solid stage, and keeping that stage in good condition. The roles that people perform, and how they choose to perform these roles upon that stage is up to the individuals provided that the platform is sound' (Seedhouse 1986: 65).

Turning to the concept of 'education', Seedhouse (1986: 83) contrasts it with 'training', which he equates with 'indoctrination' and 'which involves imparting a single set of ideas'. He proposes a theory of education which contrasts with that espoused by the biomedical model. Seedhouse regards education as having two principal aims: first, 'To provide the learner, either directly or indirectly, with all relevant information about a subject area'; second, 'To instil a childlike curiosity ... to encourage a questioning attitude, a confidence to select and to criticise; to promote the sense that the information that is being presented is what we have now – it is not the final word; and to encourage the idea that each of us is part of a continuing inquiry' (Seedhouse 1986: 83). To suggest that all our knowledge is tentative, provisional and changing and that everyone (professional and layperson alike) is engaged in an on-going enquiry is to challenge the fundamental premises upon which the biomedical model is based. This challenge, in itself, is liberating and therefore empowering.

Seedhouse's concept of health education is derived from the synthesis of his ideas on health and education. He contends that health education 'should not indoctrinate' or be 'a propaganda exercise' (Seedhouse 1986: 84). Its aim should be: first, 'To ensure that all people have a good standard of general education', and second, 'To develop people's powers of conceiving, and so to enable them to make the most of the information they have' (Seedhouse 1986: 85–86). Seedhouse identifies what he believes to be the benefits – to both professionals and lay people – of a health education programme which embodies these aims and exhorts the health professionals to strive towards them (Seedhouse 1986).

3.5.1 IMPLICATIONS FOR PRACTICE

Some of the implications of adopting Seedhouse's philosophy need to be identified. These seem to fall into two broad categories: those associated with personal attitude change and those related to the practical aspects of health care and the manner of its delivery. With reference to the former category, it behoves all of us to undertake a regular re-examination of our metaphysical and ethical beliefs in relation to our role as health care workers. How we conceive of 'health', 'health education' and 'persons' will determine the quality of our services. For example, many of us regard the patient–therapist relationship as central to clinical practice without ever questioning either the underlying assumptions associated with these concepts or, more fundamentally, our own frame of linguistic reference. That language reflects ideological beliefs and attitudes is confirmed by the periodic need to revise dictionaries. The language we use to describe the world, however, also defines the framework within which we perceive that world. Thus the very use of the terms 'therapist' (agent) and 'patient' (passive recipient) dictates how we conceive of this relationship, and may, indeed, contribute to the perpetuation of that attitude. The fact that these terms continue to be used supports the contention that many professionals wish to preserve the inherent inequalities that characterize their relationships with members of the general public. Had there been a genuine wish to eliminate this inequality and establish a relationship founded on egalitarian principles, the traditional nomenclature would surely have been replaced by terms deemed to reflect these ideals. It therefore seems to be necessary to introduce a new linguistic frame of reference in order to precipitate an attitude change that has hitherto been slow to evolve. Interestingly, it has been suggested by a music therapy colleague that the terms 'researcher' and 'co-researcher' deserve serious consideration as contenders. Within this frame of reference, 'education' for 'health' would be a socially shared goal, a collective enterprise, with each participant demonstrating mutual respect for personal autonomy reflected in a willingness to engage in the processes of both teaching and learning.

To focus briefly on the second category concerning the various aspects of health care delivery, many physiotherapists currently seem to encounter numerous extrinsic as well as intrinsic barriers to good practice. Lyne & Phillipson (1986: 10) catalogue a number of these barriers and identify 'the pressure of acute referrals' as being 'the most significant barrier to health education'. They cite other problems associated with workload and work organization and lack of resources (see also Leathley 1988) and report that 'problems of professionalism' and 'communication between professions' further militate against educational activities. Whitehead (1989) echoes these problems and identifies additional obstacles to good practice. The first of these 'is almost certainly inadequacies in pre-service and in-service training' which is often 'treatment orientated'.

Whitehead (1989: 32) alludes to the unsatisfactory practice of ' "crisis" treatment' and the fact that some professionals do not consider 'educational work' as 'their role', some report 'lack of confidence in educational skills, and lack of support from managers who may give the impression that it is not a legitimate activity for their staff'. The results of a survey undertaken by Sluijs et al (1993) reveal that those therapists with high expectations about the effects of educational compliance paid more attention to the education of their patients and that those who spent more time with their patients had a better relationship with them.

3.6 CONCLUSION

How, then, are we to effect attitudinal and organizational change? How are we to overcome these various obstacles to the establishment of good practice? As Whitehead (1989: 43) laments, 'the over-riding impression … is one of health educators attempting to swim upstream, against the current of forces which have operated to damage health or undermine educational efforts'. Her report of lay participation in community health projects, however, provides an encouraging example of what is surely good practice of the kind in which more physiotherapists could become increasingly involved, given opportunities and encouragement to do so by their managers. Furthermore, Whitehead's account of community-based health education illustrates that change, although a difficult process to manage, is possible, given the initial commitment among professional health workers. And this is the crucial point. In order to establish and maintain good practice, physiotherapists must be genuinely committed to this ideal; they must find the energy to examine and evaluate their knowledge, skills and attitudes on a regular basis and be receptive to new perspectives. Where possible, they must initiate and manage change within both the educational and clinical context and, perhaps most importantly, they must work to dismantle interprofessional barriers.

If these exhortations are summarily dismissed as the incoherent ravings of an inveterate idealist, it is difficult to find a rational argument that might serve to combat such a reaction. The only hope, perhaps, lies in directing the reader to Mary Warnock's writings on educational practice and, in particular, to her valuable observation that 'it is the function of an ideal to be unattainable. It is no argument against adopting an ideal, therefore, to show that it is impossible to attain it' (Warnock 1977: 31). To aim for the establishment of physiotherapy practice based on Aristotelian principles does not, therefore, imply a naive belief that this aim will be fully realized; rather, it demonstrates a genuine commitment to those principles and a serious intention to strive towards their realization.

Chapter 4

Coping with illness

Frances Reynolds

4.1 INTRODUCTION

The purpose of this chapter is to explore and illustrate the many diverse ways in which people cope with illness. As well as increasing a sense of empathy for patients, the information may suggest ways in which patients' coping strategies and resources can be enhanced through physiotherapy. The chapter will explore a range of positive coping strategies that serve to increase subjective well-being and improve physical health. The chapter will also consider strategies that can have maladaptive consequences. Some of the factors that influence people's choice of strategy will also be examined, including personality characteristics, values and support systems.

As indicated in Chapter 11, there are close relationships between people's perceptions of illness and their coping responses. An illness or injury that is experienced as highly threatening to the person's functioning, identity or indeed life itself sets quite different coping challenges compared with an illness that is believed to be transient. These responses are partly determined by the condition itself. Acute (short-term) conditions are often regarded as relatively manageable, and a range of straightforward, problem-solving strategies may be applied such as seeking medical attention, rest, self-medication or 'lay' remedies (such as ice-packs for sprained ankles). Nevertheless, even acute conditions may provoke frustration and anxiety when valued roles and activities are interrupted. For example, an élite athlete may fear that a fracture could end his or her sporting career. Chronic illnesses and any long-term impairments arising from injury tend to give rise to a wider range of difficulties. The person in such circumstances confronts not only problems directly related to their disease or injury, such as pain, or mobility limitations, but also emotional responses, social role changes and threats to self-image. The intrusiveness of an illness into everyday life also affects coping and distress (Mullins et al 2001). Some long-term conditions, such as mild diabetes, may be relatively invisible to others, especially when controllable through effective self-management strategies. Conversely, illnesses that seriously undermine social roles and daily activities, or which profoundly affect the person's view of the future, pose different challenges for coping. Not surprisingly, individuals manage these diverse challenges in a variety of ways. In the absence of a cure, people with chronic conditions require resourcefulness, tenacity and a broad repertoire of coping strategies if they are to adapt successfully to ensuing changes in their health, identity and lifestyle, and achieve an acceptable quality of life.

4.2 WHAT IS 'COPING'?

Coping refers to actions taken to deal with and minimize harm or threat. Coping with illness involves not only dealing with physical symptoms and dysfunction, but also managing the psychological, social and financial changes that accompany illness. Some strategies are more or less consciously selected. For example, a person with increasing mobility problems due to multiple sclerosis may decide to use a wheelchair after a lengthy period of reflection and debate about the advantages and disadvantages of this option. He or she may seek information from wheelchair services and from acquaintances with a similar health condition. Friends and family may be consulted. Advantages such as easier access to shops and other facilities may be weighed against anticipated disadvantages, such as the possibility of negative social reactions. Other types of coping strategy may be determined by much less explicit decision-making processes. For example, some people respond to highly threatening diagnoses by denial, refusing to believe medical opinion. Denial appears to be a subconscious defence mechanism protecting the person against unmanageable levels of anxiety. With time, support and additional information, there may be less need for denial, and the person may gradually recognize and accept the diagnosis, and move on to other forms of coping (Kubler-Ross 1969, Davidhizar & Giger 1998).

Two vignettes follow, illustrating the way in which individuals seek to cope with their health problems.

Case study

Elaine is 61 years old. Three years ago she was treated for breast cancer. She describes herself as having had 'the full works', i.e. mastectomy, radiotherapy and chemotherapy. Lymph nodes were removed from her armpit and this surgery has left her with difficulties in raising her left arm. She arranges to have physiotherapy for this problem from time to time, and is usually conscientious about practising the exercises that she has been recommended. Elaine experienced the cancer treatment as highly stressful – 'not the best of times', she said ironically – and she took early retirement from work on health grounds. Both Elaine and her husband have occupational pensions.

Elaine recounts that she was both fearful and angry about the illness in the early days, and that she talked a great deal about her feelings to a close friend. Her husband was too upset himself to really listen to her experiences. She says that she now thinks much less about the possibility of death, and has recently decided to fulfil a life-long ambition. Last September, Elaine enrolled on a fine arts degree course. She jokes that she cannot really draw but that she is enjoying the course immensely. She decided not to tell anyone on the course about her cancer as she cannot tolerate being pitied, and would prefer others to relate to her on her own terms.

Case study

Jack is 45 years old, and is married, with 10-year-old twin boys. He has osteoarthritis, and has severe pain in his knees. He delayed seeking medical advice for several years, and self-medicated with pain-killing tablets. In the last year he has been assessed by a consultant and placed on a waiting list for knee replacement surgery. Jack is worried about losing his job as a warehouseman, and is rarely absent. He finds it difficult to talk to his wife

about his health and job worries, and she is concerned about the level of medication and alcohol that he is using. His wife thinks that his health and functioning might improve if he lost some weight, increased his fitness, and followed advice from a physiotherapist. However, Jack does not feel able to take these initiatives. He feels that working and providing for his family, despite almost constant pain, are taking up all his energy.

In reflecting on the coping strategies employed by Jack and Elaine, it is clear that Elaine was quite expressive of her feelings in the early stages of illness, confiding her fears and other experiences to a close friend. This may have helped her adjustment considerably (Stanton et al 2000). Nevertheless, she chooses whom to confide in. She maintains control over her disclosures to fellow students in order to present a positive self-image and to avoid pity, or the 'master status' that cancer can confer on a person (Charmaz 1991). Jack, in contrast, does not seem able or willing to talk about his health problems to anyone. For some time, he even delayed seeking help from medical practitioners. It is unclear whether he sees help-seeking as a form of 'weakness', that perhaps challenges his notion of masculinity. Elaine is using the opportunity of early retirement to immerse herself in an occupation that she has long been interested in – fine art. Her studies help her to develop her creative potential, and may serve to distract her thoughts away from the possibility of the recurrence of cancer. Elaine's quality of life and ability to cope with her health problems may also be enhanced through the opportunities for social contact that the course provides. She is also taking appropriate steps to manage her residual disability through physiotherapy. These are very sound strategies for living positively with a long-term health problem. Judging from her use of irony during the interview, she also seems to cope with difficulties through humour. Jack does not seem to have these resources and appears much more restricted in his choices. He is using strategies (such as self-medication and alcohol) that suppress his pain and worries, but he does not seem able to take positive health-promoting actions. His role as provider to the family is all-important to him, and is probably central to his identity. His focus on accomplishing this role leaves little room for actively managing his health problems. He appears to put his family's needs above his own. It is possible that Elaine's greater financial security, and lack of dependent children, provide her with greater choice and control over her lifestyle.

4.3 A MODEL OF COPING

While a number of distinctive coping strategies have been identified on the basis of the vignettes above, they have not been connected in any theoretical way. Lazarus & Folkman (1984) presented an influential model of stress and coping, based largely on quantitative studies using standardized scale measures. However, the model may require further development on the basis of qualitative studies that explore how people describe their personal ways of living with illness and the development of their strategies over time.

The model of Lazarus & Folkman (1984) portrays stress as more than an objective external event. Instead, the amount of stress experienced is determined by two sets of cognitive (appraisal) processes. Firstly, the person appraises the personal meaning of an event such as illness (primary appraisal), and the degree of threat that it poses. For example, a woman who has witnessed a close relative become very disabled with rheumatoid arthritis might respond with extreme anxiety to receiving a similar diagnosis herself (Donovan & Blake 2000). Patients who have not had this negative experience might feel much more reassured by receiving a medical opinion that their arthritis is mild, and controllable through medication and physiotherapy. As well as appraising the threat of illness or injury,

Lazarus & Folkman (1984) describe secondary appraisal processes. That is, individuals who confront a stressful event reflect on their coping resources, and evaluate whether these are equal to the task in hand. They may decide that they have successfully confronted similar events in the past. Confidence may also be increased if they know others who have coped well with a similar problem. For example, a person newly diagnosed with multiple sclerosis may feel more confident about coping if he or she has observed a relative with neurological disease live a satisfactory lifestyle. Coping resources also include social support and information. A socially isolated person with little knowledge about the nature of the disease or injury might feel overwhelmed by anxiety. This perspective on coping reminds us that people cope with medically similar illnesses in different ways, depending on their personal appraisal of the illness and their coping resources.

From the Lazarus & Folkman perspective, stress has both objective and subjective features, so coping reflects both strategies for managing the stressful event itself and also strategies for managing the feelings that the stressful event provokes. This leads to a differentiation between *problem-focused* and *emotion-focused* coping. For some forms of stress, this is a helpful distinction. At work, for example, a person may deal with a stressful workload by delegating tasks or through better time management. These are problem-focused strategies because they directly tackle the nature of the overload, or its causes. Alternatively, the person may take more time to unwind after work – for example, through taking physical exercise or talking with friends. Another person might adopt a less adaptive approach – for example, drinking alcohol to excess, or engaging in fantasy or wishful thinking. These strategies may be regarded as emotion-focused because they help the person to deal with the build-up of anger or anxiety that the workload is creating, rather than addressing the workload itself. Emotion-focused strategies tend to be more common in the early stages of a stressful experience such as illness, when shock, anxiety and grief reactions are uppermost. There is some evidence that emotion-focused strategies become less adaptive if they persist in the longer term. In particular, their use is associated with negative emotional states such as anxiety and depression (Felton et al 1984, Pakenham 1999). However, the distinction between problem-focused and emotion-focused strategies is not always helpful for illuminating people's ways of living with illness.

It is worth debating how to classify Elaine's engagement in art, and the role that it is playing in helping her to cope with cancer. In some senses it is the disease itself that is the 'problem'. However, given that little more can be done to cure Elaine's cancer, perhaps a variety of problem-focused and emotion-focused strategies are needed to tackle the experiences of illness, rather than the disease process itself. Elaine's illness has resulted in retirement from work and loss of roles. Art-work may therefore be a problem-focused strategy because it deals successfully with the problem of how to use time productively within the home environment. On the other hand, art may be considered as an emotion-focused strategy helping Elaine to feel more positive about her self and her abilities, and enabling self-expression. This strategy may also be a distraction or psychological escape from illness – a strategy that is not clearly problem-focused or emotion-focused (Carver et al 1989).

Such debates have led some to argue that the distinction between problem-focused and emotion-focused strategies is too coarse-grained a classification, with too many disparate strategies grouped under these umbrella headings (Leventhal et al 1997). Nevertheless, others support this classification because evidence indicates that patients who adopt problem-focused strategies achieve greater well-being. Therapists may help patients to cope more successfully with illness by encouraging the use of problem-solving strategies for dealing with the difficulties that they are experiencing. In addition, having access to a broad repertoire of coping strategies may promote greater well-being. However, rapid changes and instability in coping strategies may be detrimental and reflect greater emotional distress or desperation about a health problem (Schwartz & Daltroy 1999).

4.4 POSITIVE SELF-MANAGEMENT STRATEGIES IN ILLNESS

People adjusting successfully to long-term health problems tend to develop a variety of self-management strategies over time. These include:

- Acquiring information (about the disease, treatment options, benefits and services)
- Health promotion strategies (improving nutrition and physical exercise, practising relaxation and developing meaningful occupations that promote well-being)
- Goal-setting and pacing
- Increasing social support (e.g. joining organizations for people with similar health problems)
- Personal growth strategies – altering priorities and finding meaning
- Humour.

4.4.1 ACQUIRING AND USING INFORMATION

Patients' needs for empowering information about their condition should be recognized by everyone working in the multidisciplinary team. Bennett (1993) refers to the obligation of health professionals to provide 'informational care'. Knowledge enables patients to manage their anxiety through being better able to interpret their symptoms and needs, to make informed choices about treatment options, and to experience an enhanced sense of control, even in the context of serious progressive disease (Earll et al 1993). Such experiences are vital for combating depression, and for increasing commitment or adherence to treatment, thereby maximizing health. There is evidence that knowledge can affect measurable outcomes. For example, patients who have information before surgery that helps them to interpret their postoperative symptoms tend to be less anxious, use less analgesic medication and sometimes have shorter hospital stays (Schuldam 1999). Therapists can help patients gain relevant information through referring them to books, leaflets, internet sites and patients' support organizations.

However, they need to be aware that patients' anxiety about their illness often interferes with their processing of information, especially in the early stages of treatment (Hammond 1998). Vital information may need to be repeated several times. Therapists need to pass on not only information about the disease or injury, but also evidence about treatment effectiveness, to harness the patient's motivation to adhere to recommendations (Abbott et al 2001). Some patients become very knowledgeable about their condition and treatment options, and have many questions and opinions about their treatment programme. Rather than responding defensively, Wilson (1999) argues that health professionals need to harness patients' expertise positively in the rehabilitation process.

4.4.2 HEALTH PROMOTION STRATEGIES

Health promotion strategies can also increase the person's self-efficacy (sense of confidence) for managing their health problems (Stuifbergen & Rogers 1997). Physical health and well-being are maximized by good nutrition and physical exercise. The person adopting positive health behaviours may also benefit psychologically from feeling in greater control of his or her health condition. Physiotherapists can have an important role to play in advising people with acute and chronic conditions about safe exercise that will help to maintain health, strength and mobility. Sleep, rest and a graded or paced approach to daily activity are also important for restoring well-being, and for managing fatigue and pain.

Meaningful occupation also contributes to well-being, although it has been a neglected area of health promotion. Illnesses commonly restrict work and leisure activities, leaving people with not only empty days, but also a loss of enjoyment and self-esteem. People who retain (or acquire) work and leisure pursuits during illness may be better able to resist 'mastery' by their illness (Charmaz 1991), and achieve a better quality of life (Lundmark & Branholm 1996, Reynolds 1997). Work and leisure counselling requires a multidisciplinary approach, involving occupational therapy, health psychology and others, and may facilitate an important means of coping with ill health (Drummond & Walker 1995).

4.4.3 GOAL-SETTING AND PACING

Some people cope with chronic conditions, such as back pain, by setting manageable, meaningful goals. Indeed, this approach is foundational to most pain management treatment programmes. Goals may be both short-term and longer-term. Pacing valued activities around one's limitations enables a sense of accomplishment (Mannerkorpi et al 1999) and helps the person to maintain morale and hope. Evidence of reaching interim goals is valuable for demonstrating progress. Having active task management strategies helps to counteract the sense of helplessness that might otherwise give rise to depression. Goals need not necessarily relate to physical accomplishments, such as walking a certain distance. Well-being may be maintained, for example, through setting a goal of widening one's social circle, or finishing a creative product such as a painting or tapestry (Reynolds 1997).

4.4.4 INCREASING SOCIAL SUPPORT

Social support is vital for most people with pain and long-term health problems, partly because it appears to protect against depression (Brown et al 1989b). Initially, therapists and others within the multidisciplinary team may offer an important source of support. Family and friends may also provide practical and emotional help, although some people find that their willingness declines over time (Lackner et al 1994). Coping may also be boosted through making contact with people who are in similar circumstances. Many patients' support organizations provide face-to-face support through local branch meetings, as well as indirect support via newsletters and websites. Therapists can help patients develop such support networks through having the appropriate addresses and telephone numbers of local organizations available (for example, for people with multiple sclerosis or cancer).

Meeting with others who have a similar health problem helps to reduce feelings of isolation and rumination on questions such as 'Why me?' Support groups often share coping strategies and information, thereby empowering more appropriate choice and reducing the individual's sense of powerlessness. Members often value the opportunity of being simply 'themselves', when they are used to the burden of having to put on a brave face to avoid distressing family and friends (Lackner et al 1994). Practical as well as emotional help gained through joining a group may make a considerable difference to the person's quality of life (for example, help with shopping or gardening). Some people feel more positive about their own circumstances by recognizing that others are coping successfully with more advanced or serious forms of the illness. Support is also a two-way process. Many people find that through offering support to others within a group they gain a strong sense of satisfaction and self-esteem (Schwartz & Sendor 1999). This issue leads on to considering personal growth strategies for coping with illness.

4.4.5 POSITIVE GROWTH STRATEGIES

While most people anticipate that serious illness would be a wholly negative experience, studies are showing that some people interpret the illness experience as having had certain positive effects on their lives (Holahan et al 1996). Crossley (2000) found that more than half of the people she interviewed with HIV/AIDS described their health condition as the catalyst for a more authentic, more intense way of living. One man said:

> Before this diagnosis I think I would have lived in the future, looking to the future, but I think since I have had this diagnosis I'm much more living in the present, here and now, today and tonight … I think it is [a good thing] because it means I am getting the most from every moment as it is actually unfolding (Crossley 2000: 144).

Mohr et al (1999) found that a substantial subgroup of people with multiple sclerosis had found benefits within the illness experience, such as deepening social relationships, increasing spirituality and an enhanced appreciation of life. Studies such as these show that confronting illness and mortality sometimes leads to a radical reappraisal of values and priorities. Former lifestyles may be rejected as shallow and unthinking. Instead, people may embrace more meaningful occupations, or embark on life-long ambitions. Even people with very debilitating illness such as amyotrophic lateral sclerosis (a type of motor neurone disease) sometimes interpret their illness in positive terms. Indeed, one man taking part in a study by Young & McNicoll (1998) described his illness as a 'blessing', because it had enabled him to adopt a more authentic way of life. Reynolds (1997) found that some women with long-term health problems had taken up art-work in the aftermath of diagnosis, to cope with empty time, worry and pain. Ultimately their creative occupations had made such a positive impact on their quality of life that many did not regret the illness that had prompted their new lifestyle. Such findings require more research, but they indicate that 'coping' involves more than illness management. If valued occupations can be maintained, despite illness, then the person will continue to derive satisfaction, self-esteem, social contacts and a sense of purpose.

4.4.6 HUMOUR

Humour may signify an emotional distancing that is helpful to coping with unpleasant experiences. Several authors have argued that distancing and humour are vital resources for living positively with difficult life circumstances and transitions (Lefcourt & Davidson-Katz 1991, McGuire & Boyd 1993, Young & McNicoll 1998). Reeves et al (1999) noted how participants living with HIV infection made liberal use of humour. However, humour may only be an option for those enjoying a secure sense of self, and strong social support.

4.5 NEGATIVE STYLES OF COPING

Not surprisingly, for some patients, the stress of illness provokes a number of responses that could be considered dysfunctional or definitely harmful. These include:

- Prolonged denial
- Disengagement and helplessness
- Adoption of the sick role
- Abuse of non-prescription medication (for example, painkillers) and consumption of alcohol, and illicit drugs.

When used over time, these more passive strategies appear to be associated with increasingly severe depression (Brown et al 1989a).

4.5.1 DENIAL

Denial is not uncommon in the initial stages of illness, and represents a failure or refusal to recognize the true nature of the diagnosis or prognosis (Reeves et al 1999). From a psychodynamic perspective, denial is self-protective and allows the patient time to develop, below the threshold of conscious awareness, more adaptive coping strategies (Davidhizar & Giger 1998). However, if denial persists, unfortunate consequences may follow. For example, if the patient continues to ignore serious symptoms of disease, any eventual treatment is likely to be less successful. Opportunities to discuss important matters with the family may also be lost, with the result that the patient fails to participate in important decisions (for example, about home or hospice care in terminal illness). Prolonged denial may also prevent the patient from acquiring useful information and social support. This form of coping may also underpin the demands that some patients make for exhaustive investigations and multiple medical opinions. These in turn may lead to unnecessary surgery or medication, particularly in the case of chronic pain. Several authors have suggested that acceptance of illness improves self-management, whereas denial and avoidance behaviour are associated with treatment non-compliance (see, for example, Mayer 1991, Abbott et al 2001).

4.5.2 DISENGAGEMENT AND HELPLESSNESS

Where patients regard their illness as uncontrollable, and their treatment options as ineffective, they may feel overwhelmed by feelings of helplessness. Bennett et al (1999) found that patients treated for a first myocardial infarction who had low confidence in their ability to carry out exercise and negative beliefs about its effectiveness were less likely to report behavioural change in the subsequent 3 months. In turn, their rehabilitation and recovery could be impeded. Some of the people with fibromyalgia pain and fatigue interviewed by Mannerkorpi et al (1999) described how their lives had become dominated by illness symptoms that they could not cope with. Such responses are clearly detrimental to rehabilitation and quality of life.

4.5.3 ADOPTION OF THE SICK ROLE

Initially the concept of the sick role was not negative, and described the status, rights and obligations of the patient (Parsons 1951). By adopting the sick role, the person was entitled to abdicate usual responsibilities, and withdraw from work and other roles. In return for this lightened load, the patient focused on complying with treatment and recovering. The meaning of the sick role has shifted somewhat over time, and now it is often associated with excessive dependence. For example, a person suffering chronic pain or mobility problems may gradually perform fewer duties within the home. Many daily occupations may be curtailed, particularly when the patient's family unwittingly reinforces passivity through over-protection, and by taking over the person's usual roles and responsibilities. Even if the pain eventually subsides or becomes more manageable, the sick role behaviour is likely to continue, because it has been learned and rewarded over time. This process can lead the patient into an increasingly constricted, unsatisfying lifestyle, in which illness symptoms continue to be the main focus of attention.

4.5.4 ABUSE OF ALCOHOL AND ILLICIT DRUGS

Men seem to be somewhat more likely than women to use alcohol and illicit drugs when stressed (Gianakos 2002). This way of coping may be encouraged by prevailing cultural notions of masculinity, which inhibit men from expressing emotions and help-seeking (Lengua & Stormshak

2000). Alcohol abuse during current stress is more likely to occur when stress has previously been managed through alcohol consumption (Holahan et al 2001). In addition to its direct impact on health, substance abuse indirectly jeopardizes recovery and well-being through preventing the development of more adaptive problem-solving strategies. Therapists need to be aware of substance abuse, as this is likely to impair patients' ability to monitor their condition, to recall advice and to practise exercises learned in treatment. Referral for more specialist help to manage this health risk behaviour may be required.

4.6 SOME FACTORS INFLUENCING CHOICE OF COPING STRATEGY

Leventhal et al (1997: 28) point out that relatively little is known about how and why people select certain strategies for managing illness: 'Although a multitude of studies have been published on coping with illness, we know precious little about how people select a coping procedure and how they decide if it merits long-term commitment.' A number of influential factors have been discussed in the research literature, such as:

- Personality
- Social support networks
- Spiritual or religious values
- Severity and intrusiveness of symptoms experienced
- Cultural factors
- Environmental resources and barriers.

4.6.1 PERSONALITY

It appears that coping strategies may reflect long-standing personality traits and learned habits. These include traits such as hardiness (Wallston 1989), sense of coherence (Antonovsky 1990) and self-efficacy (Holahan et al 1996). These variously named traits all tend to be associated with a strong sense of control, meaningfulness and optimism. Carver et al (1989) propose that some people are by disposition optimistic whereas others are pessimistic, although it is unclear whether these traits or dispositions are genetically inherited or learned from early life experiences. Pessimists tend to expect the worst, and are prone to highly negative thoughts (which may take the form of catastrophizing; see Section 8.5.2). There is abundant evidence that patients whose thoughts dwell on the negative tend to be more depressed and tend to fare less well in rehabilitation. For example, Keefe et al (1989) showed that initial level of catastrophizing among people with rheumatoid arthritis was highly predictive of poorer rehabilitation outcomes 1 year later, even when other significant variables were controlled for. Conversely, optimism and a 'fighting spirit' seem on balance to promote well-being and adherence to treatment (Abbott et al 2001). Given this evidence, it appears important for therapists to help patients to resist pessimism. For example, a hopeful outlook may be encouraged through gently challenging the patient's pessimistic statements (such as 'I'll never do ... again'), by carefully grading exercises and treatment programmes to minimize the possibility of failure, and by demonstrating objective improvement to the patient (for example, through showing records of present and past performance in rehabilitation).

4.6.2 SOCIAL SUPPORT AND FAMILY DYNAMICS

Coping strategies and lifestyle choices are rarely a matter for the individual in isolation (Maes et al 1996). Family support or rejection have major influences on the person's choice of coping strategies. High levels of practical and emotional support are associated with adherence to treatment, positive emotional states and successful rehabilitation outcomes. But there is also some evidence that people cope less successfully with illness when exposed to a highly critical family context (Manne & Zautra 1989). Therapists need to be aware that chronic illness and serious injury (such as head injury or spinal cord injury) all too often precipitate the breakdown of marriages and partnerships, creating stress and loss of resources at the very time when support is vitally needed. People enjoying a wider social network also tend to have more diverse social roles (as colleague, friend, brother, etc.). This diversity is thought to be protective of well-being (Wethington et al 2000).

4.6.3 SPIRITUAL/ RELIGIOUS VALUES

Finding meaning in adversity is an enormous resource for coping with stress and achieving a better quality of life. Antonovsky (1990) argues that people with a strong sense of coherence are more likely to find such meaning. Strong religious or spiritual values help to provide people with a sense of meaning or purpose, as well as enhancing their experience of emotional support during serious illness. A number of qualitative studies have found that people describe long-term illness as clarifying their spiritual values, and as providing them with a sense of a higher power. Such a perspective may help the person to perceive illness as a journey towards the unknown, a journey shared by all living beings (Stuifbergen & Rogers 1997, Mohr et al 1999, Reeves et al 1999, Schwartz & Sendor 1999).

4.6.4 SEVERITY OR INTRUSIVENESS OF SYMPTOMS

It is not surprising that severe symptoms present more of a challenge to a person's coping resources. Hence, coping strategies may change in relation to exacerbations and remissions of illness. Among people with neck and low back pain, for example, more severe pain is associated with use of more passive coping strategies. In turn, passive coping relates to depression and poor general health (Mercado et al 2000). Maladaptive coping strategies also seem to be linked to more severe pain and activity limitation among people with rheumatoid arthritis (Zautra et al 1995). However, the direction of cause and effect is debated. While it is possible that maladaptive strategies encourage a greater preoccupation with pain and other symptoms, it is important to recognize that severe chronic discomfort can lead people into abandoning constructive strategies through despair and hopelessness.

4.6.5 CULTURAL FACTORS

Social and cultural belief systems determine the extent to which specific illnesses are stigmatized. Stigmatized illnesses are particularly stressful because it is more difficult for sufferers to be open about their health problems, or to gain social support. For example, Heckman et al (1998) compared the experiences of people with HIV infection living in urban and rural areas of the US. They found that rural dwellers reported much greater social discrimination in relation to their illness, experienced more anxiety and loneliness, and used more maladaptive coping strategies.

4.6.6 ENVIRONMENTAL RESOURCES AND BARRIERS

The availability of physical and environmental resources also affects coping. For example, positive policies towards illness and disability in the workplace may help some people to continue in work for longer, whereas negative attitudes and policies may lead to earlier enforced retirement. Given that financial security empowers choice (for example, enabling the purchase of suitable aids and adaptations in the home, or private physiotherapy), such enabling and disabling factors in the person's environment have a great impact on coping strategies and quality of life. For people with mobility problems, living successfully with illness depends in part upon transport – for example, whether the person has an adapted car, a companion who can drive, or a reliable local bus service for disabled users. Many unemployed disabled people find that social security benefits are set so low as to deny meaningful choices over housing, transport and leisure. Health professionals need to be aware of these powerful social and environmental barriers to successful coping.

4.7 COPING AS A DYNAMIC PROCESS

It is rare for people to cope with illness in a static way. Instead, early responses to illness are more likely to be emotion-focused, or may involve denial. A process of grieving for lost physical health may ensue. With greater experience of the illness or impairment, and increasing exposure to information and social support, the person may successfully tackle the stressful nature of illness through a range of active strategies. Some strategies manage the illness itself, or the feelings that it arouses, and some strategies promote health and quality of life more generally. In some cases, the person has too few personal, social and financial resources, and may become entrenched in maladaptive ways of dealing with illness. The arrival of additional stressors (such as loss of job or carer) may also change the person's previous ways of coping with illness. So too, changes in the nature of the disease (for example, the appearance of a new symptom such as incontinence) may challenge existing coping strategies and disrupt the psychological equilibrium previously established.

4.8 CONCLUSION

In this chapter, coping has been described as any strategy taken to deal with and minimize harm or threat. Coping with illness, particularly chronic conditions, involves more than managing symptoms. Role and identity change, and restrictions on work and leisure are all stressful parts of the illness experience. Some theorists have suggested that problem-focused coping strategies are more adaptive than emotion-focused strategies. In stressful situations where objective events can be altered, this statement is well supported by evidence. However, the distinction between problem-focused and emotion-focused strategies is more blurred in relation to coping with illnesses that have no cure. It is clear that people develop over time a variety of coping strategies. Some strategies relate directly to managing symptoms. For example, the person may find ways of performing daily tasks despite mobility limitations, or may practise exercise and relaxation to improve physical functioning. Other strategies deal with the wider stressors of illness, such as having unstructured time following retirement from work on health grounds. The person may explore activities that provide interest and satisfaction. Such activities may also help to motivate physical activity, maintain self-esteem and provide opportunities for participating in the community. Some strategies relate more to values and lifestyle. For example, illness for some people prompts a more authentic lifestyle and a deeper commitment to religious and/or humanitarian values. Maladaptive coping strategies tend to suppress feelings and awareness, and thereby offer little help in the longer term. The model developed by Lazarus & Folkman (1984) emphasizes that coping draws on particular resources, including personal skills, knowledge, personality traits, social support and environmental context. Therapists have a considerable role to play in helping patients to develop a wide, adaptive repertoire of coping strategies that serve to maximize health and promote a satisfactory level of well-being.

Chapter 5

Ageing in a social context: implications for health and social care

Paul Kingston

Old age is a stage in our lives, and like all other stages it has a face of its own, its own atmosphere and temperature, its own joys and miseries.

(Hesse 1976: 269; originally published 1952)

We believe that the joys, fears, sufferings, and mysteries of ageing can be successfully explored with humility and self-knowledge, with love and compassion, with a sense of the sacred, and with acceptance of physical decline and mortality.

(Cole & Winkler 1994: 12)

5.1 INTRODUCTION

Older people are an important part of the work of those engaged in rehabilitation in general and physiotherapy in particular (Pickles et al 1995, Lewis 2002, Squires & Hastings 2002). The aim of this chapter is not to focus on specific issues within the rehabilitation process, but to examine the social context of an ageing population, and to analyse the way in which ageing is constructed within social and medical discourse. More specifically, the chapter will first briefly outline the dominant medical discourse constructed by the medical profession around an ageing population in the middle of the twentieth century. Second, it will outline the emergence of a debate that considers 'old age' as a social construct, outlined by the theoretical positions of political and moral economy. Third, the emerging area of cultural studies within a gerontological framework will be analysed. Fourth, reference to ageism will be considered alongside the implications of all four frameworks for therapeutic work with older people.

5.2 PERSPECTIVES ON AGEING

5.2.1 THE EARLY GERONTOLOGICAL LITERATURE

Perhaps one of the enduring themes noted in both early literary texts and certainly found in the general political discourse around an ageing population is ambivalence. It has been argued that 'it is possible to detect two polarized views [of old age] ... So, while extremes are noted – from ridicule on the one hand to respect on the other – history generally suggests a less than positive view of old age' (Kingston 1999: 1).

Ambivalence was manifest in its most extreme form in early fictional writing, where euthanasia was considered as a social policy option for an ageing population. For example, Anthony Trollope, in *The Fixed Period* (Trollope 1993; first published 1882), described a British colony that attempted to change the law so that euthanasia through the use of chloroform was imposed at the age of 65. Similarly, a play written by Thomas Middleton in 1618, *The Old Law*, tells of the Duke of Epire, who institutes a policy whereby all women who have reached 60 and all men who have reached 80 are put to death (see Barker 1958). Even more astounding were the comments by Sir William Osler (a world-famous early geriatrician) during his valedictory before leaving Johns Hopkins University for the University of Oxford at the turn of the nineteenth century: 'I have two fixed ideas ... The first is the comparative uselessness of men above 40 years of age. My second fixed idea is the uselessness of men above 60 years of age.'

Comments from politicians have also expressed a negative attitude towards old age: 'It is dangerous to be in any way lavish to old age, until adequate provision has been assured for all other vital needs' (Beveridge Report 1942: para. 236).

These comments and illustrations can, in retrospect, be understood as early articulations of the 'generational equity' thesis, first noted in the 1980s. The concept of 'generational equity' is based on the thesis that 'the nation [USA] is squandering its wealth on entitlements to the elderly while children remain impoverished' (Quadagno 1990: 631).

Medical writing in the 1940s and 1950s also reflected anxieties about the economic resources required to provide an adequate health and welfare response for an ageing society (Kingston 1998: 5). The tenor of this early literature constructed an ageing population as a social problem. For example, the word 'problem' was frequently found in the title of many early publications: *Medical Problems of Old Age* (Exton-Smith 1955); *Social and Medical Problems of the Elderly* (Hazell 1960). Howell's comments reinforce a highly negative view of an ageing population: 'Of course, the basic fact is that old people consume more of our national wealth than they produce...This tends to diminish the standards of living for the remainder of the population. In fact, from the economic point of view, most old people are "parasites"' (Howell 1953: 13).

Further retrospection suggests that such negativity concerning an ageing population can be seen as setting the ground for what Robertson (1991) was to term some 40 years later 'apocalyptic demography'. This theoretical perspective suggests increasing numbers of impaired elderly people using a disproportionate percentage of the gross national product for their care and welfare in old age. Robertson's paper opens: '...catastrophic projections of the burden to society of an increasing ageing population abound' (Robertson 1991: 135). It is important to note that, while Robertson uses the term 'apocalyptic demography', her thesis contests the fallacy of such a construction around an ageing population.

Hagestad & Dannefer (2001: 5) have argued that such a 'misery perspective' (Tornstam 1992) may stem from good intentions: 'focusing on troubled segments of the older population in order to give decision makers a basis for making socio-political changes or aiding medical professionals'. More recently, Phillipson has argued that the way in which the concept of old age developed in the mid twentieth century was fashioned by two distinct trends: 'First, there was what Estes & Binney (1989) described as the "bio-medicalisation of ageing". The focus was on individual organic pathology and medical interventions...A second... feature...concerned the crucial role of the pharmaceutical industry in predetermining the "problem" of old age' (Phillipson 1998: 33). In summary, it is noted that, irrespective of the focus of the historical social construction of an understanding of an ageing population, it has rarely been possible to detect a positive discourse.

While such historical negativity is noted in such stark terms, it is still apparent that contemporary key debates are taking place concerning the economics of an ageing population, especially in relation to pensions, welfare spending and health and social care costs. It is suggested that ambivalence is still prevalent, and continues to materialize in debates about the relative societal cost of an ageing population. Clearly, the legacy of such a despondent view of an ageing population had not entirely disappeared in the late twentieth century. For example, the title of a publication from the World Bank (1994), *Averting the Old Age Crisis*, constructs and reinforces the apocalyptic demography view of an ageing population. It is argued that this title continues to frame the way in which an ageing population is socially constructed as a 'burden', and in particular this view appears to be operationalized in a variety of forms of institutionalized ageism, for example health care rationing.

From the late 1950s onwards and following Sheldon's (1948) classic, *The Social Medicine of Old Age*, studies began to analyse old age within the frame of reference of the family; see also Townsend (1957) and Shanas et al (1968). Alongside such debates, pensions and retirement took centre stage. By the 1970s the recognition that an ageing society was a health and social policy success was beginning to emerge within the literature.

5.2.2 POST–MODERN CONSTRUCTIONS OF AGEING

By the early 1970s a range of gerontological literature published in North America had travelled the Atlantic. Textbooks included the *Handbook of Aging and the Individual: Pyschological and Biological Aspects* (Birren 1959) and the *Handbook of Social Gerontology: Societal Aspects of Aging* (Tibbitts 1960). By the early 1980s, social gerontology was emerging as a credible academic discourse in the UK and by 1988 Masters Degree courses started to materialize across the UK. However, both in the US and UK there still appeared to be a preoccupation with the biology of ageing. Friedan (1993) reports how, at a gerontological conference in 1988, she ran into David Gutmann, who was doing his annual count of papers dealing with irreversible disorders of age, such as Alzheimer's dementia, compared to functional problems that could be treated or solved. The ratio was two to one: '"For every paper on life span development, there are now seven on incontinence", he said. "Death is big this year." He is full of black humour. "Elder abuse is coming on strong." Of course as he pointed out, incontinence and elder abuse are easier for graduate students to measure than, for instance, wisdom' (Friedan 1993: 126).

5.2.3 THE POLITICAL ECONOMY PERSPECTIVE

By the 1970s a shift of emphasis from 'microfication' – that is, the increasing attention and spotlight on the psychosocial characteristics of individuals (often from a decrementalist standpoint) – was noted. In particular, Hagestad & Dannefer (2001) have argued that alarm about the absence of theoretical rigour in the social scientific study of ageing forced social theorists to reconsider ageing from a 'macro-level structural perspective'. The rejoinder was the emergence of what has been coined the 'political economy of ageing' (Estes 1979, Phillipson 1982). Estes (1999: 18) has argued that work on the political economy of ageing has begun to 'specify how the meaning and experience of old age and the distribution of resources to the ageing are directed by economic, political, and socio-cultural factors'. The considerable importance of this perspective was to locate old age within the post-modern capitalist economy. In many ways, the previous constructions of apocalyptic demography and intergenerational equity can be seen as the precursors to the focus on physical debility and physiological decline that are outlined in the political economy thesis as social constructions. The argument follows that the structured dependency for many older people, particularly in welfare terms, had been 'constructed', and is not determined by objective facts related to the reality of ageing.

Perhaps one of the significant developments at the latter part of the twentieth century has been gerontological studies emerging from the humanities. However, such developments were considered seriously suspect in certain academic gerontological circles. In her fascinating analysis *The Fountain of Age*, Betty Friedan (1993) points out that a group of North American scholars, including James Birren, Rick Moody, Robert Kastenbaum, Nancy Data and David Gutmann, had attempted to set up a division of humanistic studies of ageing. However, 'The gerontological establishment had refused to let them set up a division ... it was dismissed as "not scientific"' (Friedan 1993: 123).

Perhaps the logic of 'political economy' and the strength of the arguments (principally the economic arguments around structured dependency) allowed little room for manoeuvre for the humanities. However, Estes (1999: 27) suggests that the 'classical opposition of culture versus structure has given way in the 1980s and 1990s to an understanding of the importance of the interplay of structural and cultural factors' (see Griswold 1994).

Such insights have allowed theorists to argue that 'levels' of analysis, while individually absolutely necessary, should also include 'bold attempts to grasp connections across micro- and macro-levels' (Hagestad & Dannefer 2001). This is not a new perspective; in 1990 Elder & Caspi (1990) suggested that macrolevel change creates new opportunities or constraints at meso and micro levels, such as community and family, in turn; these microconditions affect individual development.

5.3 THE HUMANITIES AND OTHER PERSPECTIVES

An emerging area of research and scholarship that offers important insights into how individuals attempt to understand changes across the life-course can be found in sociological theory variously described as 'career' or 'status passage narrative'. A status passage narrative is generally conceived of as being an account of the way in which an individual has undergone, might undergo, or even conceptualizes changes in their 'status' relative to other points in their life-course development. It has been suggested that such narratives, whether they are about middle age or old age, are seen as 'frames through which we organize our lives' (Plummer 2001: 192). Such a life-course approach has again been offered as a method of offering a micro-level perspective that is complementary to the political economy thesis.

Many of these theories have been superimposed on the critical turning points found in old age. It is therefore no surprise to find that health status, and its impact on a life biography, has become an important area of study, especially given the prevalence of chronic illness in later life. However, very few empirical studies have tried to illuminate old age and chronic illness utilizing the theoretical framework of status passage (Glaser & Strauss 1971), although theoretical papers do offer a link between 'critical incidents' and status passage (see, for example, Kingston 2000). Unfortunately, little has been written about the positive aspects of status passage in later life.

An emerging development in social gerontology is the focus on cultural studies (see Blaikie 1999, Gilleard & Higgs 2000). In the preface to *Cultures of Ageing*, Gilleard & Higgs (2000: ix) report: 'Plans to write this book began ten years ago. At that time, ageing was still represented in academic textbooks as either the product of biology or the outcome of social policy. Since then ageing has become more evidently inserted into the cultural world.' The cultural emphasis in gerontology has partly emerged through the idea that individuals can, and do, choose their identity. Lives have become 'projects' and 'lifestyles', which can be purchased as a commodity.

Blaikie (1999: 15) points to positive ageing messages 'about the hedonistic joys of leisured retirement'.

5.3.1 STORIES OF AGEING

Invaluable insights into the meaning of old age can also be gained by reading about ageing and old age in novels. Hepworth's considerable contribution in this area is summed up in the introduction to *Stories of Ageing*:

> My main aim in writing this book is to encourage you as readers to explore fiction as an imaginative resource for understanding variations in the meaning of the experience of ageing in society and to go out and make your own selection from the increasingly wide range of novels available. If you do so then this book will have been a success (Hepworth 2000: 1).

Hepworth argues, convincingly, that it is possible, and valuable, to interweave fiction and fact 'in order to enhance our understanding of ageing'. Several gerontological textbooks over the years have achieved such a mix, for example *An Ageing Population* (Carver & Liddiard 1978) and *Ageing and Later Life* (Johnson & Slater 1993). The impact of stories is also enhanced when they are produced in visual medium, for example the work of Alan Bennett in the 'Talking Heads' series shown on UK television. Secondly, compilations of fictional abstracts and poetry focusing on ageing and the life-course are being published. For example, Kingston (2000) has previously noted that the nine chapters in the *Oxford Book of Ageing* include: Stages/Journey; Change/Metamorphosis; Generations; Solitude/Loneliness; Works; Eros/Thanatos; Celebration/Lament; Body/Spirit and Remembrance. Finally, Hepworth notes the emergence of 'literary gerontology' particularly in North America, where: 'experts in literary criticism and the history of literature have drawn on gerontological research (often from a psychological/developmental perspective) to carry out in depth analysis of particular texts or writers' (Hepworth 2000: 4).

Such powerful insights into the ageing process and ageing worlds are clearly not utilized sufficiently within health and welfare curricula. It is prudent that educators interested in gerontology open the welfare curriculum to the humanities, so that fiction can illuminate the existential world of later life.

Running almost parallel to the focus on narrative and biography is an emerging obsession with longevity. In his fascinating book *Time of our Lives*, Tom Kirkwood (1999) offers a chapter called 'Longevity records', in which he outlines what is known about longevity. For example, Kirkwood describes in detail the world record held in 1999 by Jeanne Louise Calment, 1875–1997, who died aged 122 years and 5 months. Blaikie (1999) also comments on the death of Calment; however, he attempts to argue that longevity, while in itself fascinating, carries with it history and imagery. Blaikie notes that, although Calment was proud of her feat: 'less lofty considerations excited the oldest women in the world: a week before her 121st birthday, Jeanne Calment is agitated. "I hope you've remembered to get my shampoo", she tells nursing staff in a commanding tone. "And my jewellery. I'll be needing it for the photographs"' (Blaikie 1999: 1). Similar preoccupations are outlined in Jackson's (1999) *The Book of Life: One Man's*

Search for the Wisdom of Age. The front cover suggests the book is: 'A journey in search of the oldest people in the world'. However, Jackson links the fascination with longevity with: 'A voyage of discovery, what it means to be truly alive'. In essence, Jackson has attempted the link between the success of biological longevity and the existentialist importance of understanding the meaning of old age.

Most recently, the growing significance of an ageing society, and therefore the importance of understanding the implications of the scientific and demographic changes, was outlined by Tom Kirkwood in the Reith lectures in 2001 (http://www.bbc.co.uk/radio4/reith2001/). It is important to note that ageing was chosen as a topic for the 2001 lecture series: the Reith lectures were inaugurated in 1948 with the aim of advancing public understanding about significant issues of contemporary interest. Choosing the topic of ageing has in itself promoted the importance of trying to develop a critical analysis of the continuing demographic challenges.

During the five lectures, Kirkwood explored how biomedical science is continuing to understand the ageing process alongside an analysis of the implications of an ageing society. In his first lecture Kirkwood suggested that death is not inevitable: a concept that has perhaps become a normative view in society. Of course, if that is the case, the demographic changes that we have already detected over the last century with increased longevity may well continue to increase the length of people's lives. In the second and third lectures, Kirkwood outlined his theory of biological ageing, known as 'disposable soma theory'. The implications of this theory suggest that we might, in the future, be able to understand, in significant genetic detail, the causes of certain diseases, for example Alzheimer's disease. It might also be possible to understand how certain of the bodily changes in old age might be modified. The third lecture perhaps offers greater insights into the sociology of ageing. Entitled 'Making Choices', the lecture was broadcast from a purpose-built retirement community in the West Midlands in the UK. This lecture argued that without doubt one of the major challenges for the twenty-first century will be to develop alternative forms of long-term care that offer choice and dignity and present older people with the option to remain in their own homes for as long as possible.

When the Reith lectures are considered in their totality, the main focus was clearly a biomedical understanding of the ageing process. This is undoubtedly an important aspect of the challenges of an ageing society. The biomedical perspective must, however, complement insights gained from social science and the humanities. If biomedicine is to understand how and why we age, social science/humanities must continue to generate answers that give insights into the meaning of ageing and old age. A glance at the journal of the Chartered Society of Physiotherapy from January 2000 to December 2002 reveals just five articles specific to older people, four of which take a biological perspective. The AGILE-Thames group (2002) notes that, although older people form the largest part of physiotherapists' clientele in the National Health Service (NHS), students still qualify without having had any experience of working with this age group.

5.4 AGEISM

The first usage of the term 'ageism' appears in Butler & Lewis (1973), as follows:

> Ageism can be seen as a process of systematic stereotyping of and discrimination against people because they are old, just as racism and sexism accomplish this for skin colour and gender. Old people are categorized as senile in thought and manner, old-fashioned in morality and skills. Ageism allows the younger generations to see older people as different from themselves. Thus they subtly cease to identify with their elders as human beings (Butler & Lewis 1973: 9).

Since Butler & Lewis first used the term, gerontologists and sociologists have been able to illustrate how ageism is manifest: in terms of ageist language and media typifications, stereotyping, as structural discrimination, for example health care rationing, and as social exclusion.

Undoubtedly, one of the enduring challenges for welfare policy at macro and micro level is the elimination of ageism. The importance of eradicating ageism is reinforced in the UK by the National Service Framework (NSF) (Department of Health 2001a). The NSF sets out a 10-year programme of action, based around eight standards:

> The National Service Framework for Older People is an action plan to improve health and social services for older people. It sets new national standards and service models of care for all older people whether they live at home, in residential care or in hospital. It focuses on:
>
> - Rooting out age discrimination;
> - Providing person centred care with older people treated as individuals with respect and dignity;
> - Promoting older people's health and independence.

It is important to note that the first standard within the NSF tackles ageism: the aim being 'To ensure that older people are never unfairly discriminated against in accessing NHS or social care services as a result of their age' (Department of Health 2001a: 16). Action includes an audit of policy followed by: 'Analysis of the levels and patterns of services for older people, in order to facilitate comparisons across health authorities and establish best practice benchmarks based on health outcomes and needs' (Department of Health 2001a: 22). However, an additional task will be to challenge and modify professional attitudes around ageing. Research evidence consistently points towards ageist attitudes found across a variety of health and welfare practitioners (Bytheway 1995, French 1997).

There can be little doubt that the legacy of a twentieth-century literature that promoted disability, decline and decrement as the focus of old age, is still to be found in certain professional circles. Such a legacy is also perpetuated by the media, in the form of 'apocalyptic demography', and intergenerational conflict. Nevertheless, a cultural shift is emerging, partly linked to the 'new consumerism' in later life. However, complacency should be avoided; it will need significant changes in attitudes alongside the 10-year NSF before any measured success in eradicating ageism and discrimination can be announced. Physiotherapy education needs to tackle the issue of ageism in every possible way, including the direct input into physiotherapy courses of older people themselves.

5.5 CONCLUSION

Over the last 100 years the theoretical framework in which old age has been socially constructed has changed beyond recognition. The very early gerontological literature constructed a largely decremental focus. The construction argued that older people either were moving through a period of both physical and psychological deterioration, or were a demographic nightmare with burdensome implications for society in terms of fiscal costs and health care demands in particular. In most cases the two phenomena were linked together; hence, titles like *Social and Medical Problems of the Elderly* (Hazell 1960).

By the 1970s, theorists had begun to argue that the socially constructed dependency of old age, especially pensions and institutional care, was a post-modern manifestation of the capitalist economy. The latter part of the twentieth century incorporated a more balanced epistemological perspective, which focused both on the political economy of ageing and social structures and on the existential meaning of ageing from the perspective of older people. This included a call for the use of the humanities, which included literature and other media, in an attempt to understand later life. However, it is argued that the nihilistic inheritance of perceived deterioration and decline in old age has left a legacy that is frequently and consistently played out in the media. Moreover, ageism remains a potent discriminator, in both health and social care services. One of the implications is to use the arts, including novels and poetry, in physiotherapy education to broaden perspectives and to break down stereotypes.

The challenge for health and social care professionals is to balance the existing political, psychological, economic and medical knowledge developed thus far with an appreciation of the lived experience of old age. For example, Blaikie (1999) argues that it is possible to resolve the dualism of structure (political economy, etc.) and agency (the existential world of ageing) by paraphrasing Karl Marx: 'ageing people make their own histories, but not under circumstances of their own making. The answer would appear to lie in theorising a dialectic between the life-world and the social structure' (Blaikie 1999: 5; see also Giddens 1979). Most importantly, older people need to be able to tell their own stories, to explore their own desires and aspirations. The ability to continue to have control over one's own destiny appears also to be vitally important to older people.

However, there is a danger that the pendulum will swing too far in the direction of particular theoretical frameworks. Phillipson (1994: 8) outlines his anxieties: 'we must guard against the reinventing of gerontology which, in elevating personal meaning and the inventiveness of everyday life, ignores the basic social divisions which continue to disempower significant groups of elders'. Physiotherapists have many important skills to offer older people that can help to maintain their desired lifestyles and meet their aspirations. In order to do this successfully, however, it is necessary for physiotherapists to respect each older person as a unique and valued individual within their particular social and cultural context. Treatment goals need to be set with the older person, and their dignity and autonomy should be respected. Physiotherapy skills may sometimes need to be adapted to address the needs of older people and good communication, both with the older person and with other members of the multi-disciplinary team, is essential for good practice.

SECTION 2

The psychosocial context of health and illness

Chapter **6**

Sex, gender and health care

Helen Roberts

6.1   INTRODUCTION

Women spend more time looking after other people's health than do men, and they do this work both professionally and in the home. Women go to the doctor more often than men, take more medicines than men, and are likely to spend more time on health-promoting behaviours on their own behalf, and on behalf of those they care for, than men (Foster 1995). On the other hand, on average, men in the UK die earlier than women, although the mortality gap may be narrowing. We need to recognize that the extent to which men and women fare differently depends on which aspect of health is being measured (Annandale 1998: 159).

The organization of health care and the care of sick people have a long history of sex differentiation. This is true on a routine, day-to-day basis, as well as in acute and chronic illness and disabling conditions. It is not only in the gender structure of service delivery that we can see differences between men and women. As McPherson & Waller (1997: 3) have pointed out, there have always been differences between the health problems of men and women. Even in early hunter–gatherer societies, the major causes of death are likely to have been different according to gender.

This chapter falls into three sections. The first describes some differences between the sexes in morbidity (ill health) and mortality (death) and then discusses sex differences in the work force of the medical profession and the professions allied to medicine. Of course, the vast majority of health care and the care of sick people is not performed by professionals at all but carried out in the home. As one child put it in a recent interview: 'I don't have a doctor I have Mum!' (Liabo et al 2002). Sex differences among unpaid carers are discussed below, as is the problematic notion of 'caring', objectifying as it does those who are 'cared for' (Keith & Morris 1995).

Statistical data give us one type of information about the health of men and women and about the relative proportions of men and women in different health care professions, but they do not tell us about the experience of good or poor health, what it is like to be a woman in a male-dominated profession or a man in female-dominated work. Some attention will be given to this, and to the differential respect accorded to 'care' and to 'cure'.

The second section of the chapter covers two areas of health care where physiotherapists are likely to have a significant presence. In the first, childbirth, women make up 100% of those giving birth (though increasing numbers of male partners play a role beyond that traditionally expected at conception). In the second, the area of spinal cord injuries, women patients are in the minority for reasons evident when one considers the sex differentiation in the kinds of activities where these injuries may arise.

The final section is speculative and focuses on the gender structure of the physiotherapy profession and the kinds of research, particularly in the area of physiotherapy, which might be fundable, feasible and useful in addressing the different needs of men and women patients.

6.2 SEX DIFFERENCES IN HEALTH STATE AND HEALTH STATUS

What kinds of data do we have on men, women and health? Physiological variation between men and women and the process of reproduction account for some of the differences between the sexes in rates of death and illness. The social contexts within which women and men live also help us to understand some of these differences. Young men, for instance, are more prone to drive fast cars and are considerably more likely than young women to be seriously injured in road traffic accidents, rugby games or as a result of violence. Men, and in particular young men, have higher suicide rates than women, though women are more inclined to self-harm.

Macfarlane's work (1990) remains one of the clearest guides to sex differences in health statistics, with examples of the main data sources available in the UK. She points out that while women can expect to live longer than men, statistics about the use of health services give the impression that women make greater use of these. Admission rates in acute non-psychiatric hospitals are higher among women than men overall, even when admissions to maternity wards are excluded. However, in people under 15 and over 45 years of age, more boys and men are admitted, and in the age group 15–44, Macfarlane (1990) shows that once admissions due to reproduction (abortions, miscarriages and so forth) are excluded, differences in admission rates between men and women virtually disappear. Sex differences in attendance at out-patient clinics are negligible.

There are a number of areas where rising levels of surgical intervention in relation to women have caused concern. One is Caesarian section: a large and increasing number of women are having their babies delivered in this way (Teo 1990, Macfarlane & Mugford 2000, Macfarlane et al 2000). Another is hysterectomy. More than 30 years ago, in a much-quoted editorial, it was suggested that 'The uterus has but one function: reproduction. After the last planned pregnancy, the uterus becomes a useless, bleeding, symptom-producing, potentially cancer-bearing organ and therefore should be removed' (Wright 1969: 562). Some 20 years later, an editorial in the *British Journal of Obstetrics and Gynaecology* on the prophylactic removal of the ovaries (oophorectomy) concluded, '[their removal] should be offered to all women over the age of forty having an abdominal hysterectomy'. Perhaps we should be thankful that the author adds:

> [It] should only be performed after adequate discussion, understanding and of course consent. The woman has the ultimate choice. If she exercises what is perhaps the only worthwhile argument against prophylactic oöphorectomy, namely *a sentimental desire to keep her ovaries* [emphasis added] then it would be a foolish and insensitive gynaecologist who would ignore this compelling argument (Studd 1989: 509).

It is interesting in this context that a legal case in the mid-1990s involving a woman of 35 who had a hysterectomy during which, without her consent, an 11-week fetus was aborted, found in favour of the obstetrician concerned (Dyer 1996). However, when the General Medical Council (GMC) heard the case in May 2002, the surgeon (who is now retired) was found guilty of serious professional misconduct on the grounds that he had failed to ensure the woman had given her 'informed consent' to the procedure. The surgeon had told the committee that he made the decision to continue with the hysterectomy even though he realized the patient might be pregnant because he thought it was in her best interests (http://news.bbc.co.uk/hi/english/health/newsid_2017000/2017021.stm). As McPherson (1997) has pointed out, many women are not aware of the degree of discretion and uncertainty underlying some procedures, and see this as a matter for their doctors.

In terms of primary health care, women consult general practitioners (GPs) more often than men, and the sharpest differences are again in the childbearing age group. Macfarlane (1990) presents data which show that, once consultations which are not for illness are removed, for instance those for contraception, the differences are much smaller, and when consultations for pregnancy, childbirth and diseases of the male and female genitourinary systems are excluded, the differences virtually disappear. In terms of minority ethnic health, South Asian and Black Caribbean men were more likely than the general population to have consulted their GP in the past 2 weeks and to have more than one consultation over this period. Standardized for age, and expressed as a ratio to the general population (1.00), the annual GP contact rate ratio for South Asian and Black

Caribbean men ranged from 1.46 to 2.64. Among women, contact rates were significantly higher for South Asian and Irish women (Bajekal 2001).

Of course, data about the use made of health services are not necessarily the best measures of health. Consultation rates and hospital admission rates tell us about the use of services, not the state of people's health. Blaxter (1985) makes the distinction between temporary states of health, 'Am I ill today?', and longer-term health status reflected in answers to the question 'Am I basically a healthy or unhealthy person?' In a survey in Glasgow, women aged between 35 and 54 years were asked to report on their health (McIlwaine et al 1989). When asked how they considered their own state of health, more than 60% replied that it was about the same as that of other women of their acquaintance. At the same time, over 50% described themselves as lacking in energy, over 40% had trouble sleeping and about 40% reported feeling depressed. In a 1988 National Survey of NHS Patients in General Practice, 55% of women patients thought it important to be able to see a GP of their own sex, and 37% thought it important to be able to see a GP of their own ethnic group. The proportion of men expressing these preferences was lower (Department of Health 2001b).

Sociologists have described how the process of defining oneself as ill, or acting on symptoms, depends in part on how common such symptoms are in a society or group. If a symptom is common, it is likely to be considered normal and therefore not defined as illness. Zola (1966), in his study of illness behaviour, found that tiredness was often considered normal. Some researchers have argued that women will report more ill health than men because they are in a better position to act on symptoms and adopt the 'sick role'. Verbrugge & Wingard (1987) have suggested that the crucial feature of women's social roles may be flexibility, but Popay (1991) points out in her study of health and health care in families with vastly different levels of income that flexibility was missing from women's daily experience of life as mother, housewife or paid employee.

What do we know about the differences in the ways health professionals view their male and female patients, and the consequences of this for their treatment? Stimson's (1976) classic study asked doctors about the patients whom they considered least and most troublesome. Among patients considered 'least trouble' were: men, those with organic, easy-to-diagnose medical problems and those who have confidence in the doctor, accept that there are limits to the doctor's skill, are cooperative, and have good homes and circumstances. Among those considered 'most trouble' were: women, those with vague symptoms, and those who do not follow advice, are unable to cope and are in poor social circumstances. More recently, there has been work indicating differences in the diagnosis and treatment given to women and men presenting similar symptoms, for instance in cardiac care, and Sharp (1998: 109) reminds us that coronary heart disease (CHD) is the leading single cause of death among women in the UK, although CHD still has a rather male image, impacting on the way in which both women and professionals view risk and symptoms.

A recent survey on general practice (Department of Health 2001b) shows that there are also differences in the ways in which men and women view their doctors, at least in general practice. Women are slightly more likely to be critical of GPs' attitudes towards their patients but the differences are not great. It was found that 46% of women, compared with 41% of men, said that during their visits to the surgery in the last 12 months, the GP had not always given them enough information about their condition or treatment, and 12% of women (and 9% of men) had not felt able to ask all the questions they wanted on their last visit to the surgery.

6.3 WOMEN AS PROVIDERS AND USERS OF HEALTH CARE

Women are both the main users of the health service, and the main providers of health care. Sex differences in the organization of both paid and unpaid health care and the care of sick people are not new, as an article more than a century ago in the *British Medical Journal* makes clear: 'In the truest interest of women it is better that they should not practise the medical profession … it is scarcely possible for a woman to go through a course of medical education without losing that simplicity and purity of character which we so much value'. In case it should be thought that this would leave women with nothing to do, the authors suggest that unpaid health care may be the solution: '[We] have frequent reason to lament that there is no spinster aunt or sister at hand to take charge of some poor invalid' (*British Medical Journal* 1977: 1149; taken from *British Medical Journal* 1877).

When the Sex Discrimination Act came into force in the mid-1970s, one consequence was that the doors of all physiotherapy schools, some of which until that time had run courses exclusively for women, were open to men. Another consequence was the opening up of medical schools to women. A week after the new law came into force, an editorial in the *British Medical Journal* suggested: 'Any woman doctor who decides to make a career in a prestigious specialty such as neurology or cardio-thoracic surgery will find that she is competing with men who give one hundred percent of their effort to their work: she cannot expect to succeed if she tries to combine her specialist training with bringing up a family herself' (*British Medical Journal* 1976: 56). In response to this, one might point to an article in *The Lancet* which notes that while women doctors who temporarily or permanently drop out of full-time practice have been studied frequently, men, who are just as expensive to train, have not, despite their disappearance from National Health Service (NHS) practice through emigration, death, alcoholism, suicide or removal from the medical register. The authors point out that, in a working lifetime of 40 years, a woman doctor with an average family is likely to do seven-eighths of the work of a doctor who has not had to carry the primary responsibility for bearing and rearing children (Bewley & Bewley 1975). While the 1976 *British Medical Journal* article did not speculate on the problems of male neurologists or cardiothoracic surgeons attempting to combine family and professional life, it is heartening to note that, in the intervening years, there has been an increasing tendency for young men in medicine to explore ways of combining family and work life. As with women attempting the same juggling act, their aspirations in this direction have frequently been the triumph of hope over experience.

Although there had been a gradual erosion of male quotas in medical school entrance in the years preceding the new law, one result of the Sex Discrimination Act of 1975 has been that the majority of entrants to British medical schools are now women. Men have not rushed into physiotherapy with quite the same enthusiasm as women have entered medicine.

How are men and women distributed within health care employment? Women make up about 80% of the NHS workforce, but tend to be concentrated in less well-paid jobs. The NHS is a major employer for women. More than a decade ago, Buchan & Pike (1989) showed that about 90% of nurses were women, 73% of chiropodists, 89% of dieticians and 76% of physiotherapists. Graham (1990) showed that overall 11% of white women in paid employment work in the health services (public and private); for black and ethnic minority women, the proportion is 17%. About a third of hospital doctors are women.

The current website of the Chartered Society of Physiotherapy (www.csp.org.uk) includes pictures of both men and women practitioners and highlights its equal opportunities policies: 'The Chartered Society of Physiotherapy, and the courses it approves, work towards equal opportunities of access. They welcome applicants regardless of their sex, age, race, ethnic or national origins, sexual orientation, social class, family responsibilities, political and religious beliefs.' Times have changed from 20 years ago when the pamphlet *How to Become a Chartered Physiotherapist* (Chartered Society of Physiotherapy 1984) referred to both short and tall stature as possible problems for physiotherapists. While the contraindication for very tall people was apparently physiological since they 'are particularly susceptible to the occupational hazard of back injuries', in relation to short stature, there was an additional problem, 'whereas small people may often acquire the strength and skill to cope with [lifting and support of heavy patients], *they must also be able to gain the confidence of patients*' [emphasis added] (Chartered Society of Physiotherapy 1984). The problem that the Chartered Society of Physiotherapy identified in 1984 was a realistic one. Some patients may lack confidence in short people, just as some patients may lack confidence in black people, or disabled people. But practitioners, irrespective of height, ethnicity, sex or physical disability, need to be taught the skills to gain the confidence of patients and to cope in a dignified way with those patients who lack confidence in their carers. Misplaced confidence by patients in treatment that has not been evaluated would be quite another matter.

In 2001, 10% of physiotherapists were men, and the website of the professional association suggested 'numbers are rising rapidly'. In a 1999 survey on equal opportunities, the Chartered Society of Physiotherapy found a third of members in the 35–44 age group and just over a quarter in the 25–34 age group, so the age profile of the profession is quite a young one. The pay for people who work in the professions allied to medicine within the NHS is not high. The management structure of the NHS does afford some relatively well-paid posts as physiotherapy managers but, by definition, these are few. The majority of practising physiotherapists are under the age of 40, and patterns of employment can be related to family formation. The Chartered Society of Physiotherapy equal opportunities survey found that around two-thirds of respondents had caring responsibilities outside work. Of course the majority of health care and a good deal of care of sick people is not performed by health professionals at all but is done in the home, usually, but not always, by women as mothers, wives and daughters. Graham (1984, 1987, 1990), who has written extensively on women's 'health work', describes and analyses some of the components of this work. Among those caring for children, about three out of every four women in households with pre-school children are full-time carers, and in single-parent households, women outnumber men by nine to one. Piachaud (1985) points out that the 'principal carers' of able-bodied children up to 2 years of age spend about 8 hours a day in health behaviours directed to their children: getting them up and dressed, toileting, feeding, bathing and so on. Women are more likely to be carers than men are – 58% of carers in Britain are women, compared with 42% who are men. Women are also more likely than men to carry the main responsibility for caring, where there is more than one person with some responsibility (www.carers.gov.uk).

While women predominate in health care, the high-status and highly paid jobs continue to be overwhelmingly occupied by men. Lower-paid and unpaid care is more likely to be undertaken by women. It is sometimes said that doctors cure and nurses care. Certainly, with the exception of surgery, those who do the 'hands-on' care tend to be the least rewarded in terms of pay and status.

6.4 WOMEN'S EXPERIENCES OF HEALTH CARE

This section describes some of the aspects of health care in two areas where physiotherapists have a significant presence. One is pregnancy, childbirth and the immediate postpartum period, which are transient physiological events, and the other, long-term disability. Different kinds of data can give us very different perspectives on the same subject. Knowing all there is to know about the physiology of normal labour, for instance, tells us nothing about what it is like to become a mother. Similarly, knowing all there is to know about spinal cord injuries does not tell us what it is like to be a healthy disabled person, and the recipient (or not) of others' caring activities.

6.4.1 PREGNANCY AND CHILDBIRTH

Kitzinger (1984) points out that it was the work of Dick Grantly-Read in the 1930s, combined with advances in obstetric physiotherapy stemming largely from the office of Helen Heardman, which formed the basis for most types of preparation for childbirth that many midwives and obstetricians today accept as smoothing the path of women in labour. In the area of childbirth, there has for some time been a level of concern about women's satisfaction with maternity services. The Maternity Services

Advisory Committee, which was set up by the Secretary of State for Social Services and the Secretary of State for Wales in 1981, was concerned with the number of consumer complaints about the impersonal nature of care in hospitals. This committee published three reports, and one of their recommendations was that the satisfaction of parents with these services should be explored at a local level.

Quantitative work in obstetrics can tell us important facts about the number of instrumental births, the number of Caesarian sections, the use of induction and drugs to accelerate labour, and so on. The maternity services have tended to be more inclined than some other clinical specialties to audit their work at a local level in order to monitor perinatal deaths, and in some cases to look more broadly at service provision. A report on midwife-led services in south-east London for instance (Allen et al 1997) showed high levels of satisfaction among women.

Women's attitudes and feelings about their experiences of pregnancy, childbirth and early motherhood are more difficult to measure, though research instruments may be used to rate on a scale of 1 to 5 whether they found a particular procedure, such as episiotomy, very unpleasant (5), unpleasant (4), neither pleasant nor unpleasant (3), pleasant (2) or very pleasant (1). Attitudinal data collected in this way are naturally simpler to analyse than open-ended questions, but important work can be done by collecting information from patients in a systematic way by talking to them (Britten 2000). Oakley's accounts of pregnancy, childbirth and the first months of motherhood, for instance, provide grounds for thinking about the sorts of maternity services which women would find helpful, and some of the problems of becoming a mother (Oakley 1981). Oakley's work is based very firmly on women's own accounts rather than on 'expert' views of how women feel or should feel. The majority of her data were obtained through careful face-to-face interviewing.

Questionnaires may also elicit some aspects of women's experiences of pregnancy; Mason (1989) describes how 'open' answers in women's own words may be used and analysed as part of a more formal survey. For readers interested in carrying out a survey into patient satisfaction, Mason's (1989) *Women's Experience of Maternity Care: a Survey Manual* is helpful reading. Some of the most important work on pregnancy and childbirth in recent years has been the move towards evidence-based medicine (a surprise to some that there was ever any other sort). The collection of data from randomized controlled trials on everything from episiotomy to looking after one's own clinical notes, and from trial labour in those who have undergone a previous Caesarian section to the prevention of premature labour, have revolutionized midwifery and obstetric practice, and given an important tool to women who want to influence the way they are treated in pregnancy and childbirth. One of the most important ways to empower people is through sharing knowledge and those working on evidence-based medicine (based in the UK at the Cochrane Collaboration in Oxford) are looking at different ways of ensuring a voice for 'users' as well as ensuring that the results of studies are well disseminated (Enkin et al 1990).

For readers with a particular interest in women's health, the Association of Chartered Physiotherapists in Women's Health is one of the clinical interest groups recognized by the Chartered Society of Physiotherapy. Originally formed in 1948 as the Obstetric Association of Chartered Physiotherapists, it has as an objective to act in the professional interest of chartered physiotherapists working in women's health (http://www. womensphysio.com).

6.4.2 WOMEN AND DISABILITY

Physiotherapists will be aware of the important distinction between impairment and disability. Broadly, impairment refers to the injury or disease and disability to the consequences of impairment within a social context. People with impairments may be disabled by poor access to buildings, the prejudices of employers and others, and enforced dependency (see Section 17.4). Lonsdale, who has written on women and disability, suggests that:

> Dependency has particular implications for women because of the important part which gender plays in determining whether someone is expected or encouraged or indeed even allowed to be independent. Since women are encouraged to play a more dependent role in society than men, disabled women often have a particular struggle to achieve control over their own destinies, although they are sometimes 'allowed' out of the passive and dependent female role (Lonsdale 1990: 10–11).

One problem for women in general, but which takes on particular salience for disabled women, is that being 'good' may mean being passive and obedient. As Lonsdale points out, being a 'bad' patient could mean demonstrating precisely those characteristics of independence and activity that are necessary for coping and surviving. Lonsdale describes how it is not unusual for a disabled woman to be labelled 'unrealistic' if she wants to live independently, especially if her plans do not conform to the expected female role. Disabled women who are mothers face not only the challenges which all mothers face, but also the challenge of being a parent in a disabling society. In some cases, these challenges will be met by a response which supports the 'carers' of the disabled parent, without providing the services which would render the parent less dependent. Keith & Morris (1995: 42) write:

> the social issue of caring has been constructed on the assumption that unpaid work within the family … will continue … Colluding with the government's position that public resources will never be adequate to replace the practical assistance given within the family (mainly by women) to disabled and older people, many researchers and campaigners have focused on services which would 'ease the burden' of caring.

As the authors point out, a statutory duty is imposed on social services authorities to carry out assessments by the 1986 Disabled Persons Act, and to meet such needs by the 1970 Chronically Sick and Disabled Persons Act. Focusing on the needs of carers may obscure the rights that disabled people have to receive services.

Sometimes, therapy can be considered more important than a disabled person's education and many disabled people have challenged this view. Before the 1981 Education Act, disabled children would usually be educated at ordinary schools only if they had very insistent parents. One of the respondents in Lonsdale's study describes how physiotherapy disrupted her education at the special school she attended. She writes: 'If you are going to be disturbed from your Maths class to go to physiotherapy, that's wrong. Physiotherapy and hydrotherapy should be a separate thing from school. It shouldn't affect your education … It's bad enough being disabled but to have no qualifications either, then you're going into the world of work with nothing' (Lonsdale 1990: 93).

A book based on interviews with women with spinal injuries describes some aspects of their quality of life as workers, mothers, lovers and patients, after an accident or illness resulting in paralysis. One writes: 'I had regular physiotherapy and did occupational therapy, but there was no-one to discuss problems and personal feelings with, and no sort of counselling to help with the present or future. It seemed as if one was expected to be cheerful and "keep one's chin up" all the time' (Morris 1989: 24). The book describes the problems women have in coping with the emphasis in spinal units on sport, competition and physical achievement, and suggests that this may be directly related to the fact that rehabilitation programmes have been geared primarily towards men with spinal cord injuries. This can mean people being pushed into an approach to physical achievement that they experience as oppressive and inappropriate. One woman wrote: 'Excellent though the physiotherapy was, I did find later that my performance improved with exercise done to music and for pleasure. Most things were sport orientated. I hate competition and have no eye for balls or arrows' (Morris 1989: 27).

In this section, some of the qualitative research that provides us with a framework for understanding the experience of the patient as a person has been described. The translation of what can be learned from qualitative research into clinical practice may not be as straightforward as adopting a new drug which has been found effective through a randomized controlled trial, but it is as important and highlights the need for mixed methodologies in good research (DePoy & Gitlin 1998, Petticrew & Roberts 2003).

6.5 WORKING FOR CHANGE

There has been a gradual change in the health professions in recent years in the extent to which they are willing to consult patients and to see them as whole people rather than 'a tib and fib' or 'the paraplegic in bed five'. Some health professionals embrace this change while others are pushed more or less willingly towards it. The previous section described some of the ways in which we may begin to learn more about patients' needs and perspectives and how our differing views of men and women may affect the ways in which they are treated. We have different expectations of patients according to gender, and should be encouraged to question these and develop services in ways in which patients can describe to us if we listen. There are huge reservoirs of untapped knowledge among 'lay' people which professionals have been slow to access (Roberts et al 1995) and which we would do well to explore further (Beresford & Croft 1995). The current UK government has made clear its commitment to patient/user/consumer involvement.

What of gender differentiation within the profession of physiotherapy? Much of the material relating to sex differences in the health professions is based on literature concerning doctors, because this profession within health care has not only been frequently studied, but has developed strong pressure groups. What are the consequences of physiotherapy being a largely female profession in terms of the labour market?

According to a report by Buchan & Pike (1989) on the professions allied to medicine, the key characteristics of the work force are the comparatively low age profile and the predominance of women. There is an increasing proportion of elderly people in our society which means that the demand for physiotherapists is also likely to increase. Given the age and sex distribution of physiotherapists and what we know about family formation patterns, however, problems are likely to arise as women take periods out of the labour market to bear and rear children. Research on female pharmacists currently working in the NHS revealed that better pay, more flexible hours and crèche facilities were frequently given as factors important in the recruitment and retention of workers (Bevan et al 1989).

There are recruitment crises in a number of areas of the NHS, including physiotherapy where there are large numbers of vacancies together with unmet projected needs. The equality agenda and the recruitment and retention agenda have a number of areas in common (Buchan 2000, Department of Health 2000b). The Department of Health has made a number of recommendations aimed at the retention of staff. The Institute of Manpower Studies, which has considerable expertise in employment and training matters, reports that data are lacking on the extent to which these initiatives have been taken up. Meager et al (1989) point out that where they have been taken up, in the area of job sharing for instance, there is some evidence that the increase has been as a result of pressure from individual employees rather than policy-led management initiatives. Issues such as these, the European market and the organization and management of health provision within the NHS and the private sector are likely to shape the way in which physiotherapy develops into the twenty-first century.

6.6 CONCLUSION

Female-dominated professions have a number of strengths, although they tend to be short on industrial muscle. Ironically enough, some of these strengths relate to 'feminine' characteristics of caring, empathy and patience brought to the professional lives of many women through their female socialization. If men are to be encouraged into physiotherapy in greater numbers, it is important that these qualities are not lost. At the same time, it will be interesting to monitor the extent to which senior posts in physiotherapy are differentially occupied by men and women in proportion to their overall numbers in the profession, and for women to learn from men some of those characteristics which make them inclined to apply for, obtain, and function in those senior positions from which it is possible to have a wide-ranging influence on the way in which physiotherapy is practised.

In terms of service provision, we do not know exactly what patients need unless we ask them, and listen to their answers. Research need not be done in an academic library or a laboratory. Oakley (1981: 308) points out that 'experience does alter the way people (experts and others) behave: this is part of the scientific method, that theories should be tested empirically, not just once under artificial conditions, but constantly in the real world'. Much of research is 'finding out' and physiotherapists, including students, are often in a position to find out from their patients and clients what their needs are, what they find satisfying about a particular service and in what ways they feel the service might be improved. Not all suggestions patients make have massive resource implications, and at a time when consumer satisfaction is said to be important, there should be management sympathy for carrying out this basic research.

ACKNOWLEDGEMENT

I am grateful for information provided by Caroline Miller, Senior Information Officer at the Chartered Society of Physiotherapy.

Chapter 7

Health care for people from ethnic minority groups

Karl Atkin, Sally French and Ayesha Vernon

7.1 INTRODUCTION

After many years of neglect, there has been increasing interest in meeting the health care needs of minority ethnic groups living in the UK. Like many other health professionals, physiotherapists can sometimes be confused about how best to engage with minority ethnic populations. At best, this means the perspectives and needs of minority ethnic people do not adequately inform service delivery. At worst, it means service support is informed by racist myths and stereotypes. This chapter offers a preliminary introduction to the current themes informing debates about health care for minority ethnic groups. It aims to provide physiotherapists with the confidence to engage with these often complex and politically charged debates and to be able to apply this understanding to their own practice. The chapter begins by providing the context for our discussion by exploring the nature of the UK's minority ethnic population and the relationship between ethnicity and health. It then moves on to a detailed discussion about institutional racism and, in particular, its value in making sense of the disadvantages faced by minority ethnic groups in relation to health care. The chapter then explores various initiatives that could improve existing provision.

7.2 MINORITY ETHNIC GROUPS LIVING IN THE UK

Ethnic minorities comprise approximately 6–7% of the UK population. This total figure, however, disguises the diversity of the minority ethnic populations. According to the 1991 census, the largest minority ethnic group is of South Asian origin (2.7%), which is made up of Indian (1.5%), Pakistani (0.9%) and Bangladeshi (0.3%) people. Those of black Caribbean descent make up 0.9% of the UK population and those classified as Chinese comprise 2.1%. There is also a growing number of people who claim mixed ethnic origin (in the region of 0.5%).

The main immigration into the UK occurred from the British colonies in the 1950s and 1960s (Law 1996), encouraged by the government as a way of rebuilding the infrastructure of the UK following the Second World War (Mason 2000). In the post-war period, citizens of what was then the British Empire were given the right to enter the UK, work and settle with their families. Increasing numbers of migrants arrived, first from the Caribbean and then from India, Pakistan and parts of Africa. Today, over 40% of what are currently regarded as ethnic minority populations are born in Great Britain and their lifestyles are subtly different from those of their parents and grandparents (Atkin et al 2002). This reflects further diversity in the different experiences and expectations of the respective generations – an issue to which we will return.

People from ethnic minority groups are more plentiful in some parts of the UK than in others and are more likely to live in urbanized and densely populated areas. In Greater London, for example, about a quarter of the population classify themselves as being from ethnic minority groups (Modood et al 1997). The distribution of individual ethnic groups varies considerably across the UK (Owen 1993). People identifying themselves as black Caribbean are more heavily concentrated in London and the West Midlands. People of Indian origin are more likely to be found in London, the West Midlands and the East Midlands. Pakistani populations are less strongly represented in London but have large populations in West Yorkshire, Greater Manchester and the West Midlands. They also make up the largest minority ethnic group in Scotland. Bangladeshi people are more likely to be found in London and to a lesser extent in the West Midlands. People falling into the Chinese category are more evenly distributed across the UK, whereas those classified as 'other-other' form the largest ethnic minority group in Merseyside and Wales, suggesting a high incidence of people of mixed-race origins in these areas.

The history of migration also means there are differences between the gender and age structures of minority ethnic populations and the general population (Mason 2000). Many of the early migrants to Britain were men (Cashmore & Tronya 1990). The numbers of women increased as a result of family reunification, however, and initial gender imbalances became increasingly equalized (Mason 2000). Nevertheless, differences remain, and among 'White', 'Black-Caribbean', and 'Black-other' populations, women are in the majority, whereas among South Asian groups, men predominate (Owen 1993). The lowest ratio of males to females is seen in the 'Black-Caribbean' population (949 males per 1000 females). Among South Asian populations the ratio is 1013 males to 1014 females, with the most striking excess of males to females found in Bangladeshi populations (1090 males to 1000 females).

Differences are also evident when discussing age structures. Minority ethnic populations are in general younger than the general population (Mason 2000). According to the 1991 census, less than 3% of minority ethnic populations are over 65 years old. However, the proportion of older people from minority ethnic populations is growing. Comparing different age cohorts between the 1981 and 1991 censuses suggests that the largest percentage growth for minority ethnic groups has been in people over 65, at 167% (Butt & Mirza 1996). More generally, demographic trends indicate an imminent steep growth in the numbers of African-Caribbean and South Asian (especially Indian) descent over the next 10 years. These figures suggest the numbers of minority ethnic older people can no longer be dismissed as being too small to impact on policy and practice (Atkin 1998).

7.3 HEALTH AND ILLNESS

It has been shown that illness and impairment are positively correlated with low socioeconomic status, including poor housing and higher rates of unemployment (Nazroo 1998). People from ethnic minority groups are disproportionately represented in this section of society, and thus their level of illness and impairment is often higher than that of the majority population (Kurtz 1993, Hill 1994). Asian people, for example, have a higher incidence of diabetes (Nazroo 1998); African-Caribbean people have a higher incidence of stroke (Beevers & Beevers 1993); and the babies of women from many ethnic minority groups are smaller than average, predisposing these infants to impairment and life-threatening events (Jacobson et al 1991). There is, however, considerable variation in the level of illness and impairment among the ethnic minority groups, with Bangladeshi, Pakistani and African-Caribbean people being particularly adversely affected (Butt & Mirza 1996).

As well as the link with poverty, there are a number of disorders that mainly affect people from specific ethnic minority groups; one of these conditions is sickle cell disorder, which is transmitted genetically and largely affects African and African-Caribbean people in the UK (Anionwu & Atkin 2001). It is estimated that 1 in 10 people of African-Caribbean origin carries the gene, and 1 in 500 has the condition. The disorder is, however, also present in people of Mediterranean, Asian and Arab origin and the incidence among other ethnic groups – including white and mixed race – is rising. At the present time there are at least 15 000 people in Great Britain with a sickle cell disorder, thus making it Britain's most common genetic illness. Another genetic condition largely found among South Asian and Greek-Cypriot populations is thalassaemia. There are about 700 people with thalassaemia living in the UK (Anionwu & Atkin 2001).

There is also a higher than average incidence of tuberculosis, rickets and osteomalacia among Asian people, and specific eye conditions which can lead to severe visual impairment are more common in some ethnic minority groups than others (Mason 2000). Diabetic retinopathy, for example, is particularly common among Jewish people, and cataracts are prevalent among Asian people. White people are, of course, similarly affected with a high incidence of specific conditions, for example cystic fibrosis and breast cancer. Any tendency, therefore, to view the health needs of people from ethnic minority groups in terms of 'problems' is unjustified and should be avoided. We will return to this later in the chapter.

This high incidence of illness and impairment is offset by the relatively low percentage of older people from ethnic minority groups in Britain, due to the fact that many people emigrated after the Second World War when they were young. Many will reach old age within the next few years and their health and social needs will become more urgent (Atkin 1998).

Despite these variations it must be borne in mind that low socioeconomic status, often resulting from racism, and leading to poor housing, diet, and unemployment, is far more influential than ethnic origin or cultural difference with regard to the incidence of illness and impairment (Nazroo 1998). The higher incidence of conditions such as tuberculosis, rickets and osteomalacia is often the consequence of socioeconomic disadvantage. Average weekly household incomes of minority ethnic populations, for example, fall below that of white households, for example 82% of Pakistani and 84% of Bangladeshi households have incomes below half the national average. This compares to 45% of Indian families, 41% of African-Caribbean families and 28% of white families (Modood et al 1997). Such inequalities continue into old age, with 85% of older people from minority ethnic groups being solely dependent on means-tested benefits, compared to 25% of the white population (Butt & Mirza 1996). In the past, cultural differences have been used to explain inequalities in health and access to health care. We are now beginning to understand how socioeconomic position is a more important variable in explaining the disadvantages faced by minority ethnic groups. Socioeconomic status is also emerging as important in explaining differences between minority ethnic groups and, in particular, the poorer health of Bangladeshi and Pakistani people, when compared with Indian populations (Nazroo 1998). At the same time, however, people from ethnic minority groups should not be stereotyped as poor, unemployed and disadvantaged. The enormous differences in terms of language, religion and social customs among people from different ethnic minority groups should also be remembered. Minority ethnic groups do not form a homogeneous group and the majority population may resemble some ethnic minority groups in terms of culture more than the ethnic minority groups resemble each other.

Services for people with illnesses and impairments specific to their ethnic minority status have been neglected. Grimsley & Bhat (1988) point out that uncommon conditions which affect white people, such as phenylketonuria, are screened, implying that more common conditions such as sickle cell disorders would be screened if they affected the majority population. In general, provision for those with sickle cell disorders and thalassaemia remains under-resourced and poorly coordinated, especially when compared to services for those with cystic fibrosis and haemophilia (Anionwu & Atkin 2001). Tuberculosis, which is also more common in certain ethnic minority groups, has, in contrast, had a high profile, probably because of its perceived threat to the majority population (Bhopal & White 1993). The lack of knowledge of conditions that specifically affect people from ethnic minority populations can easily interact with racist attitudes concerning illness behaviour, leading to a lack of belief in symptoms, such as pain, of which a person is complaining. This is a common experience of people with sickle cell disorders, where – as we shall see – they may be stereotyped as drug addicts or as people with low pain thresholds (Anionwu & Atkin 2001).

7.4 INSTITUTIONAL RACISM AND HEALTH CARE

The MacPherson inquiry into the death of Stephen Lawrence introduced the idea that institutional racism was rife in UK organizations. Health and social care services were not immune from such criticisms. This was further substantiated with the introduction of the amendment to the Race Relations Act in April 2002, which makes statutory agencies responsible for introducing strategies that tackle institutional racism within their organization. Institutional racism, however, is not a new idea and had been around for at least 20 years (Glasgow 1980). Conceptually, it has been a helpful and productive idea in making sense of health inequalities as well as inappropriate and inaccessible service provision (Law 1996). Institutional racism is often called camouflaged racism, meaning that it is not immediately obvious, but is embedded in the taken-for-granted assumptions informing organizational practices. In effect, institutional racism occurs when the policies of an institution lead to discriminatory outcomes for minority ethnic populations, irrespective of the motives of individual employees of that institution (Mason 2000). Institutional racism, however, has become something of a buzz-word – little more than a fashionable term that is in danger of losing its meaning. It is, therefore, helpful, with the use of empirical examples, to re-examine its usefulness in making sense of the experience of minority ethnic populations as they try to gain access to appropriate health care. This is especially important for physiotherapy, which as an occupational group has found it difficult to engage with these debates.

7.4.1 CONSTRUCTING NEED: IGNORING DIFFERENCE AND DIVERSITY

Perhaps the heart of the problem, and fundamental to an understanding of institutional racism, is the idea that the same service for all equates with an equal service for all. Consequently, services sometimes obscure their failures to meet the needs of minority ethnic people by assuming they treat everyone the same. In reality this means that services are organized according to a 'white norm', which does not recognize difference and diversity and assumes that policies, procedures and practices are equally appropriate for everyone (Atkin 1996). When talking of the UK National

Health Service (NHS), Weller (1991: 31) states: 'this service remains essentially geared to the attitudes, priorities and expectations of the majority population which is considered as white, middle class and nominally Christian.' Such practices legitimate non-recognition of the care needs of minority ethnic communities and disregard, for example, the dietary, linguistic and cultural needs of minority ethnic groups. Most health care professionals feel ill-equipped to respond to cultural differences (Anionwu & Atkin 2001) and they rarely understand the lifestyles, social customs and religious practices of people from ethnic minority groups (Admani 1993a, Farooqi 1993). Special bathing aids, for example, may be completely inappropriate for people whose washing methods are different from those of the indigenous population. Childcare practices may vary, and ways of coping with terminal illness and death may differ (Green 1989a, 1989b, 1989c, 1989d). It may be totally unacceptable for people from some ethnic minority groups to be treated by a person of the opposite sex or in view of other patients, in the hydrotherapy pool or gymnasium.

The most obvious example of this failure to recognize cultural diversity is the inability of the NHS to provide adequate support for those whose first language is not English (Robinson 2001), and this of course has particular implications for physiotherapists. It is worth exploring this further as it illustrates the complex nature of institutional racism and its consequences for minority ethnic populations. Interpreters are often in short supply and difficult to get hold of (Robinson 2001). This is why, when a person cannot speak English, family members are sometimes used as interpreters and, although acceptable to some people, others object to the practice (Atkin et al 1998). In some cases young children are required to act as interpreters of complex medical information, often about sensitive or potentially embarrassing issues (Anionwu & Atkin 2001). Women have pointed to the problems their husbands have faced in simultaneously translating distressing information and coming to terms with it themselves. Husbands' accounts confirm these problems, and report particular difficulties in deciding how much they should tell their non-English-speaking wives; often they have wanted to protect their wives from information deemed upsetting. However, this has left women without important information about their health or the health of their child – information important for understanding, coping and caring (Anionwu & Atkin 2001). In other cases, people did not want their health problem to be shared with other family members, but often felt they did not have a choice because of the lack of language support.

Difficulties may occur even when interpreters are used (Chamba et al 1999). Most interpreters, for example, have little specialist knowledge and face difficulties in interpreting clinical information and procedures, sometimes with unfortunate consequences. This has meant that people have often gained misleading and erroneous information about their illness or impairment (Atkin et al 1998). Patients and their families have also pointed to the problems of communicating through a third party. This, they felt, made it difficult to ask questions, and, more generally, take part in a discussion with health professionals. Not surprisingly, patients and their families express dissatisfaction with the process (Chamba et al

1999, Bhakta et al 2000). Many practitioners, for their part, share these concerns about the shortfalls in interpreting services. For example, interpreters are often either unavailable or else difficult to organize. For these reasons, many health professionals prefer to use family members (Atkin et al 1998). Even when interpreting services are available, practitioners have still identified problems. Several practitioners have remarked that there are often differences in the language or dialect spoken by the interpreter and that spoken by the patient. Others have questioned interpreters' skills in interpreting genetic information as well as their own competence in working with interpreters (Chamba et al 1999). Thus barriers are created to effective communication (Atkin et al 1998). Barriers to communication, however, are more than language-specific and evoke cultural differences (Walker & Ahmad 1994), particularly since ethnic and cultural misunderstandings, myths and stereotypes can undermine the communication process. Understanding this is another important aspect of institutional racism.

7.4.2 MISREPRESENTING THE HEALTH CARE NEEDS OF MINORITY ETHNIC GROUPS

Health and social services often identify minority ethnic health and social 'problems' as arising from cultural practices (Walker & Ahmad 1994). This results in service organizations blaming minority ethnic communities for the problems they experience. Minority ethnic people, for example, are frequently characterized as in some way to blame for their own needs because of deviant and unsatisfactory lifestyles (Cameron et al 1989). Indeed, there is a history of defining health problems faced by minority ethnic communities in terms of cultural deficits where a shift towards a 'Western' lifestyle is offered as the main solution to their problems; examples include the discussion on maternity and child health (Rocherson 1988). Recently, impairment, and more generally 'poor birth outcome', among Asian communities have often been attributed to consanguineous marriages (Ahmad et al 2000). Darr, for example, notes that in relation to thalassaemia major in the Pakistani community, health professionals often relate the condition explicitly (and less often implicitly) to consanguineous marriages, and therefore consider it to be self-inflicted and located in these communities' presumed cultural and biological pathology (Darr 1997). The relationship between consanguineous marriage and the incidence of impairment and poor health is, of course, complex (Ahmad et al 2000). What is important to note, however, is that the preoccupation with cultural practices, such as consanguineous marriage, in explaining impairment means that other important explanations – for example, the role of poverty or of services – are rarely mentioned. Such an approach also carries an implicit criticism of Asian cultural practices and further creates mistrust between health professionals and their patients (Ahmad et al 2000).

As part of this preoccupation with culture, minority ethnic groups also have to contend with inappropriate generalizations of cultural practices and the use of simplistic explanations for their behaviour. Introductory notes on minority ethnic communities, present in most training material for service practitioners, often follow this pattern. One would not, for instance, attempt to summarize a Western approach to child-rearing practices in one paragraph, yet this is what minority ethnic people are subjected to. Cultural myths also explain why prenatal diagnosis is sometimes withheld from Muslim families, because it is assumed that termination is unacceptable to them. However, as with other sections of the population, termination is acceptable to some Muslim families but not to others (Atkin et al 1998). Assumptions held by practitioners sometimes deny these families choice about their health care (Anionwu & Atkin 2001).

Other myths contribute further to this failure to recognize the support needs of South Asian families. A convenient stereotype is that these families virtuously 'look after their own'. Health and social care agencies use this as a reason for not planning or providing services for disabled or chronically ill individuals or their families (Walker & Ahmad 1994). The assumption that Asian people live in self-supporting extending family networks is simplistic for a number of reasons; see Walker & Ahmad (1994) for a detailed account of these reasons. Household structures, for example, are changing as well as the expectations that inform family obligations. None the less, the assumption that Asian families have the necessary material, emotional and social resources to cope with chronic illness with limited professional support is at best misguided and at worst a racist denial of their support needs (Atkin & Rollings 1996).

Generally, neat cultural packages identifying key characteristics of minority ethnic people do not solve the problems facing community care services and are likely to perpetrate and reinforce cultural stereotypes and myths (Butt 1994, Culley 1996). This is not to dismiss the role of cultural identity in informing people's service needs but to challenge accounts that seek to pathologize and simplify cultural practices. Simple one-page summaries of how Hindu, Muslim or Sikh people are likely to respond to ill health are unlikely to solve the difficulties in providing sensitive and appropriate care to these populations. This comes to represent an important struggle facing minority ethnic groups.

Finally, before leaving this discussion of institutional racism, reference should be made to the potential effect of racist attitudes held by some front-line practitioners. These attitudes can deprive minority ethnic communities of their rights to services, especially since health and social service professionals exercise considerable discretion in their day-to-day work (Lipsky 1980). Racist attitudes on the part of service practitioners have been reported in a number of studies in health and social services (see, for example, Ahmad 1993). For instance, practitioners working in local authorities often list minority ethnic people as 'high-risk' clients, 'uncooperative' and 'difficult to work with'. Similarly, evidence suggests that racism within the NHS affects minority ethnic people, with common stereotypes portraying them as 'calling out doctors unnecessarily', being 'trivial complainers', and 'time wasters'. These attitudes become manifest in ideas about the 'passivity' of Asian families and the 'lower pain thresholds' of African-Caribbean patients, thereby denying the minority ethnic populations the support they need.

The treatment of pain among African-Caribbean people offers another important example of how institutional racism comes to deny people access to the care they need. Health professionals often feel those with sickle cell disease are over-reacting and exaggerating their pain (Atkin et al 1998), because of ideas about lower pain thresholds of African-Caribbean people. Lack of treatment can, however, also be justified by yet another racial myth. The control of pain often requires powerful painkillers. Some doctors worry about their black patients becoming dependent on drugs and this can contribute to the significant under-treatment of pain. There is no evidence to suggest that addiction to powerful pain-killing drugs is a more significant problem among African-Caribbean people than among any other ethnic group. The inability of services to deal with pain contributes to the vulnerability of individuals and their families and means they remain unsupported during one of the most difficult and demanding times of their life.

7.5 IMPROVING POLICY AND PRACTICE

Institutional racism provides a framework to make sense of the discrimination and disadvantages faced by minority ethnic groups as they try to gain access to appropriate health care. This, however, is only one aspect of the problem of providing sensitive and equitable service provision for minority ethnic groups. Analysis of the problem is one thing; doing something about it is another. Accounts of institutional racism tend to focus on the unfair structuring of opportunities. The critical emphasis of the literature is perhaps understandable and has successfully highlighted the negative consequences of racism, marginalization and unequal treatment (see Ahmad 1993). None the less, by focusing on disadvantage there is a danger of adopting a 'victim-orientated' stance. Maulana Karenga described the dilemma:

> How does one prove strength in opposition without overstating the case? Diluting criticisms of the system and absolving the oppressor in the process? How does one criticize the system and state of things without contributing to the victimology school which thrives on litanies of lost battles and casualty lists, while omitting victories and strengths and the possibilities for change inherent in both black people and society? (cited in Jeyasingham 1992: 1).

Constantly highlighting the negative consequences of service provision does little to advance thinking and practice (Levick 1992). Focusing on the needs of minority ethnic groups is not the same as meeting those needs. Action is required. The disadvantages experienced by minority ethnic groups are not inevitable and change is possible. Commitment to change and empowerment is the key. It is, therefore, worthwhile to explore some potential strategies than could improve the health care of minority ethnic groups.

7.5.1 RACE EQUALITY TRAINING

Health professionals are predominantly white and non-disabled, and receive very little training concerning the needs and difficulties of ill and disabled people among ethnic minority groups (Vousden 1987). It is almost impossible to be entirely free of racist beliefs and attitudes when brought up in a society such as our own. Some of these attitudes and behaviour patterns may be conscious while others are submerged. It may be that we attend to people from ethnic minority groups a little less than other people, that we do not expect as much of them, or that we give them a little less of our time. In many ways the more subtle and submerged racism becomes, the more difficult it is to deal with. Read (1988: 52) believes that 'white people have to learn that, although it is not their fault, they are racist, however well intentioned they are, but that they can learn to change their behaviour'.

Race equality training, when skilfully carried out by people from ethnic minority groups, can help people to become aware of their attitudes and behaviour in a relaxed and non-threatening environment. It is no longer acceptable to treat people from ethnic minority groups 'just like everyone else' or to take a 'why can't they be like us?' approach. The authors of *Double Bind* (Confederation of Indian Organisations 1987), talking of Asian disabled people, state: 'True integration is recognising that disabled Asians may have special needs. Treating everyone the same is not equality, because it does not take into account these needs. This would be assimilation and not integration' (Confederation of Indian Organisations 1987: 19). Ill and disabled people from ethnic minority groups must be sought and actively involved in the education of health professionals.

There also needs to be greater awareness and understanding of the cultural diversity of people from different ethnic minority groups and a sensitivity to these differences when communicating with and treating them. Physiotherapists, for example, should have a working knowledge of their likely health beliefs, dietary needs, religious practices and social customs, but above all should be prepared to learn from their patients and clients. As we have seen, however, attempting to understand cultural differences must not lead to simplification and stereotyping.

7.5.2 INTERPRETERS

There is an urgent need for more trained interpreters. In the London borough of Tower Hamlets, for example, the 1981 census recorded 172 languages (Wilson 1989). A register of bilingual staff is helpful and can give rise to a dramatic uptake of services (Baxter 1988), but Chaudbury believes that interpreters should ideally be independent of the organization. In relation to the education service, she states: 'Interpreters who see their role as interpreting the LEA's [Local Education Authority's] wishes to the parent can very easily slip into putting pressure on to parents to go along with what is being proposed' (Chaudbury 1990: 10). Ellis (1993) makes the point that interpreters are frequently used to pass on unpalatable information or to negotiate difficult decisions, rather than to facilitate understanding.

It would also be helpful if more written information was translated into minority languages, although this should not be regarded as a 'cure-all'. Ley (1988) cites evidence, concerning patients and clients generally, that the written word is not always a very effective way of communicating information. Kroll (1990) contends that pamphlets should be used only to consolidate information that has been given orally, and Bahl (1993) believes that people from ethnic minority groups should be involved in producing their own health education literature to ensure its accessibility.

7.5.3 EMPLOYMENT OF HEALTH PROFESSIONALS FROM ETHNIC MINORITY GROUPS

In a survey of racial equality in the social services, it is stated that 'without equal employment opportunities it is unlikely that there will be equal opportunities in service delivery' (Commission for Racial Equality 1988: 11). There is considerable evidence of lack of opportunities for training and employment for minority ethnic workers in the health services (see Baxter et al 1990, French 1992, Admani 1993b, Gerrish et al 1996, Darr & Bharj 1999), which can be viewed as a form of racism.

The appointment of an Asian worker in a social service respite team brought a dramatic increase in the number of Asian people using it (Holden 1988). In *Double Bind* (Confederation of Indian Organisations 1987), it is recommended that outreach teams, comprising people from the Asian community, should attempt to reach Asian disabled people and their families who are not using statutory services. The authors believe that outreach teams should be of the same cultural background as the target groups.

In today's climate of 'equal opportunities', it is to be hoped that more health professionals from ethnic minority groups will be recruited. Hugman makes the point, however, that equal opportunity policies can serve as a form of image management and that equal opportunity statements can be used 'as a smokescreen behind which racism remains intact' (Hugman 1991: 158). Darr & Bharj (1999) demonstrate how, despite a formal equal opportunity policy in colleges of health, the recruitment of South Asian people into the nursing profession remains a serious problem. They conclude that the failure to employ a multicultural workforce limits the ability of the NHS adequately to address the health needs of minority ethnic groups.

Employing a multiethnic workforce has particular implications for physiotherapy. According to a survey undertaken by the Chartered Society of Physiotherapy (CSP), 98% of physiotherapists describe themselves as 'white', with the largest minority ethnic representation found among 'Indian' people (0.5%). Only 0.08% of physiotherapists described themselves as of 'Pakistani' or 'Bangladeshi' descent. More encouraging, however, is the intake of students training to be physiotherapists. For the past 3 years, minority ethnic students have made up just under 10% of the total intake. Of these students, 1.4% describe their ethnic origin as 'Indian' and 1% describe themselves as 'Black-Caribbean'. 'Bangladeshi' students, however, are still under-represented (0.05%). None the less, the CSP recognizes the problem and is aware that, as a profession, physiotherapy does not meet a key criterion of the NHS plan, which emphasizes that staff working in the NHS are representative of the communities they serve. The CSP is seeking to address these problems and has established an Equal Opportunities Working Party (Kate Morgan, personal communication, 2002).

In order to provide appropriate and culturally sensitive services to people from ethnic minority groups, it is essential to consult the people concerned, and their organizations, at every stage of service planning and implementation. It is very important to avoid tokenism, whereby just one or two people from ethnic minority groups (perhaps those already working in the organization) are asked for their opinions. The service should be regularly evaluated and an accessible complaints procedure put in place. More generally, consultation involves a fundamental shift in power between health professionals and the people to whom they offer support (Bhopal & White 1993).

7.6 CONCLUSION

It is clear from the above account that, although progress is slowly being made, a great deal still needs to be done to provide people from ethnic minority groups with sensitive and effective health care. The attitudes and behaviour of individual practitioners are vitally important in bringing about change, but management backing and the development of policy relating to resources, staff recruitment, and working practices must be made at every level of the organization if meaningful progress is to be achieved.

Unfortunately, policy makers and practitioners still remain unclear about how best to engage with the communities they serve. Despite considerable research activity, we still have little indication about what types of policies and interventions actually work when providing accessible and appropriate support for minority ethnic people. Examples of good practice, for instance, are rarely disseminated and seldom subjected to rigorous evaluation, which would help us understand why they work. Accounts of the experience of minority ethnic populations tend to focus on the unfair structuring of opportunities and on unmet needs. The critical emphasis of the literature is perhaps understandable and has successfully highlighted the negative consequences of racism, marginalization and unequal treatment. Constantly highlighting the negative consequences of service provision, however, does little to advance thinking and practice. There is, therefore, a need to develop a strategy that enables us to explore interventions that meet the needs of minority ethnic populations. This is the challenge facing health care professionals, which of course includes physiotherapists, in the first decade of the twenty-first century.

ACKNOWLEDGEMENTS

We would like to thank Kate Morgan from the Chartered Society of Physiotherapy for providing data on the ethnic breakdown of the profession. We would also like to thank Angie Ryan, from the Centre for Research in Primary Care, University of Leeds, for collecting material for inclusion in the chapter.

Chapter **8**

The psychology of pain

Tamar Pincus

8.1 AIMS AND SCOPE

Psychology is 'the science which uses introspective and behavioural evidence to understand the internal processes which lead people to think and to behave in the ways they do' (Eysenck 1998: 2). As such, the study of the psychology of pain incorporates everything that affects the pain experience and the response to it, with considerable overlap with the sociology of pain and psychophysiology, among many other branches of behavioural medicine (see Ch. 9). One of the most common approaches to answering questions in psychology is the development of a theory, followed by extraction of hypotheses, to be tested under more or less rigorous scientific conditions. This in turn has sometimes resulted in important breakthroughs in treatment. For example, the development and testing of cognitive models of pain, which are discussed at length throughout this chapter, have led to cognitive-behavioural therapy for chronic pain (see Ch. 18), which has proved not only successful, but also superior to purely physical interventions (Morley et al 1999).

In modern health science, pain is often defined as a multidimensional experience consisting of sensory, cognitive–evaluative, and affective–motivational dimensions. It is more common than not for social, cultural and environmental factors to be ignored; however, these aspects are addressed in Chapter 9. This chapter will concentrate on the psychological aspects of the pain experience, i.e. the cognitive–evaluative and the affective–motivational dimensions. The literature on the neurobiology of emotion in general and in reference to pain will therefore not be covered, and for this the reader is referred to current reviews elsewhere (Derryberry & Tucker 1992, Chapman 1995). In addition, this chapter makes reference to pain behaviour. Pain behaviour is defined as overt expressions that communicate pain and distress to others (Turk & Okifuji 1999). These include vocalization (moans, complaints), expressive motor behaviour (grimacing, gait, posture, movement), help-seeking (medication consumption, consultation), and functional changes (resting, reduced activity, work loss).

Recent years have seen a shift in the outcome targeted in psychological pain interventions, especially in chronic pain. Interventions seldom attempt to alter the intensity or even the frequency of pain episodes as their primary target. Instead, the focus is on disability: the impact of pain on the ability to carry out normal behaviours, including moving, working, taking care of oneself and maintaining regular daily activities. Pain behaviour therefore includes also return to work and work absenteeism, utilization of health services, and medication consumption. These translate into the main components of the cost of pain to individuals, work and health organizations and governments. Changing pain behaviour depends on individuals' wish to change (motivation), on whether they believe they can, and should, change (beliefs and attributions), and on their emotional state not only before trying to change but also throughout the period of change, and following it. Psychological interventions that have considered these elements have proved successful (Morley et al 1999). These are described in detail in Chapter 18.

Many factors associated with these aspects are discussed elsewhere, including illness perception (Ch. 11), the effect of pain on self identity (Ch. 9), the effect of having an explanation for pain on distress and behaviour (Sections 4.4 and 18.4), and the impact of the quality of communication between clinicians and patients (Ch. 14). These concepts are closely related both to the psychology and to the sociology of pain, and have been included elsewhere. This chapter centres on the 'inner side' of the pain experience;

on processes that take place within an individual, sometimes even without awareness. The aim of the chapter is to introduce readers to psychological models, to describe the evidence for and against these models, and to discuss the implications for clinicians and patients.

Initially, two modern models of pain will be briefly described. Both models suggest that emotions and cognitions have a profound effect on the pain experience. The next section is concerned with describing the evidence, and it is divided into three sections.

First, emotions, and their complex relationship with pain, have been studied in depth, especially in reference to depression and anxiety. In this chapter, the definitions of these concepts will be challenged, and the tools used to measure them criticized. The approach that seeks a linear (if possible, causal) relationship between emotional distress and pain will be questioned. The main focus will be on depression.

Second, theories of personality, including personality characteristics as risk factors, have been a focus for investigation. This evidence will be reviewed, and the implications of the findings for clinicians and patients will be discussed.

Third, cognition has become a central theme for research in the psychology of pain. Cognition is defined as a 'generic term embracing the quality of knowing, which includes perceiving, recognizing, conceiving, judging, sensing, reasoning and imagining' (*Stedman's Medical Dictionary* 1976). Cognitive psychology is 'concerned with … mental processes, including those involved in perception, attention, learning, memory, problem solving, decision making and the use of language' (Eysenck 1998: 11). These processes might be available to our consciousness, so we can describe them, and debate them in our thoughts. Attitudes, for example, often belong in this category. Other processes are automatic, such as, for example, selective attention. In the psychology of pain, both conscious and automatic processing can affect the experience of pain and our response to it, so it is no wonder that the study of cognition in pain has formed such a major part of the psychology of pain. Self-reported cognitions and their effect on pain behaviour will be discussed, with a special focus on fear-avoidance and catastrophizing. In addition, new paradigms allow the testing of processing biases using more objective measures, and the findings from these studies have resulted in deeper understanding of the relationship between perception, emotion, self concept and pain suffering. This evidence will be described.

Finally, a hypothetical model that attempts to synthesize the evidence and suggest direct implications to clinicians will be outlined.

8.2 METHODS IN THE INVESTIGATION OF PSYCHOLOGICAL FACTORS IN PAIN

Psychological investigation has to a great extent owed its methodology to the philosophy of science. Research has often attempted to be as objective as possible, by limiting the influence of the investigator on the data collection process, and by attempting to quantify the variables measured. In recent years there is some change in this approach, as more qualitative methods become acceptable, and other philosophies, including phenom-enology, have become influential (Smith et al 1995). The majority of research in the psychology of pain, however, is still quantitative in its approach, whether using questionnaires in quasi-experiments and observational studies, or within a fully experimental design.

8.2.1 THE VALUE OF THE EXPERIMENTAL APPROACH

An important aspect added by psychological research is an emphasis on the experimental paradigm. Observational methods, in which variables are measured and their relation to other variables examined, are limited in the interpretation of the findings. Many researchers argue that causal links between factors cannot be established. A good example of this is presented below in the discussion of depression and pain and the possible causal links between the two. Even the use of complex statistical procedures, such as path modelling (see Section 8.4.5), should not be construed as establishing cause and effect. Experimental methodology, on the other hand, allows investigators to study the direct effect one variable has on another, by manipulating the variables in a controlled fashion. In the study of pain such controlled manipulation is very common, most often in the form of randomized controlled trials.

8.2.2 DRAWBACKS TO THE EXPERIMENTAL APPROACH

Psychological research has added small-scale studies, which test both the effect of psychological factors (for example, fear) on pain, and the effect of pain on psychological factors (such as concentration on a task). The drawback of these experimental approaches is that, although their findings are easier to interpret, they are often limited in their scope, and might tell us little about real life experiences. The origin of this approach is in psychophysics, and it is perhaps best represented these days in the work of Donald Price (Price 1999), whose research into the measurement of pain has allowed the standardized quantitative comparison between different treatments (Price & Harkins 1992a, Gracely 1999).

The psychology of pain includes:

- Studies using induced pain in otherwise healthy groups
- Studies using induced pain in people who have an illness or a painful condition
- Studies carried out in groups with a clinical pain condition.

Sometimes the findings from one of these groups are inappropriately generalized to another group. For example, Greene & Hardy (1958) found that the thresholds in healthy individuals to heat producing a pricking pain was reduced over 13 minutes by a whole degree (cited in Price 1999: 27). Should we conclude that, over time, pain threshold is reduced in patients with chronic pain? In fact, such generalizations are dangerous. Experimental studies inducing pain in undergraduate students tell us little about the experience of chronic pain. This is an important point, since *pain is always defined by its meaning to the individual.* Price (1999) points out that eating chillies, having a mouth ulcer and having mouth cancer might produce, at a given moment, a similar sensation in terms of its location, intensity and duration. However, the *meaning* of the experience is completely different. The burning sensation associated with chillies might not be experienced as pain at all. The degree of unpleasantness experienced by someone worried about the long-term effects of cancer will exceed that of the person with the mouth ulcer.

At the end of the day, undergraduates participating in an induced-pain experiment can get up and go home free of pain. What is more, they know they can. Most patients take their pain home with them.

8.3 MULTIDIMENSIONAL MODELS OF PAIN

Pain is a universal but intensely individual phenomenon. Over the past decade researchers and clinicians have come to realize that focusing on intensity, location and time course is a limited way of defining pain. Dimensions of affect (emotion and feeling), contextual and personal meaning and cognition are also fundamental components of the pain experience. Patients suffering from long-term pain conditions probably knew this all along.

8.3.1 THE GATE CONTROL MODEL OF PAIN

There are several influential multidimensional models of pain, all of which owe an acknowledged debt to the gate control theory of pain (Melzack & Wall 1965). The scope of this chapter does not allow for a review of the gate control theory, except for noting the crucial breakthrough in the proposition that psychological mechanisms can affect pain perception. This proposition was a historical break away from the conventional medical model, which suggested that affect followed the experience of pain (i.e. pain could result in anger and fear), but could not impact on it (for example, high levels of fear reducing pain thresholds). Melzack & Wall suggested descending neural 'messages' from the brain, which could increase or inhibit the pain signals (reviewed in Melzack & Wall 1982). The following models are considered as theoretical constructs within the gate control model, rather than models attempting to replace it.

8.3.2 LEVENTHAL'S PARALLEL PROCESSING MODEL

Multidimensional models of pain are typically complex, and it is not easy to extract testable hypotheses from them. One of the most complex models is described by Leventhal and colleagues (Leventhal & Everhart 1979, Leventhal et al 1983, 1990). Leventhal was particularly interested in the interaction between emotion, cognition and the pain experience. He suggested that pain is processed through two separate but interacting 'channels':

1. A sensory channel processes information about the sensory components of pain, such as intensity, location and sensory properties such as temperature, and pressure.

2. An affective channel processes components about the affective component of the pain, including elements of unpleasantness, fear and suffering.

Although pain is processed in parallel through both channels at all stages of the pain experience, one channel is considered to be dominant. Thus, if attention can be shifted *away* from the affective components of the pain towards the sensory components, suffering should be reduced overall. This is a major departure from theories of distraction, which promote the diversion of attention from the experience of pain altogether (see Section 18.10). There is some evidence to support the idea that focusing attention on sensory components can reduce distress (Johnson 1973), but there is far more evidence to support distraction as a strategy for pain control, providing the pain intensity is low or moderate and relatively constant (Eccleston et al 1997).

8.3.3 PRICE'S SEQUENTIAL PROCESSING MODEL

Another important description in Leventhal's processing model is a hierarchical set of processing. This includes the conceptual level, which includes the individual's beliefs, reasons, attributions – in short, the processing that people can report when they describe their thought processes (for example, 'I'm terrified of going to the dentist because I hate the sound of the drill'). A different level is the 'schematic' level of processing. A schema can be defined as a consistent internal structure, used as a template to organize new information (Williams et al 1997). This level of processing can impose selective filtering on incoming information, so that information congruent to the schema will be selectively processed. This idea is important, as it has led to a wealth of evidence on information processing biases in pain, described later.

Note that, despite the fact that schemata operate at an automatic level, so people may not be aware of their content or the result of the selective processing effect, they can have a profound effect on the pain experience. An example borrowed from research in patients with spider phobia illustrates this point nicely. Individuals who are afraid of spiders often suffer constant fear and anxiety to the extent that their well-being is compromised. Unintentionally, they scan the environment for spiders, therefore detecting more of these small objects of fear, and reinforcing their misconceived fears that spiders are all around. In an experiment that demonstrated this automatic processing towards information congruent with spiders, spider-phobic individuals were shown selectively to shift attention from a neutral task towards words associated with spiders, such as 'crawling', 'hairy', etc. (Watts et al 1986). These individuals were not aware of, and could not control, this selective shifting of attention, since it operates at the schematic level of processing, at a pre-conscious level.

The important message to clinicians is that patients' emotions and cognitions operate at levels that the patients cannot always describe. This is quite different from being unwilling to describe – it is an absence of awareness of the operation of a selective process.

In contrast to Leventhal's parallel processing model, a sequential model of processing has been described by Price (Price 1999). This is an evidence-driven model, based on a series of psychophysiology experiments, mostly using induced pain procedures, in both healthy populations and people with painful conditions. Despite reservations about generalizing from these populations to clinical groups, and especially to people with chronic and progressive pain (see Section 8.2.2), Price's model is probably the best supported by data. Price defines pain as 'a somatic perception containing (1) a bodily sensation with qualities like those reported during tissue-damaging stimulation, (2) an experienced threat associated with this sensation, and (3) a feeling of unpleasantness or other negative emotion based on this experienced threat' (Price 1999: 1). This definition does not require the clinician or the patient to demonstrate any tissue damage. Instead, it focuses on perception and processing, thus placing it firmly within psychology of pain.

Other important aspects of Price's model are:

1. Price introduces the concept of a 'self' (a 'home base' interior to the body). Perceived threat to the self has a profound impact on pain processing as it results in the perception of the unpleasantness of pain.

2. The unpleasant component of the pain experience is seen as separate from pain intensity. Both dimensions, nociceptive sensation and unpleasantness, are necessary to produce pain.

3. Although affect is perceived as part and parcel of any pain experience from the onset, the model is sequential. Affect in the very first onset of pain is considered to be an arousal-related fear experience. Later, a more evaluative affective processing 'kicks in', which might include anxiety, frustration and anger. However, with time, as reflection on the impact of pain becomes more elaborate, despair, hopelessness and depression develop.

Most people are familiar with the affective dimensions in the later stages of pain. It should be remembered that there is an affect involved even in the earliest stages. I once saw a 3-year-old child strike her forehead against the corner of a window frame. Her howls were resounding, despite the fact that the injury was minute and fast disappearing. When asked, she explained that the window 'hurt her feelings'. Her fear, surprise and sense of unfairness were part and parcel of the pain. As adults, we might use more rational explanations to comfort ourselves, but our immediate response to unexpected pain is still the same: there I was minding my own business, not hurting anyone, and the world bit me.

8.4 PSYCHOLOGICAL FACTORS AND PAIN: REVIEW OF THE EVIDENCE

8.4.1 PERSONALITY AND PAIN

Personality theory occupies a broad spectrum within psychology. It is generally agreed that it refers to individual differences at the emotional and motivational levels. The most contentious assumption behind most of the theories and the measurements is that people's behaviour is consistent over time, and that this behaviour is significantly affected by the individual's long-standing characteristics, otherwise known as traits. Most people are familiar with the terms 'extrovert' and 'introvert', coined to describe personality dimensions that relate to willingness, ability and desire to engage in social contact (Eysenck 1967). Another well-known description is neuroticism, a dimension that, at the high end, tends to be associated with tension, anxiety and depression. Being labelled 'neurotic' can be a difficult experience, especially for patients. The tendency to respond emotionally to situations is no doubt amplified in the presence of pain, and high emotions through treatment sessions can be daunting, exhausting and even irritating to clinicians. There is not yet adequate training for most pain clinicians to assist them in dealing with both the patient's emotions and their own. Sometimes, it seems that instead of concentrating on helping people cope with and manage these emotions, science has been used to try to scapegoat patients for having them.

Among people with pain, the study of personality factors has been carried out almost exclusively using the Minnesota Multiphasic Personality Inventory (MMPI), which was developed, validated and updated in psychiatric populations. Patients with chronic pain have been demonstrated to score highly on hypochondriasis, depression and hysteria on the MMPI (Love & Peck 1987, Wade et al 1992a, 1992b, Gatchel 1995a, 1995b). On other non-psychiatric measurements they appear to score highly only on neuroticism, which represents negative affectivity (Costa & McCrea 1985). Neuroticism might, therefore, be an expression of distress and depression, rather than a personality trait. Indeed, in many patients these profiles are subject to change after intervention (Fernandez & Turk 1995). There are a few studies that have used scores on the MMPI to predict which patients will respond well to different types of treatment (Wiltse & Rocchio 1975, Smith & Duerksen 1980), but other studies have found contradictory evidence (Waring et al 1976).

Some of the evidence for the 'pain personality' has now been challenged (Main & Spanswick 1995, Gatchel & Epker 1999). The commonly used MMPI has been criticized for criterion contamination when applied to pain populations (Pincus & Williams 1999, Main 2000). Some items on the hypochondria/hysteria scales have been demonstrated to reflect symptoms of physical disease, thus artificially inflating the scores of individuals with physical disorders (Pincus et al 1986). Ahles and colleagues (1986) found that the proportion of patients labelled psychiatrically disturbed was considerably decreased when they used the new updated personality norms. Comparisons with other groups of people with chronic physical disorder, instead of healthy populations, have challenged the assumption that patients with chronic pain are more disturbed than other groups (Gardiner 1980). A recent systematic review of the evidence for psychological risk factors, measured at the acute stage of low back pain, predicting poor outcome found that, despite the wide citation for significant evidence, the findings failed to achieve statistical significance (Pincus et al 2002).

There is an on-going debate about the stability of personality traits (Krahe 1992). However, if traits and combinations of traits are stable components of personality, many people feel strongly that this avenue is not beneficial to patients, clinicians and the macro world of health providers. They argue that this research path could prove punitive to patients, without offering an avenue for change, since personality traits are considered difficult if not impossible to alter. The strongest criticism of this approach is that the use of psychiatric measurements in pain studies is based on a false premise of distinguishing between real/organic and functional/psychogenic pain (Williams 1999). An excellent review of research and theory in this area is presented by Gatchel & Weisberg (2000).

In conclusion, does personality affect pain? Common sense tells us it does. Personality style will affect interaction with others, including clinicians. It will affect the way in which individuals elicit help from others. It will impact on the way others respond. The consulting room is never a sterile laboratory, and both the patient's personality and that of the clinician have an effect on healing and on health. The current understanding of personal characteristics of patients and clinicians and their influence on pain experience and pain behaviour are limited. Even if the evidence was robust, and both the concepts and the measurements deemed valid, the implications for clinicians would be complex. Should clinicians aim to 'screen' for certain personality types? Should they aim to change certain traits? There are complex ethical dilemmas attached to these questions. The promising aspect of this approach is in the growing realization that personality – whatever this might be – is part of the clinician–patient interaction. Clinicians cannot leave their own personality outside the consulting room door, and many people believe they should not strive to do so. The study of the clinician's personality and its effect on patients' pain experience is an exciting new area, currently little researched. It might come to form an important part of an audit trail and, through reflective learning, part of career development, increase satisfaction in both patients and clinicians. Acknowledging the impact that personal characteristics have on health interactions means that clinicians must see themselves (rather than what they advise and do to patients) as active agents in the pain experience of their patients.

8.4.2 EMOTIONS AND PAIN: FOCUS ON DEPRESSION

In this chapter, I have chosen to concentrate on depression and distress in terms of the affective component of pain. We know that fear, anger, frustration and indeed joy, happiness and excitement also play a role in the pain experience. The research on these, however, is much less clear and the findings are limited. Depression and distress, on the hand, have been investigated in depth.

Almost every modern model of pain includes affect as an important dimension of the pain experience. None the less, research in practice has often been unwilling to acknowledge this dimension, and especially to address the hypothesis that affect is integral to the pain experience, rather than a response to it, or a vulnerability factor that compromises adjustment. Thus, despite clear evidence-based guidelines (Gracely & Dubner 1981, Price & Harkins 1992a, 1992b) about the necessity to measure pain intensity and pain distress (unpleasantness) separately, the majority of randomized controlled trials for pain relief fail to measure pain distress.

Another research focus has involved the attempt to separate and categorize patients with chronic pain into those who score high on depression/distress from those who score low. Researchers have asked: 'Does having a long-term painful condition cause depression or does a tendency towards depressive thinking result in poor coping with pain, or even in maintaining pain?' (Gamsa 1990, Banks & Kerns 1996, Wade et al 1996). Others have asked: 'Is depression in patients with chronic pain the same as in other depressed groups (in terms of its prevalence and its qualities) and if so, can it be treated by the same methods, including the prescription of antidepressants?' Very few have asked: 'What is the emotional component in the experience of pain, how does it affect perception and behaviour, and can it be changed?' (Banks & Kerns 1996, Pincus & Williams 1999). Each of these questions will be addressed in the following section.

8.4.3 PREVALENCE OF DEPRESSION IN PAIN

Chronic pain can be a devastating experience. It is often inescapable, resulting in a sense of hopelessness and helplessness, and it has a profound impact on every level of quality of life, from the interaction with family members to work status and daily activities. It is not surprising, then, that the prevalence of depression in groups with chronic pain is often quoted as being as high as 50% (Romano & Turner 1985, Geisser et al 1994). However, there is a marked discrepancy between the figures reported in different studies, even in groups with the same diagnosis (DeVellis 1993). Some of the discrepancy can be explained through sampling bias. People who are recruited at work (for example, Epping-Jordan et al 1998) will differ significantly from people recruited at a pain management programme (such as those reviewed in Morley et al 1999), where many people are no longer in employment due to their pain. However, some of the discrepancy is also due to measurement error.

8.4.4 MEASUREMENT OF DEPRESSION IN PAIN

The diagnosis of clinical depression as a mental disorder is usually carried out in an interview by a qualified professional (for example, Structural Clinical Interview for DSM Diagnosis, SCID; Spitzer et al 1989). The diagnostic criteria for depression include depressed mood, loss of pleasure or interest, appetite disturbance, sleep disturbance, loss of energy, cognitive impairment, and thoughts of suicide (Sullivan et al 1992). However, the study of depressed mood in pain populations has typically been carried out using self-report measures. The most common of these are the Beck Depression Inventory (Beck et al 1961), the Center for Epidemiological Studies Depression Scale (Radloff 1977), the MMPI Depression Scale (Hathaway & McKinley 1951), the distress scale on the General Health Questionnaire (Goldberg 1978), the depression scale on the Symptom Check List-90 (Derogatis 1983), and the Hospital Anxiety and Depression Scale (Zigmond & Snaith 1983). There are also instruments developed specifically for particular groups, such as the depression subscale in the Arthritis Impact Measurement Scales (Hawley & Wolfe 1993) for individuals with rheumatoid arthritis, and the modified Zung Depression Scale (Main et al 1992) for low back pain populations (see Table 8.1).

Almost all the instruments listed in Table 8.1 have been criticized for inflating depression scores by including so-called 'somatic' items (Pincus et al 1986, DeVellis 1993, Williams & Richardson 1993, Pincus & Williams 1999, Wesley et al 1999). Such items ask about fatigue, appetite, sleep

Table 8.1 Scales for the measurement of depression and other psychological factors

Concept	Common measures	Implications
Depression	Beck Depression Inventory (BDI; Beck 1961) Center for Epidemiological Studies-Depression (CED-D; Radloff 1977) General Health Questionnaire (GHQ; Goldberg 1978) Modified Zung Depression Scale (Waddell & Main 1984) Hospital Anxiety and Depression Scale – Depression (HADS; Zigmond & Snaith 1983)	High scores on the affective component – consider referral. High scores on the somatic component may be due to pain
General anxiety	State and Trait Anxiety Inventory (STAI; Spielberger et al 1970) Hospital Anxiety and Depression Scale – Anxiety (HADS; Zigmond & Snaith 1983)	Explore gently, and if appears disabling and constant, refer
Self-efficacy	Self Efficacy Scale (SES; Kaivanto et al 1995) Pain Self Efficacy Questionnaire (SEQ; Nicholas 1989) Arthritis Self Efficacy Scale (ASE; Lorig et al 1989)	Low self-efficacy can be increased through activity. Set achievable goals together
Coping and catastrophizing	Coping Style Questionnaire (CSQ; Rosentiel & Keefe 1983) Pain Cognition List (PCL; Vlaeyen et al 1990) Pain Related Control Scale (PRCS; Flor et al 1993)	Pain-specific catastrophizing can be reduced through gradual exposure to activity Generalized catastrophizing – explore gently, and if appears disabling and constant, refer
Fear avoidance/ fear of pain	Tampa Scale for Kinesiophobia (TSK; Kori et al 1990) Fear Avoidance Beliefs Questionnaire (FAB; Waddell et al 1993) Pain Anxiety Symptoms Scale (PASS; McCracken et al 1992)	Reduce through gradual exposure to the activities that are the focus of fear
Locus of control	Multidimensional Health Locus of Control (MHLC; Wallston et al 1978) Beliefs in Pain Control Questionnaire (BPCQ; Skevington 1990) Pain Locus of Control (PLC; Main & Waddell 1991) Survey of Pain Attitudes (SOPA; Jensen & Karoly 1992, Jensen et al 1994a)	Can be shifted through discussion and contracting
Personality traits	Minnesota Multiphasic Personality Inventory (MMPI; Hathaway & McKinley 1951) Eysenck Personality Questionnaire (EPQ; Eysenck & Eysenck 1975)	Of limited use

quality and libido. These factors are considered to be important elements of depression in clinically depressed groups. However, in individuals suffering from chronic pain, they may well reflect levels of pain rather than of mood.

8.4.5 THE SEARCH FOR A CAUSAL LINK BETWEEN DEPRESSION AND PAIN

There is robust evidence to suggest that people who are distressed at early stages of the pain experience are more likely to become disabled in the long term. In patients with low back pain, high scores on depression at the acute stage (up to 3 weeks) have been shown to predict disability 12 months later, particularly in primary care (Dionne et al 1995, Cherkin et al 1996, Thomas et al 1999). Most importantly, this effect was independent of clinical factors such as pain and function at baseline (Pincus et al 2002). There is also evidence to suggest that, within the population at large, people who are distressed are more likely to develop back pain (Linton 2000). In addition, the prevalence of depression in chronic pain populations is significantly higher than in pain-free healthy individuals. It seems that the presence of pain can result in the development of depression, and that the presence of (or the tendency towards) depression can result in an increased risk for the onset of musculoskeletal pain.

It is sometimes assumed that pain without an identified organic cause is an expression of depression (Blumer & Heilbronn 1982, 1984). It is further suggested that depression in patients with painful conditions is therefore best treated by antidepressants (Mathews & Steptoe 1988). This might hold true for a fraction of individuals, but can also result in mistrust between patients and clinicians. In fact, syndromes in which pain is purely of psychological origin, such as a delusional or hallucinatory cause, are estimated at less than 2% of patients with chronic pain who do not have lesions (Craig 1999). The idea that in the absence of an identifiable organic cause pain must be 'in the head' is not only insulting to patients, it is patently incorrect. As described in the models above, the experience of pain does not require an identified organic cause (Melzack & Wall 1982).

Several excellent studies have examined the causal path between pain and depression by measuring both at two time points, and applying a complex statistical procedure called structural equation modelling (path analysis) to the data (Gamsa 1990, Wade et al 1996). Two comprehensive reviews of the evidence have concluded that there is better evidence to suggest that the experience of pain leads to the development of depression than vice versa (Romano & Turner 1985, Gamsa 1990, Banks & Kerns 1996). On average – that is, across the whole group – the better fit was provided by the path that hypothesized that pain resulted in depression, rather than vice versa.

However, some researchers have argued that the search for a causal path is misleading, at it presumes that depression and pain are two orthogonal (independent) experiences (Pincus & Williams 1999). In a review of this subject, they argued that 'research into the role of depression in chronic pain is unlikely to clarify matters until the concept of depression in a pain context is better defined. Once the concept is clearer, new measurements can be developed and the process can be investigated' (Pincus & Williams 1999: 211).

8.4.6 THE CONCEPT AND QUALITY OF DEPRESSION IN PAIN

Depression, even in the absence of pain, is poorly understood. Perhaps the most influential cognitive theory of depression was suggested by Beck and colleagues (Beck et al 1979, 1985). The theory described how schemata influence people's perceptions, interpretations and memories. These schemata act to distort information towards negative views of the self, the world and the future. This process can result in anger turned towards the self, and subsequently self-blame, guilt and self-hating. Key features are perceptions of oneself as guilty, shameful and unlovable (Greenberg & Alloy 1989).

The nature of depression in the majority of individuals who are described as 'depressed' in chronic pain groups is qualitatively different. Elements of self-hate, guilt and shame are far less common. These features are not common in chronic pain, because most patients do not perceive themselves as responsible for their suffering (Pincus & Morley 2001). Anger is common, but is usually turned towards external agents that are perceived as contributing to the suffering; these can include health services, work, or even government policies. This anger is often justifiable, and should not automatically be considered a pathological feature.

The quality of depression in chronic pain seems to include features of helplessness and hopelessness, and focuses around the feeling of being tortured, punished and caused to suffer, without a sense of possible escape. This qualitative difference between depressed pain patients and clinically depressed groups was tested experimentally in a selective memory task (Pincus et al 1995). Patients with chronic pain were divided into those who scored high on a depression measure, those who scored within normal range, and a control group. They were presented with words associated with classical clinical depression (guilty, shameful, unlovable), words associated with suffering (suffering, tortured, disabled) and neutral words. A surprise memory test showed clearly that only the depressed pain patients differed from the control group, and that they selectively recalled the suffering words, but not the clinical depression words. Another important finding was that the recall bias was specific to words that people related to themselves, indicating that their self-schema included elements of suffering (Pincus & Morley 2001).

8.4.7 CONCLUSION ON PAIN AND DEPRESSION

Negative emotions, often described as depression but probably better conceptualized as suffering and distress, are common in individuals who suffer from pain syndromes, especially if the pain is long-term and has a large impact on their life. The main features in this type of suffering are a sense of hopelessness, helplessness, lack of control and direct threat to integrity of the self. However, there are common misconceptions about depression and pain. These include the idea that depression is a homogeneous experience, which can be treated identically across groups, environments and settings. Another misconception is the idea that depression is independent of pain. It is impossible to 'treat the body', while leaving it to someone else to deal with the mind. Suffering is an integral part of the pain experience (see Ch. 9). Clinicians who attempt to ignore it are poor clinicians. On the other hand, when patients' suffering and distress are particularly high, a wise clinician should recognize his or her own limitations and refer the patient for appropriate professional help.

8.5 COGNITION

8.5.1 SELF-REPORTED COGNITIONS: COPING

In recent years, pain behaviour has become a focus for interventions and research in general. It is widely acknowledged that changing pain behaviour depends on whether people believe they can change, and believe they should change. These beliefs in turn will depend on the degree to which people think they can control their pain and their life in general.

Health beliefs in chronic pain have been investigated in depth, and the evidence for the effect of beliefs on behaviour will be discussed. In addition, cognitions about pain, including coping style, are addressed. Coping is described as the person's cognitive and behavioural efforts to manage (reduce, minimize, master or tolerate) the internal and external demands when they perceive these as taxing or exceeding their resources (Folkman et al 1986a, 1986b; see also Section 4.2). It is generally agreed that coping and beliefs have a strong relationship with adjustment in pain, and therefore need to be addressed by clinicians (Jensen et al 1991b). Coping styles in pain are usually measured by the Coping Style Questionnaire (CSQ; Rosenstiel & Keefe 1983). Patients are asked to endorse strategies they use, which include diversion of attention, positive coping self-statements, praying and hoping, increased activities, reinterpretation of pain sensations, ignoring the pain, and catastrophizing. Some of these strategies are considered 'passive' or 'helpless'. The helpless factor on the CSQ has been found to account for 50% of the variance of distress in people with chronic low back pain (Keefe et al 1990b). This chapter will now describe and critique the evidence on catastrophizing, which is broadly considered a maladaptive coping style.

8.5.2 CATASTROPHIZING

Catastrophizing is a cognitive style, which may be general, or specific to physical symptoms. It includes negative thoughts and self-statements about the present and the future, and typically includes three factors: rumination, magnification and helplessness (Rosentiel & Keefe 1983, Chaves & Brown 1987). Individuals who are high on catastrophizing are the most disabled and do worst in conventional treatment for their pain (Sullivan et al 1998). There is also experimental evidence to suggest that catastrophizing amplifies somatosensory information and primes fear mechanisms (Crombez et al 1998a).

Catastrophizing has also broadly been described as an exaggerated orientation towards pain stimuli and pain experience (Sullivan et al 1985). It is of great interest as a risk factor for the transition from acute to chronic pain (Pincus et al 2002), and has been described as an explanatory construct for variations in pain and depression in chronic pain (Keefe et al 1989). However, it is difficult to tease apart – both in concept and in measurement – depression and catastrophizing (Sullivan & D'Eon 1990). This hinders the interpretation of evidence.

Unfortunately, the majority of research suggesting that catastrophizing 'predicts' disability and pain independently of depression is based on cross-sectional studies (Sullivan et al 1998). There are, however, some excellent prospective studies indicating that catastrophizing affects functional impairment in rheumatoid arthritis (Zautra & Manne 1992, Keefe et al 1997). A recent systematic review (Pincus et al 2002) found that there is moderate evidence from a study in primary care osteopathic treatment (Burton et al 1995) for catastrophizing in acute low back pain as a risk factor for developing long-term disability. In their excellent review of fear avoidance in pain populations, Vlaeyen & Linton (2000) discuss catastrophizing as an important agent in the development of pain-related fear.

8.5.3 HEALTH BELIEFS: SELF-EFFICACY

Coping well and self-managing chronic pain depend on people believing they are capable of doing so. This concept is known as 'self-efficacy', and is described by Bandura (1977). Self-efficacy clearly determines how much motivation patients will have, which in turn will affect adherence and cooperation. The impact of the way we see ourselves, mentioned throughout this chapter, is a key element to all our experiences and behaviours, and should not be underestimated. Self-efficacy has even been shown to affect the body's endogenous opiate and immune systems (Bandura et al 1987, 1988, Wiedenfeld et al 1990). In acute pain produced under laboratory conditions, self-efficacy has been demonstrated to predict pain tolerance (Dolce et al 1986b). The best way to increase self-efficacy in people with chronic pain appears to be actual physical activity (Dolce et al 1986a). This has clear implications for physiotherapists.

While the evidence for self-efficacy as a risk factor for the development of chronic pain is not convincing (Pincus et al 2002), the evidence of its impact on success of treatment is extremely robust (Council et al 1988, Kores et al 1990, Jensen et al 1991a, O'Leary & Brown 1995). People with high self-efficacy believe they can relieve their pain, and subsequently are more likely to get up and do something about it. Self-efficacy in health is usually measured using the Self-Efficacy Scale (Bandura 1977). Specifically in pain populations, a less common tool, the Pain Self Efficacy Questionnaire (Nicholas 1989), has been developed.

8.5.4 HEALTH BELIEFS: CONTROL

Control over pain specifically, and health in general, has been a focus for social–medical research, because it is closely linked with behaviour and satisfaction (Chapman & Turner 1986). A key element is the division into loci of control, which typically include internal, external and chance. These are generally measured by the Multidimensional Health Locus of Control (MHLC; Wallston et al 1978), although the application of this measure to pain populations has been questioned (Main & Waddell 1991), and a less-used but more valid measure exists for pain populations specifically (Skevington 1990).

Internal locus of control is considered an adaptive coping style. Patients who believe the responsibility and the control over their pain are in their own hands do better than those who believe in others' control over their health or in chance alone (Crisson & Keefe 1988, Harkapaa et al 1991, Spinhoven & Linssen 1991). However, some of the evidence on locus of control is difficult to interpret, partly because the three domains (internal, external and chance) are considered independent, so it is possible to score highly on all three.

There also appear to be some circumstances in which high external locus of control can be beneficial (Affleck et al 1987). Perhaps the belief that powerful others are responsible for one's pain increases the placebo effect, or perhaps relinquishing control protects from perceived failure. Despite the popular perception that internal locus of control should always be encouraged, there are circumstances in which this has proved dysfunctional. This is especially the case if in reality patients have little control over their pain, or their control will be usurped due to circumstances beyond their control (Deci 1980, Taylor et al 1984). In addition, a very high internal locus of control can result in reduced negotiation with clinicians, and increased risk behaviour (Burish et al 1984). Although originally considered steady personality traits, health beliefs and locus of control are now considered to change over time and circumstance (Skevington 1995).

Locus of control is a fluid and changing process, and through careful contracting and negotiating can be used to reduce and balance the burden of management between patient and clinician.

A final reminder: clinicians also have shifting loci of control, which in turn affect not only their clinical decisions, but how they feel about themselves and their patients.

8.5.5 FEAR AVOIDANCE

Fear increases arousal, and in turn somatic perception is increased (Crombez et al 1999). But what exactly is meant by fear? General anxiety is associated with sensitivity to pain (Hill et al 1952, Kent 1986), providing it is anxiety about pain. General anxiety, which is not pain-specific, has even been found to reduce pain, by distraction (Klaber Moffett & Richardson 1995). The value of receiving appropriate, clear and accurate information for reducing anxiety is discussed elsewhere (see Sections 4.4 and 20.2). However, patients who continuously demonstrate increased generalized high anxiety should be offered a referral to appropriate professionals.

The study of fear of pain, and specifically of fear avoidance, has yielded extremely promising results, and is directly relevant to manual therapists and physiotherapists in general. The concept of fear avoidance refers to the avoidance of movement or activities based on fear of increasing the pain or causing damage, and the research has been carried out almost exclusively in back pain populations (Vlaeyen & Linton 2000).

Fear avoidance is often referred to as kinesiophobia, and is commonly measured either by the Fear Avoidance Beliefs Scale (FABS; Waddell et al 1993) or the Tampa Scale for Kinesiophobia (TSK; Kori et al 1990). There are also non-self-report measures, such as observation, that attempt to measure fear avoidance (reviewed in Vlaeyen & Linton 2000), but, as usual in cases when external behaviour is considered a marker for internal processes, their validity should be questioned.

The model of fear avoidance was developed to account for the development of chronic musculoskeletal pain from apparently 'healed' acute injury. It has gained considerable support in recent years (Waddell 1998). The model is truly multidimensional, as it incorporates behavioural, physiological and cognitive aspects of learning, and the evidence to support it comes from experimental and clinical groups (Vlaeyen & Linton 2000).

Fear avoidance has been tested in laboratory conditions, and has been found to correlate with range of motion (McCracken et al 1992), lifting time in a lifting task (Vlaeyen et al 1995), knee extension–flexion (Crombez et al 1998b) and trunk extension–flexion and weight-lifting (Crombez et al 1999).

It seems that, independent of pain intensity, fear-avoidance beliefs are associated with avoidance of physical activities. An extremely important extension of these findings has been that fear avoidance concerning work activities is associated with work loss and reported disability (Waddell et al 1993, Linton & Buer 1995).

Considering the importance of this concept, the evidence from prospective studies is remarkably poor. That is not because studies have yielded negative findings, but rather because there have hardly been any that included fear-avoidance measurement at baseline (Pincus et al 2002). One study that did measure fear avoidance in acute low back pain did not find a significant relationship with disability at 12 months (Burton et al 1995). This may be because the study was conducted on a small sample, and suffered from loss to follow-up that reduced the statistical power considerably. Catastrophizing and depression, both significant predictors, might have masked the effect of fear avoidance. In a large study set in the general population, fear avoidance beliefs were found to double the risk of developing a pain complaint (Linton & Ryberg 2001).

Most manual therapists are aware of the impact of fear avoidance on adherence and recovery. The scope of this chapter does not allow for a discussion of treatment targeting fear avoidance, but readers are referred to Section 18.4.

8.5.6 SUMMARY AND LIMITATIONS OF SELF-REPORT MEASURES OF COGNITIONS

Beliefs, coping and catastrophizing are closely linked to behaviour and disability in people with chronic pain. In a recent study, Turner et al (2000) found that beliefs about pain significantly (and independently of pain intensity scores) predicted both disability and depression in patients ($n = 169$) entering a pain management programme. Catastrophizing predicted depression, and other coping strategies predicted disability. Limited by its cross-sectional design, the study none the less suggests that targeting cognitive factors in treatment of pain is essential. The study of fear avoidance has become a focus for clinicians and researchers in musculoskeletal pain.

The study of health beliefs and catastrophizing has depended almost exclusively on self-report from patients. However, there are problems and shortcomings associated with individuals' ability and willingness to report their internal states. Firstly, the emotional component of pain is often vague and diffuse, and extremely difficult to express (Melzack & Dennis 1980). It is also dynamic in nature, changing in quality and flow, and almost impossible to reduce into language (Craig 1999). Secondly, some patients are reluctant to share their experiences, present discordant descriptions of their pain (Keefe et al 1992), or even purposefully misrepresent it (Craig et al 1999). In addition, emotional processing at a schematic level takes place at a pre-conscious level, so individuals may not be aware of biases taking place (Williams et al 1997).

8.6 EXPERIMENTAL PARADIGMS IN THE STUDY OF COGNITION IN PAIN

The final section on evidence of cognition and the role it plays in pain processing comes from a novel approach adapted from clinical cognitive psychology, called information processing biases. The idea behind this approach is to measure experimentally the products of cognitive processing (such as selective attention), rather than trying to measure concepts (such as catastrophizing). The approach is model-driven, in that hypotheses are extracted from theories and then tested experimentally, but so far no single model of pain processing can account for all the findings. The general principle behind the methodology is schema theory: the idea that, at a pre-conscious and automatic level, people select and sift incoming information. Within this context lies the suggestion that if people in pain pay more attention to pain stimuli, selectively interpret ambiguous stimuli as pain-related, and preferentially recall information associated with pain, they may maintain pain conditions for longer and exacerbate their distress. The scope of this chapter does not permit a full discussion of the approach and readers are referred to Williams et al (1997) for a general review in relation to emotional disorders. There is now a growing body of knowledge (Pincus 1998, Pincus & Morley 2001) to suggest that cognitive bias occurs in pain populations, although the complexity of selection bias in pain is not well understood.

8.6.1 THE EVIDENCE FOR COGNITIVE BIASES IN CHRONIC PAIN

Patients with chronic pain have been demonstrated selectively to recall sensory pain words in comparison with other types of words (Pearce et al 1990, Edwards et al 1992). In these tests, patients are compared to a control group, usually matched for age, gender and vocabulary. After seeing or hearing a list of words that includes sensory words, individuals are asked to recall them unexpectedly. The bias demonstrated in these studies could be the result of patients simply being more familiar with pain words than the control group. However, subsequent studies indicated that people with chronic pain did not remember all the pain words equally well, but that the bias was specific to words they thought of as describing themselves (Pincus et al 1993, 1995). In addition, the bias appears to be stronger in people with pain who are distressed. This self-referential bias, which starts to link self-image, distress and pain, is particularly interesting, because it suggests that, at deep levels of processing which cannot be controlled by individuals, their self-schema is changed in the presence of long-term pain. Whether this relationship results in distress, or only happens in patients who are distressed already, is a key question for future research.

The results in studies on attention bias have been less successful. Intuitively, one would assume that patients with pain who have a tendency to shift their attention towards anything associated with pain would be particularly vulnerable to distress. Early studies showed contradictory findings (Pearce & Morley 1989, Pincus et al 1998). An important breakthrough in recent years suggests that when such an attention bias does take place, it is associated with fear of pain, rather than the experience of pain itself (Crombez et al 2000, Keogh et al 2001). This seems to suggest that it might be linked with fear avoidance. What is clear is that the two selective biases (memory and attention) are independent of each other. This suggests that the mechanisms behind them are different, and might give clues to focus interventions.

8.7 A PRACTICAL SYNTHESIS: THE STRESS–DISTRESS MODEL OF COGNITION AND EMOTION IN PAIN

So far, evidence has been described that suggests that at every stage and level of pain, psychological factors play an important role. The literature on depression, fear of pain, health beliefs, coping strategies, self-efficacy, and catastrophizing has been reviewed. These are only the tip of the iceberg. Readers may well raise their hands in despair, thinking: 'which of these am I supposed to identify? When? And what should I do about it?' The following section is an attempt to synthesize the evidence about some of these factors and discuss the clinical implications.

8.7.1 THE STRESS–DISTRESS EMBEDDED MODEL

Both fear and depression are important parts of the pain experience. But they can also be conceived of as fundamentally different: fear is associated with heightened arousal and shifting of resources towards the external world, while depression involves reduced arousal, and shifting of resources away from the external world, into the self, through rumination. Based on this observation, a model of stress and distress in pain is proposed.

The model hypothesizes two hierarchical constellations of embedded states. The constellations are relatively independent of each other. Individuals can manifest symptoms from the highest level of one constellation, while showing none, or little, of the other. The constellations are characterized by different cognitive processing biases, have different processes acting as catalysts, and may require different focused interventions.

The *stress constellation* consists of three states. At the lowest level, individuals suffering from repeated experience of pain will show fear avoidance, or specifically, fear of movement that is perceived as a danger that will result in increased pain and further injury. A large proportion of people with pain will experience this state. Many adjust over time and through necessity. Information and education packages may suffice as interventions at this level. Some patients may require simple behavioural interventions, such as those studied by Vlaeyen and colleagues (Vlaeyen & Linton 2000). Gradual exposure to activity, with constant monitored feedback, has been shown to be effective and to reduce fear. Cognitive bias at this level will consist of selective attentional processing of sensory information, but only in patients who are high on fear.

At a higher level, fear of pain is generalized to health. At this level, individuals will start experiencing and manifesting symptoms of stress. This includes catastrophizing cognitions, somatization and some physical symptoms associated with stress, such as panic attacks, dizziness, shortness of breath and such like. Pain, at this level, has been generalized to be perceived as a threat to health and well-being. Attention bias at this level will probably be towards health-related information. Cognitive-behavioural interventions are required.

A small proportion of patients may manifest symptoms at a higher level yet. At this level, anxiety becomes further generalized, and severe stress is evident. Symptoms associated with general anxiety may be present. Individuals who suffer from generalized anxiety syndrome, when combined with prolonged exposure to pain and injury, may be particularly vulnerable. Somatic symptoms at this level are highly prevalent. This state may require pharmacological interventions as well as cognitive-behavioural treatment.

The *distress constellation* also consists of three states. At the lowest level individuals will experience loss and frustration directly associated with compromise of daily activities due to pain. The majority of patients will experience these emotions, which will be enhanced in groups where an explanation for the pain is not obvious, and therefore justification for suffering is an unresolved issue. At this level, recall bias for sensory information will be manifested. Many patients will adjust to the restrictions in their lives, or find ways of overcoming them. Reassurance, positive social support and maintenance of daily activities will reduce distress at this level. Information and education packages will also be useful.

At a higher level, distress increases, as the representation of pain and illness becomes enmeshed with self-schema (Pincus & Morley 2001). This involves processes in which past concepts of the self are compared with potential future self. This results in an experience of distress and loss, and increases the emotions of helplessness and hopelessness. Processing biases will show a marked recall bias for illness information as well as sensory information, and this will be particularly strong in self-reference. Cognitive-behavioural intervention is indicated, to increase activities that are not associated with pain, thus 'restructuring' the self-schema. Acceptance and management of normal life in the presence of pain are the key to reduction in distress.

At the highest level, symptoms of depression are manifested as hopelessness and helplessness, generalized to more aspects of self and daily living. Emotions of loss, guilt and despair will be present. Individuals with a history of depression will be particularly vulnerable to develop this state in the presence of chronic pain. Cognitive bias is further generalized to negative processing, indicated by recall bias for negative information, including typical depressive stimuli (feeling guilty, unlovable, etc.) as well as illness-related stimuli. At this level pharmacological intervention may be required, as well as cognitive-behavioural treatment.

The model contextualizes somatization within stress, threat and anxiety. It also differentiates the distress experienced by the majority of those with chronic pain from clinical depression. Further, it accounts for numerous findings of cognitive biases in these patients. Finally, it indicates clear and differing interventions for patients, depending on the state they are indicated to be in, both by self-report and by tests of cognitive bias. It also suggests a way forward from the 'throw the full bag of tricks at them' scenario, in which multidisciplinary programmes employ a battery of cognitive-behavioural approaches, because it is not known which of them would help which patient. A recent review of such interventions found that the more techniques were used, the stronger the effect, but more research is needed to tailor treatment to individual needs (Morley et al 1999).

8.8 CONCLUSION

The key points can be summarized as follows:

1. Pain always includes a component of 'unpleasantness', 'suffering' , and 'negative affect'. These are part and parcel of the pain experience, rather than a response to injury and sensation.

2. Self is a super-structure that organizes mental processing. Good clinical practice therefore includes addressing the patient as a 'self' and must acknowledge this and the clinician's own 'self' as agents in the healing process.

3. However, although many people with chronic pain appear depressed and report being depressed, the depression is usually qualitatively different from that of psychiatrically depressed individuals. It is usually a response to loss, combined with a sense of helplessness and hopelessness about the pain. In the context of chronic pain, caution is advised about any psychiatric labelling.

4. High levels of distress (anxiety and depression) may, in some patients, be the result of long-term inherent vulnerability. These patients would benefit from a referral to appropriate professionals. Specifically, watch out for repeated expressions of guilt, shame and self-loathing.

5. Some emotions, even if negative, are a healthy and normal response to pain.

6. Some cognitions have been identified as contributors to poor outcome. The strongest evidence is for the role of fear avoidance and catastrophizing.

7. Some cognitions operate without people's awareness, but can still affect pain, distress and behaviour. Attention, interpretation and memory bias towards pain and illness information have been found in people with pain.

8. Finally, pain cannot be treated independently of social and psychological contexts. But contracts can be reached between patients and clinicians in which the activities of both result in the reduction or the removal of pain.

Chapter 9

The sociology of pain

Julius Sim and Marion V. Smith

9.1 AIMS AND SCOPE

This chapter will examine a number of sociological aspects of pain in relation to health care in general and physiotherapy in particular. As such it is intended to complement Chapter 8.

Benign pain, principally of musculoskeletal origin, is a major cause of morbidity and loss of work. It also accounts for a major part of the work of physiotherapists. In the UK in 1998, the direct health care cost of back pain has been estimated at £1362 million (Maniadakis & Gray 2000). Each year, an estimated 10.9 million sessions of physiotherapy, and 7 million sessions of osteopathy or chiropractic, are provided in the UK for back pain alone (Maniadakis & Gray 2000). Compared with other categories of chronic disease, musculoskeletal conditions – in which the predominant symptom is generally pain – are characterized by particularly low quality of life (Sprangers et al 2000).

Meanwhile, there has been an increasing emphasis in the therapy literature on pain (O'Hara 1996, Strong 1996, Wittink & Hoskins Michel 1997, Strong et al 2002). Within this body of literature, the focus is principally on the physiological mechanisms of pain and clinical aspects of its management. It is important, however, that therapists understand the psychosocial aspects of pain, as these are central to its origin, severity and perpetuation (Waddell & Waddell 2000, Pincus et al 2002), and strongly influence the way in which pain is managed, either by health care providers or by the person in pain him- or herself. The previous chapter examined relevant aspects of the psychology of pain; this chapter will focus on sociological issues around the nature of pain and its impact on the social lives of individuals. The early sections of the chapter will examine the ways in which pain is defined and conceptualized, and its relationship to language and concepts of the body. Pain and pain beliefs will be set within a sociocultural context, in terms of its experience, expression and management. The chapter will then shift its focus to the ways in which people respond to and deal with pain, drawing in particular upon the literature on chronic musculoskeletal pain, and the attitudes and beliefs of health professionals will be discussed.

9.2 DEFINING PAIN

The nature and definition of pain have been a matter of debate and contention throughout history (Merskey 1980, Rey 1995). Attempts to define pain persist to the present day. In some accounts, pain is defined largely in terms of a sensation (for example, Hervey 1984). Others have in addition defined it in terms of tissue damage (for example, Fields 1987). These are essentially physiological definitions, and consider pain as a largely unidimensional phenomenon. Moreover, the link proposed in such definitions between pain and tissue damage is not a straightforward one (Wall 1995). The International Association for the Study of Pain Subcommittee on Taxonomy offers the following definition of pain: 'An unpleasant sensory and emotional experience associated with actual or potential tissue damage or described in terms of such damage' (International Association of the Study of Pain 1986: 217). Sanders (1985: 3), meanwhile, refers to pain as a 'sensory and emotional experience of discomfort, which is usually associated with threatened tissue damage or irritation'. These two definitions indicate that pain has an emotional dimension to it and acknowledge the fact that tissue damage is not a precondition for pain. Importantly, however, while the emotional component of pain is here characterized as unpleasant, this is not necessarily the case; the pain experience may be pleasurable, or may even be emotionally neutral (Trigg 1970).

It is clear that pain is more than just a sensation. Indeed, its sensory element is just one way of defining pain. Broadly, pain can be characterized as a multidimensional construct, consisting of sensory, affective, evaluative, cognitive, and behavioural elements (Fig. 9.1). The *sensory*

Figure 9.1. The dimensions of the pain experience (adapted from Sim & Waterfield 1997; copyright Taylor & Francis Ltd: http://www.tandf.co.uk/journals).

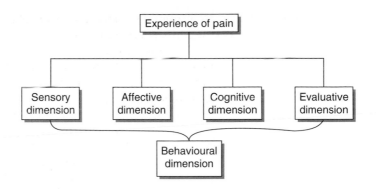

dimension of pain is simply what the individual perceives at the level of the nociceptive system. The *affective* dimension refers to the emotional associations of the sensory experience – whether it is pleasant, unpleasant, troublesome, anxiety-provoking, and so forth. It is worth noting that unpleasant emotional experiences are sometimes referred to as 'painful', suggesting that pain can be emotional in terms of its source as well as its impact, and with little or no reference to the physicality of the body.

The *cognitive* dimension refers to pain beliefs (Section 8.5.4), whereas the *evaluative* dimension of pain concerns the way in which pain is interpreted in the context of the individual's situation, for example judgements as to the significance of pain and the nature and extent of its impact on daily life. Finally, the *behavioural* dimension embraces the actions that people perform to indicate that they are in pain, or as a response to being in pain. Hence, Fordyce (1988: 278) refers to pain behaviour as quite simply: 'the things people do when they suffer or are in pain' (Fordyce 1988: 278). This covers the coping mechanisms that people adopt and the adaptations that they make to their daily lives in the face of pain (Section 9.6.5).

Although these dimensions of the pain experience are analytically distinct, they are not necessarily distinct at the level of experience. The sensory dimension of pain is, for example, normally inseparable from the affective dimension for the individual in pain.

9.2.1 PAIN AND HEALTH

Many states of ill health are characterized by pain, of either an acute or chronic nature. Indeed, pain is a defining feature of many conditions. It does not follow from this, however, that a person in pain is thereby unhealthy. Theories of health that define it simply in terms of the absence of disease, impairment, disability, or indeed of pain, provide an inadequate explanation of the ways in which health is conceptualized and experienced (Sim 1990b). In contrast, a definition of health such as that of Seedhouse makes it clear that the experience of pain is not incompatible with being healthy: 'A person's optimum state of health is equivalent to the state of the set of conditions which fulfil or enable a person to fulfil his or her realistic chosen and biological potentials. Some of these conditions are of the highest importance for all people. Others are variable dependent upon individual abilities and circumstances' (Seedhouse 1986: 61). Chapters 3 and 4 provide further discussion of notions of health.

9.2.2 CAPTURING THE PAIN EXPERIENCE

By virtue of its multidimensional nature, pain is an overall experience rather than an isolated sensation, emotion or physiological response. The precise nature and content of this experience will vary from situation to situation (for example, between acute and chronic pain), and from individual to individual. Furthermore, the nature and location of an individual's pain may fluctuate over time (Peolsson et al 2000).

Although pain may manifest itself in certain objective, external indicators – such as changes in EMG recordings, heart rate, and skin conductance measures, and other physiological and behavioural phenomena (which may be either innate or learned) – it is ultimately an internal, subjective phenomenon. Other people cannot know a person's pain directly; they can at best infer it from the individual's words and actions. However, the complexity of the pain experience does not lend itself readily to a verbal description. A further complication to the verbal description of pain is that the way in which it is experienced and subsequently described is mediated by complex linguistic and cultural factors (Zborowski 1952, Fabrega & Tyma 1976, Lipton & Marbach 1984, Waddie 1996, Smith 1998). These issues will be examined more fully later (Section 9.5).

As well as classifying pain in terms of its elements, as in Figure 9.1, a distinction can be drawn between primary and secondary aspects of the pain experience. In this connection, Fordyce (1988: 278) describes *nociception* in physiological terms as 'mechanical, thermal, or chemical energy impinging on specialized nerve endings'. This nociception may or may not bring about *pain*, which is the individual's apprehension of nociception. In contrast to these primary 'input' phenomena, *suffering* is an affective or emotional response to pain, and is an 'output'. Equally, *pain behaviour*, as defined above, is an output of the pain experience.

There is a degree of independence between the inputs and outputs of the pain experience. Not every person who experiences severe pain necessarily 'suffers' from it, and people may differ considerably in their behavioural response to apparently similar levels of nociception or pain.

The difficulty inherent in defining pain is identified by Melzack & Wall (1988: 46): 'The diversity of pain experiences explains why it has been impossible, so far, to achieve a satisfactory definition of pain. The word 'pain' represents a *category* of experiences, signifying a multitude of different, unique experiences having different causes, and characterized by different qualities varying along a number of sensory, affective and evaluative dimensions.'

It follows from the foregoing discussion that pain has three fundamental characteristics. First, it is, at least partially, *incommunicable*; that is, the person in pain cannot fully convey the nature of this essentially private experience to others:

> Nobody will ever understand 'my pain' in the way I mean it, unless he suffers the same headache, which is impossible, because he is another person … Just as 'my pain' belongs in a unique way only to me, so I am utterly alone with it. I cannot share it. I have no doubt about the reality of the pain experience, but I cannot really tell anybody what I experience. I surmise that others have 'their' pains, even though I cannot perceive what they mean when they tell me about them (Illich 1976: 147).

Almost paradoxically, while it is extremely difficult for others to grasp another's pain, for that person it is almost impossible *not* to grasp the pain that he or she is experiencing (Scarry 1985).

Second, and linked to this, pain is *imperfectly measurable*. As that which is measured is in an important sense public, whereas the pain experience is always to a large degree private, the measurement of pain cannot hope to capture the totality of the pain experience. In particular, attempts to measure pain intensity alone are necessarily incomplete: 'It is clear … that to describe pain solely in terms of intensity is like specifying the visual world only in terms of light flux without regard to pattern, colour, texture, and the many other dimensions of visual experience' (Melzack & Wall 1988: 37).

Third, pain is *incontestable*. Dennett (1981: 226) argues: 'It is a necessary condition of pain that we are "incorrigible" about pain: i.e., if you believe you are in pain, your belief is true; you are in pain.' Consequently, the idea of 'unfelt' or 'imagined' pain is self-contradictory (Trigg 1970), and a statement such as 'Some persons complain of pain when, indeed, no pain is experienced' (Hardy et al 1952: 299), makes no real sense. Equally, the charge of 'faking' pain or 'malingering' (Chang et al 2000) is ultimately impossible to substantiate. Furthermore, the conspiratorial and adversarial connotations of the notion of malingering are likely to be unproductive in the business of helping patients to deal with their problems.

9.3 PAIN AND MIND/BODY DUALISM

The notion of dualism has been explored in Chapter 3. Broadly, dualism refers to any theory that proposes the existence of two fundamentally different kinds of thing, which can never be reduced to each other. There are a number of such divisions that interest different disciplines (for example, 'things' versus 'ideas'; statements of fact versus value judgements; 'nature' versus 'nurture'), but the dualism that concerns us here is that of body and mind. The arguments over the relation between body and mind, whether they are irreducibly separate realms, one 'material' and the other 'immaterial', and what exactly mind is, are longstanding.

9.3.1 CONNECTION TO DESCARTES

Body/mind dualism as discussed in the health professions is often referred to as 'Cartesian', in deference to its treatment in the philosophy of René Descartes (1596–1650). The perceived mind/body split of modern Western thinking and science is often traced back to Descartes's interest in the differences and division between the intangibility of the mind and the materiality of the body. He characterized the distinction as between consciousness, which is something infallibly knowable (consciousness proves existence), and extension, or the body's occupation of space, which is only fallibly knowable, as we can only apprehend it as our sensory capacities allow. His writings are seen as decisive, or as representing a decisive moment in history, from which stemmed the increasingly detailed and eventually technological investigation of the body conceived more or less mechanistically, and most crucially its disjuncture from the mind (see, for example, Scheper-Hughes & Lock 1987, Fairhurst 1998).

There is a continuing interest in reviewing Descartes's work and in assessing his contribution to current conceptions of the relation between body and mind (see, for example, Rozemond 1995, 1999, Yandell 1999, Yardley 1999, Duncan 2000, Switankowsky 2000). Indeed, Duncan argues that '[r]ecent attempts by medical thinkers to overcome organic reductionism in favor of a more holistic representation of disease and health *routinely* begin by attacking Cartesian dualism' (Duncan 2000: 485–486; emphasis added). But, however it came about, a separation between body and mind is seen as pervasive in modern Western life (not just medical practice), such that modern selfhood incorporates a freedom of mind from body (Gordon 1988; see Smith 1998). In recent years, this independence has become increasingly questioned, with greater advocacy of a more holistic understanding of the person (Riches 2000).

9.3.2 DUALISM AND MEDICAL KNOWLEDGE

Biomedicine is widely perceived by medical and sociological theorists as flawed on dualistic grounds: it treats the body in isolation from an adequate therapeutic engagement with the person:

> The physical machine-like body is assumed to be extrinsic to the essential self. This paradigm has been successful in many ways. The body-as-machine is susceptible to mechanical interventions; it can be divided into organ systems and parts which can be repaired, removed or technologically supplemented; it can be tested experimentally, and so forth. Nevertheless, the paradigm is incomplete (Toombs 1988: 201).

Alongside this is the tendency for patients not to be perceived as informed commentators on their bodies' inner events. With the ever-increasing detail and sophistication of biomedicine's ability to monitor the body's workings through scans and tests, the person of the patient is inevitable but barely relevant. This is tied up with social changes in the practice of medicine over time. Lupton writes that by the beginning of the twentieth century: 'the views of patients had lost their relevance and power in the medical encounter, and the responsibility for discovering and labelling illness had become the preserve of the medical practitioner. The disease had become more important than the person who harboured it' (Lupton 1994: 86).

A different view of the relation between medical practice and mind/body dualism sees it as an opportunity for practice to move away from a reductionist or mechanistic treatment of the patient, and towards the addition of a humanistic component. Switankowsky (2000) makes a case for an underpinning of 'interactive dualism' as beneficial in allowing the health professional to work with body and person in tandem.

Body and mind are fundamentally interactive, and the state of one has a real bearing on the state of the other. Illness does not merely affect (part of) the body, but has repercussions through all aspects of the person's life. By engaging with what these repercussions are for any individual, as well as the bodily manifestations, the practitioner can not only make better-informed diagnostic judgements, but also enhance the efficacy of treatment by the extension of care to the person as well as to their body.

Thus, the same division into body and mind that allowed an isolated focus can, according to Switankowsky (2000), be conscripted to argue for a dual focus on body *and* mind to the advantage of both practitioner and patient.

9.3.3 DUALISM AND PAIN

Pain has always occupied a key position in arguments around body/mind dualism. As an enigma physiologically, neurologically, and psychologically, pain tests our understanding of the relation between body and mind no less today than in the seventeenth century. For Descartes, pain served 'as evidence for his overall thesis of mind and body as conjoint, but different, substances' (Duncan 2000: 489), although he has often been represented as disbelieving any possibility of interaction between body and mind, or a more holistic apprehension of human beings (see, for example, McMahon 1975). Descartes did indeed describe the physiology of pain in mechanistic terms, for example using the idea of a cord to portray the connection between a peripheral site of damage and the brain. None the less, according to Duncan (2000), he was well aware of the ambiguities surrounding pain as a test for the body's existence. He noted that phantom limb pain shows that pain cannot always and simply prove the existence of the body or part of the body. Pain is experienced by the mind as coming from somewhere, wherever in fact the point of excitation along the nerve pathways begins, even if that is within the brain itself: 'But the fact that we feel a pain as it were in our foot does not make it certain that the pain exists outside our mind, in the foot' (*Principles of Philosophy*, Descartes 1985: 217). Descartes also referred to the role of the emotions as part of pain experience, and opened the way for an exploration of the personal and social contexts of pain: 'we sometimes suffer pains with joy, and receive titillating sensations which displease us' (*The Passions of the Soul*, Descartes 1985: 361).

Despite these problems and others of a more philosophical nature, Descartes did use pain as a cornerstone in his argument for the close union of body and mind, although he maintained their difference.

The biomedical view of pain can be seen as stemming from the Cartesian view of separation between body and mind, but without due attention to the problematic ambiguities which Descartes confronted. The biomedical focus on body parts and processes finds pain useful insofar as it can be a symptom of pathology, but has no interest in pain as in part a manifestation of individual and cultural history and meaning.

The International Association for the Study of Pain definition of pain, with its emphasis on the basic psychological nature of the event, and the development of Melzack & Wall's (1988) gate control theory of pain encouraged the evolution of the biopsychosocial model of pain, which seeks to incorporate the person with pain and his or her sociocultural context. Duncan (2000) reports this as stemming directly from difficulties and frustrations in the treatment of chronic pain and pain-related disabilities. He writes: 'It is now considered wrong to attribute disability associated with chronic pain solely to bodily impairments and pathology. Instead, the person's psychological and behavioral responses to pain are seen as integral to the problem. Furthermore, any theory of chronic pain must include the familial, cultural and socio-political context of the pain sufferer' (Duncan 2000: 494). This appears to be a decisive move towards overcoming dualism, at least as regards chronic pain. However, there is still an overwhelming emphasis on diagnosis 'teasing out' the physical *and* the psychological origins of pain. An example of this, to which we shall return, are the twin dangers of biological reductionism and psychological reductionism in the treatment of chronic pelvic pain (Grace 1998).

9.3.4 PHENOMENOLOGY AS AN ALTERNATIVE TO DUALISM

A third approach to pain, operating outside the tradition of dualism, comes from the perspective of phenomenology. Essentially, phenomenology is a philosophical theory that regards the notion of experience as central in making sense of daily life. The world that we experience, rather than what are deemed to be objective facts of the world, is what counts. Furthermore, such experience is the object of reflection: 'Rather than straightforward, unreflective absorption in the objects of experience, the phenomenological approach involves reflection *upon* experience' (Toombs 1993: xii; original emphasis).

The phenomenological model of the body sees it as the 'center and carrier of experience … [every person] both *has* and *is* a body' (Steen & Haugli 2000: 584; original emphasis). Maurice Merleau-Ponty (for example, 1996 [1945]), a key figure in the recent history of phenomenology, argued that the experience of 'being' cannot be split into a body and a mind. We are all simultaneously subject and object, simultaneously seeing, hearing, touching, and being seen, heard, touched. We exist in the relation between the two. Steen & Haugli (2000) argue that a phenomenological underpinning to health care enriches the understanding of disease and the approach to treatment, incorporating the experiences, fears and beliefs of the patient. The ways in which pain is defined, assessed and managed are determined by the way in which it is experienced by the patient. Similarly, criteria for treatment success hinge upon changes in the patient's experience of pain. Hence, the patient achieves greater importance and significance in the whole process.

9.3.5 DUALISM AND HEALTH CARE PRACTICE

The biopsychosocial model of pain, touched upon earlier, attempts to take account of psychological and social aspects of pain (emotion, learning, cultural beliefs and expectations) as well as the physical processes of nociception and pathology. It could, therefore, be argued that it is a non-dualistic model that can encompass a truly integrated and dynamic view of whole-person experience of pain. This remains its potential. However, Duncan (2000) finds more than a hint of implicit dualism in practice. Clinicians are likely to look for physical *and* psychological factors in pain as separate contributors, which should be treated separately. Indeed, at worst the biopsychosocial model may allow medically unexplained pain to be shifted too readily to the domain of psychiatry. Chronic non-specific back pain is one example of a condition where this happens; Duncan (2000) quotes Fordyce (1995) in support of this. Another condition where psychiatric factors rapidly reach the medical foreground is chronic pelvic pain without identified organic pathology (Grace 1998). Grace does not discuss chronic pelvic pain specifically in relation to a biopsychosocial model of pain, but she does find a major thrust in the more recent literature on chronic pelvic pain treatments towards the importance of involving multidisciplinary teams in evaluation and diagnosis. However, she concludes, 'attempts to integrate understandings of the psychological and the organic and to replace a monocausal with a multicausal model are systematically thwarted while authors retain the medical conception of identifiable organic pathology as a distinct etiological classification' (Grace 1998: 144).

The problem with mind/body dualism from a treatment perspective is that 'the body with pain is externalized from the person's production of meaning and from relations between people' (Steen & Haugli 2000: 587). Steen & Haugli also point out that there are dangers here involving the patient's trust. Not only may a restricted focus on body *or* mind lead to ineffective treatment and frustration all round, but the power and prestige of biomedical opinion may persuade the patient that this focus is correct despite his or her own intuitions, leading to self-doubt and anxiety. The discovery of a physical problem legitimates pain in a way that a psychiatric diagnosis does not. The stigma attached to mental illness is powerful and the illness itself may never escape associations with hypochondria, malingering and attention-seeking.

Steen & Haugli (2000: 597), writing from a phenomenological viewpoint, conclude that health professionals who are interested in patients holistically can effectively engage with them in the 'search for the possible hidden meanings in painful muscles'. Grace (1998: 147) concludes that multidisciplinary teams that maintain discrete interests are 'not going to achieve the radical deconstruction of the organic/psychological, body/mind dichotomy that is at the root of biomedical and medical thinking and practice'. The need for a truly integrated model of mind/body is maintained strongly in both these papers: neither, presumably, would find Switankowsky's (2000) 'interactive dualism' a satisfactory solution.

9.4 PAIN AND THE SOCIOCULTURAL CONTEXT

In everyday life and normal health, we are usually unaware of our bodies for extended periods of time. As Leder (1990: 82) says, when 'functioning well, this body is a transparency through which we engage the world'. In contrast, when we suffer serious pain, our attention becomes inescapably focused upon it and our sense of agency in the world is restricted. However, what we become so aware of is never simply physical. The body is simultaneously a physical and a social environment. Turner (1984) refers to the social location of the body, such that social reality is (literally) embodied, so that our bodies are in some sense an arena for social structure and cultural meanings. The point, therefore, is that pain is not simply a biophysical event: it takes place in a sociocultural and psychological context, and is understood, evaluated, and responded to accordingly. Pain has an effect on relationships, roles, goals, and the identity of the person in pain. Severe pain, and particularly chronic pain, hence give rise to a universal alteration not just in coping with daily life and patterns of lifestyle, but more fundamentally in one's perception of oneself, and one's essential unity. Leder (1990) comments on the power of pain to separate body and mind. Because this overwhelming aspect of the pain experience does not appear in the medical model of pain, there is a danger that needs of people in pain may not be adequately met within customary clinical practice (Sullivan 1998).

Pain clearly has an impact on the life of the individual within his or her sociocultural context. However, the sociocultural context is also part of the pain. Areas of the body and different problems associated with them have meanings and values attached, so the site of the pain, the circumstances of its onset, who the individual in pain is – including past experiences, sociocultural background and pain beliefs – will all form part of the experience. This is an active process in which significance and meaning for the individual concerned become intimately incorporated into the biological event. There is no unmediated physical component to pain (Melzack & Wall 1988, Wall 1999); the physical aspect of pain is inseparable from the psychological, social and cultural aspects. Morris (1991a: 14) describes pain as 'always saturated with the visible or invisible imprint of human cultures' and points out that we 'learn how to feel pain and learn what it means'.

9.4.1 ETHNIC VARIATION IN PAIN BEHAVIOUR

Although pain is an intensely personal experience, a research field focusing on sociocultural aspects of pain behaviour and attitudes grew up in the second half of the twentieth century. A major study involving patients at a New York veterans' hospital compared Italian-Americans, Jewish-Americans, and mainly Protestant Americans of several generations' standing for their reactions to the presence of pain (Zborowski 1952, 1969). The last of these groups (the 'Old' Americans) tended to describe their pain with an air of detachment and reserve, taking the view that becoming emotional does not help either them or the staff. The Italian- and Jewish-Americans, however, tended to be very emotional and to respond to their pain with an air of drama and concern. Although administering analgesics allowed the Italian-Americans to forget their suffering – their focus therefore appearing to be on the immediate aspects of their situation – analgesics did not have the same effect on the Jewish-Americans. They continued to be concerned not only for the future of their health and welfare, but also about the possible continuation of the underlying disease unnoticed under the analgesia. From this study, Zborowski drew conclusions not only about the varying patterns according to ethnicity in responses to pain, but also about the different functions and beliefs that may underlie apparently similar patterns.

Zola (1966) also studied Italian-Americans, but in comparison to Irish-Americans. He was interested in what patients (subsequently matched for complaint and severity) initially brought to medical attention. The

Irish-Americans tended to report dysfunction rather than pain, whereas the Italian-Americans had pain as a feature of their presentations, and reported significantly more symptoms spread over greater or more areas of the body. Zola (1966: 630) commented that 'the very labelling and definition of a bodily state as a symptom or as a problem is, in itself, part of a social process'. The presentation of pain, and the selection of symptoms or recognition of symptoms as reportable, are learned within social contexts and so will be subject to sociocultural influences (for further discussion in an anthropological context, and of cultural aspects informing the decision to report pain, see Helman 2001).

Although this kind of research continues (see, for example, Calvillo & Flaskerud 1993, Bates et al 1997, Lee & Essoka 1998, Moore et al 1998b, Rosmus et al 2000), a second strand of pain research has since grown up, partly as a reaction to what has been seen as the more deterministic and stereotyping aspects of this earlier research. The focus of this second strand is the uniqueness of individual pain experience within a culture, rather than the reductionistic notion of the ethnic generalization: 'The peculiar qualities of ... pain affecting a particular person – with a unique story, living in a certain community and historical period, and above all with fears, longings, aspirations – are washed away in the ethnic stereotype' (Kleinman et al 1992: 2). Research following this remit tends to take an in-depth, qualitative approach to a single person's pain, or to a small number of people experiencing pain, and to draw out aspects of selfhood, alteration, and disrupted biography (see, for example, Frank 1995).

There is also a considerable body of research devoted to testing for ethnic variations in the experience and/or reporting of pain under laboratory conditions (see, for example, Nayak et al 2000). A common theme to these studies is the variation in pain threshold or tolerance according to ethnicity. However, experimentally induced pain does not have the same impact on people as other sorts of pain (Wall 1999). An experimentally induced pain can be 'turned off', and does not carry the same burden of fear and anxiety as unexpected and uncontrolled pain arising spontaneously; experimental pain is 'safe' and is administered with the recipient's permission. These studies are not conclusive, and have not adequately addressed the problem of teasing out physical and cultural elements in subjects' responses under local experimental conditions. It should also be borne in mind that results could be an artifact of research that sets out to find a cultural difference in an area where subjectivity is so important. People come from vastly different social backgrounds *within* a culture, and have very different personal experience. It is not unreasonable to expect considerable variation within an ethnic grouping.

9.4.2 'APPROPRIATE' PAIN BEHAVIOUR

One aspect of pain experience that is more likely to be influenced by learning and culture is knowing how it is appropriate to behave. It is often surprising how painful an apparently trivial wound or knock is, but we all – perhaps health professionals in particular – have ideas about what is a suitable display or report of pain, and make assumptions as to its diminution over time. Adamson (1997) provides an account of alternative diagnoses and treatment options in a case of inflammatory bowel disease and avascular necrosis. At one point, decisions about his care hinged critically on the specialist's inability to believe in his reported level of pain. This is a striking case; but ideas of 'normal' pain operate throughout society and have their impact on pain behaviour, including consulting behaviour. Sanders et al (2002) report the perception of painful joints as 'normal' by elderly people, despite often severe disruption of their lives, because of cultural beliefs about the relationship between ill health and advanced age. Such beliefs are not necessarily supported by practitioners (see, for example, McMurdo 2000). People who experience a lot of pain and have frequent consultations and diagnostic tests with health professionals may also learn to adapt their pain behaviour and reports of pain as they learn more about the reactions and expectations of the practitioner. Helman (2001: 132) comments: 'Clinicians should therefore be aware of this process and the difficulties it poses for reliable diagnosis'.

Health professionals too will deal with pain in different ways according to their own background and experience, and also according to the 'received wisdom' of their profession and training. It is well reported in the literature, for example, that men's pain is more readily believed (and therefore treated) than women's pain (Wall 1999, Freund et al 2003). It is not clear, however, whether this is because men and women show their pain in different ways, or because of social and/or professional stereotypes of men as tough and women as 'whingers'. The latter argument is better supported. Bendelow (1993) found little difference between men and women for meanings and definitions of pain: both included emotions and spiritual and existential notions as well as physical sensation, although men were less likely to consider emotional pain as 'real' pain.

Another aspect of health professionals' perceptions of their patients' pain that shows a gender difference lies in the relatively easier move from medically unexplained pain to psychogenic explanations as regards women. Grace (1998), for example, provides an extensive review of the literature on chronic pelvic pain without organic pathology, and argues convincingly not only for a non-dualistic approach to this problem, but also that the perception of women within biomedicine can erect a barrier to proper treatment. Lennane & Lennane (1973) provide a critical account of the persistence of a psychogenic explanation (despite evidence to the contrary) not only for chronic pelvic pain, but also for nausea in pregnancy, pain in labour and dysmenorrhoea. It is important, therefore, to: 'examine the legacy of historical myths and cultural prejudices about women's reproductive functions and child-rearing roles, to understand where this propensity for a psychogenic interpretation comes from. That the patient is termed "neurotic" or "unfeminine" does not occur in a sociocultural vacuum and this cultural context helps explain why these interpretations are so persistent' (Grace 1998: 137).

Bendelow & Williams sum up the essential dichotomy between the biomedical appreciation of pain and its experience: 'Scientific medicine reduces the experience of pain to an elaborate broadcasting system of signals, rather than seeing it as moulded and shaped both by the individual and their particular sociocultural context' (Bendelow & Williams

1995: 140). Fordyce (1997) expressed this more succinctly when he referred to pain as 'transdermal': pain is constituted by states of affairs outside the body as well as inside. It remains for health professionals to be aware of sociocultural *and* individual aspects of patients' presentations while assessing gait, limitations to movement and other pain-related behaviours.

9.5 LANGUAGE AND PAIN

The representation of pain in language is notoriously difficult (Scarry 1985, Smith 1998); indeed, Scarry argues that the resistance of pain to language, i.e. the difficulties we have in attempting to express pain in words, is central to what pain is: ultimately, it cannot be shared. Here, we want to consider two aspects of the nature of this resistance.

First, in describing pain we are attempting to use an essentially shared and therefore public system (language) to communicate an essentially private experience. In conversation, and when we use language in general, we share the meanings of the words we use because they are supported by the context we are in, and because we share the realities of the physical world and of common social experience. Pain, however, cannot be shared and does not 'appear' in the public world at all except through language and behaviour – words and non-verbal resources, such as bodily gestures (Hydén & Peolsson 2002), are all that is available to communicate this private experience. We have no direct way, therefore, of comparing a 'shooting' pain in one person with a 'shooting' pain in another: we have only the choice of the same descriptor. The difficulties we have in making the nature of pain 'appear' have been aptly captured by Dennett (1981) in his essay on why we cannot build a computer model of pain. He describes the attempt to model the pain caused by an anvil being dropped on to a left foot:

> But, says the sceptic, the program still leaves out the *quality* of the pain. Very well. We expand our theory, and concomitantly our program ... and this time we get back: There is a pain *P*, of the in-the-left-foot variety ... *P* begins as a dull, scarcely noticeable pressure, and then commences to throb; *P* increases in intensity until it explodes into shimmering hot flashes of stabbing stilettos of excruciating anguish ... C-fibres are stimulated ... (Dennett 1981: 193).

This, of course, is an account of pain, and not the experience itself. In descriptions of pain, there is always this slippage between word and experience, and the necessity of kindling the imagination or knowledge and recognition of the hearer.

Second, given that pain experience can never be shared, much of what is said to communicate pain relies on ideas of what should be said according to local and cultural practice. As we grow up, we learn how common pains are spoken of, and we learn appropriate repertoires for communicating the aches and pains of daily life. Kleinman et al (1992) cite among others Ohnuki-Tierney's (1981: 49) report of the Sakhalin Ainu of Japan as distinguishing between what they describe as 'bear headaches', 'deer headaches' and 'woodpecker headaches'; and Abad & Boyce's (1979: 34) report that Latinos in North America distinguish between 'headache' and 'brainache'. The shared part of common experiences – like being stung by nettles – is the knowledge of which words are appropriate in our language and culture. But many serious pain experiences have no such clear notions of appropriateness. Moreover, some pain words can be related to external events that can be seen – like a bad cut, or a badly bruised ankle – and some cannot. Accounts of internal pain, such as medically unexplained musculoskeletal pain, are guided only by personal and cultural background, until or unless they become influenced by health professionals. Those wanting treatment for painful conditions may well alter their accounts to fit in with the kinds of questions they are asked, the pain words the health care professional uses, and the aspects of their description that seem to be of significance to the health care professional, in their efforts to receive effective care. This role of the professional – providing words and similes – can be beneficent. Cassell (1985) argues that doctors develop a large descriptive vocabulary because of the importance of pain as a symptom, and the onus is on them to provide the patient with words to which they can respond, e.g. 'burning', 'dull', or 'Does it feel as if a balloon were being blown up in your finger?' (Cassell 1985: 61). However, it is also important that potentially significant aspects of the experience of pain do not disappear from patients' accounts because of an apparent lack of interest or understanding on the part of the health care professional. A further complication is the development of a vocabulary among health professionals that they use and a further (not necessarily coextensive) vocabulary that they expect their patients to use. Consultation can be an uneasy game of getting the words right so that diagnosis and treatment can proceed with mutual satisfaction.

One problem that follows from these aspects of pain's resistance to language, and is central to professional–patient communication, is that words may have a meaning for professionals that is not generally shared by lay people. The use of pain questionnaires, such as the McGill Pain Questionnaire (MPQ; Melzack & Katz 2001), can increase these dangers, as patients may not be given the opportunity to explain their choices of words after having completed the questionnaire. The MPQ is based upon the belief that words usually refer to one main quality, but detailed linguistic work (Smith 1989; see also Smith 1998) demonstrates that pain words are multidimensional. 'Boring', for example, appears in the MPQ group representing 'punctate pressure'. It can, however, be used to mean 'sharp and moving inwards', or 'blunt and unfocused', or 'long-term and unremitting'. 'Piercing' pain can be used to imply a brief pain or a continuous pain. 'Acute' can be used by lay people to mean 'sharp and intense', as opposed to its professional usage as 'sudden-onset, short-lived'. It is important, therefore, to build up a picture of someone's pain more broadly and discursively, in order to gain insight into how they are using language, and the aspects of the pain experience that are important for them.

Any discussion of pain is inherently metaphorical, as this is the nature of English pain words. Metaphor is a way of grasping ill-defined or alien experience in the terms of other experience that is more easily shared or understood. English pain words have a strong destructive or physical-deformative sense, and can be approached by notions of instrument or agency. A 'stabbing' pain, for example, can be understood by imagining a violent assault with a sharp instrument. 'Biting', 'gnawing', and 'drilling' carry similar connotations of destructive assault. This allows an imaginative engagement with the potential meaning of a description, but, as with all metaphorical usage, only certain elements of the pain experience are highlighted by the comparison, others are downplayed or lost. The Ainu's 'bear-headaches' mentioned above, for example, are 'like the heavy steps of a bear' (Kleinman et al 1992: 1), whereas 'woodpecker headaches' may highlight an insistence not obviously present in the idea of a bear's steps.

Any discussion beyond individual descriptors is likely to involve simile. Closs & Briggs (2002), in their study of pain descriptions following orthopaedic surgery, found that not only did patients use words that do not appear on the MPQ, they also made frequent use of what the authors refer to as analogy. Such phrases are more extended attempts to convey pain by eliciting the hearer's imaginative involvement in a scenario. A person with fibromyalgia has described the pain of the condition thus: 'Muscles feel as if they beaten [sic] with cricket bats. Joints feel as if they have been blown up by a syringe with sticky glue.' This conveys not only something about the quality of the pain and difficulties of moving the joints, but also the sense of outrage committed upon the individual by the pain experience. Söderberg & Norberg (1995: 58) report that the people with fibromyalgia in their study used similarly dramatic expressions, and 'envisaged the experience as a form of torture'. This tells us something about the person's relationship to the experience of pain, which may be of clinical value when instigating a treatment programme.

It is important to pay attention to pain language, because not only does it transform the experience into the problem presented to the health care professional, it also provides the bridge between unpleasant private experience and the social world. Peolsson et al (2000) argue that gaining linguistic control over pain should not be undervalued as a resource for dealing with pain. It remains for the health care professional to best utilize this problematical but rich resource.

9.6 THE SUBJECTIVE EXPERIENCE OF PAIN

'Pain is tiring ... it makes you want to snap at the world. It's demoralizing, it colours your whole existence. It affects me day and night; it restricts everything and governs my life. It can be in every joint and down the spine and legs. The pain is as if someone is putting in a screwdriver and turning it' (Carson & Mitchell 1998: 1244). This quotation from an interview with a person with chronic pain illustrates the potentially all-pervading impact of pain on a person's life. Pain can represent a major limitation to a person's quality of life, and confronts him or her with two main challenges:

1. Coping with oneself – making sense of the pain, dealing with its impact on one's body and its effect on everyday activities.

2. Coping with relationships – dealing with the implications of pain for one's social roles and interactions with others, including health professionals.

9.6.1 PAIN AS ILLNESS

In understanding the experience of pain, it is worth distinguishing pain as a symptom of 'disease' from pain as a part of 'illness'. The concept of disease refers to the objective facts of a state of ill health, existing at an anatomical, physiological or biochemical level. As a definition, it makes no reference to what the individual thinks or feels about this state. Illness, in contrast, refers to the subjective experience of a state of ill health (Field 1976). Illness, not disease, is what the person is aware of, and responds to in his or her behaviour and in relationships with others, including health professionals. Just as the definition of disease does not assume a sub- jective response, the definition of illness does not presuppose a biological disorder. By analogy, and as has already been noted, the experience of pain does not presuppose tissue damage.

Consequently, illness behaviour is the way in which people respond to ill health. As such, it is a purely descriptive term, and does not imply that the behaviour concerned is inappropriate, maladaptive or undesirable, as is sometimes suggested (for example, by Williams (1989)). Again, by ana- logy, pain behaviour is the behavioural response to pain, whatever form that may take (see Chs 8 and 11).

Like illness generally, 'pain is as much a social construction, as it is a result of biochemistry and psychological states' (Encandela 1993: 784). In other words, the way in which pain is defined, explained and experi- enced is conditioned by various social and cultural forces, and reflects the values and attitudes of both individuals and groups within society.

9.6.2 MAKING SENSE OF THE PAIN

Although pain is in many ways a common experience, the way in which people see themselves and their lives is not usually framed in terms of pain. Expected experiences and sensations are not painful ones, and when pain happens, it is a disruption of, rather than a part of, our taken- for-granted assumptions about how life is, or should be. The advent of pain therefore causes some form of reappraisal or restructuring of the person's life and identity. Initially, pain may be dismissed because tran- sient pain is an expected part of daily life (Hilbert 1984). However, the greater the pain, and the longer it persists, the greater is likely to be the need for change in one's life. As Baszanger (1989: 428) comments: 'The longer the illness lasts, the less it can be kept within parentheses as though it were a passing episode.'

This sense of normal meanings and experiences being overturned is particularly evident in the person's sense of his or her body: 'In most accounts of healthy individuals, the body is 'silent', very quietly perform- ing its functions without compelling moment-to-moment awareness… The lived experience of the chronic pain patient stands in dramatic con- trast: He or she is exquisitely and perpetually aware of the body' (Thomas 2000: 689–690). Linked to this heightened awareness of the body is the fact that pain has no external referent.

The person in pain is therefore faced with a potential disruption of the meaning that life holds and a threat to his or her sense of self (Aldrich & Eccleston 2000, Sidell 2001). Bury (1982) uses the term 'biographical disruption' to describe the threat to normal assumptions and patterns of daily life brought about by chronic illness and the need to reappraise aspects of the self. The fundamental choice is whether to attempt to maintain the former self in the face of pain, to try to 'suspend' the former self in the hope that it can be resumed when the pain goes, or to come to terms with a new 'painful' self. In a study of women with chronic fatigue syndrome and fibromyalgia, Åsbring (2001) found a strong sense of grief over the loss of a former identity and the activities associated with it. This was accompanied by an attempt to come to terms with a new identity. One informant commented on 'having lived a little with a "me" that is no longer the "real me", because it is a completely new person' (Åsbring 2001: 315). Similarly, in interviews with 19 women with chronic pain, Howell (1994) found expression of loss of a former self, and an attempt to construct new lives that are fulfilling despite the pain. Assuming a new identity is not, therefore, a wholly negative transition. Lives characterized by pain, even by severe pain, may none the less be rewarding and enjoyable in their totality (see Sections 4.4 and 17.3). Equally, to say that somebody has pain does not in itself say that they are not healthy – health is defined in a broader context of the individual's life (see Seedhouse 1986, Sim 1990b).

A key issue for people with chronic illness, whether characterized by pain or not, is that of uncertainty (Wiener 1975, Locker 1983, Robinson 1988, Söderberg & Norberg 1995, Adamson 1997). This uncertainty may centre on the cause of the pain, alternative diagnoses, its prognosis, or more abstract questions such as 'why me?' Those in pain characteristically experience a desire to know the reason for their symptoms (Schaefer 1995, Osborn & Smith 1998). Not only can such information provide reassurance that the pain is benign (Söderberg et al 1999), but it can also confer legitimacy on pain and provides a sense of stability on which practical coping strategies can be based (Section 9.6.5).

When seeking to assign meaning to their pain, people draw on both lay and professional explanations (Honkasalo 2000). Indeed, the meaning of pain may be the product of clinical encounters between patients and professionals, when these two explanatory frameworks come together (Baszanger 1997). This has two important implications for physiotherapists and other health professionals. First, to understand the nature of a patient's pain experience, the practitioner cannot rely solely on biomedical theories, but must try to understand the individual's own explanatory framework, rooted in a particular social and cultural background. Second, although it does not fully explain the individual's experience of pain, professional knowledge plays a part in moulding this experience. Hence, through the explanations and diagnoses that they provide to patients, professionals can powerfully influence the way in which an individual understands and experiences pain.

In Section 9.2, it was noted that pain can be emotional as well as physical in its origin. A study by Bendelow (1993) suggests that the meaning of emotional pain may be harder to comprehend and come to terms with than that of physical pain. Two of her respondents comment:

> in a way, I think [emotional pain is] worse than physical pain – that's tangible and you know what's causing it and you can put your finger on it … but emotional pain – I mean I don't think anyone can explain why human beings have emotions.

> the emotional pain goes on longer [than physical pain] – I think it's somehow worse than a physical pain because that is usually comprehensible, logical and there's a certain amount of control – you can get your head round it. I'd rather go through all the horror of smashing up my leg and all the being in hospital than two months of what I've just been through (Bendelow 1993: 281–282).

9.6.3 COMMUNICATING PAIN AND ISSUES OF LEGITIMACY AND STIGMA

One of the problems faced by people with pain is providing an account of themselves to other people. At a basic level, they may wish to communicate to others what their pain is like. However, as has already been noted (Section 9.5), this can be extremely difficult. The resources of language are ill-suited to the description of pain, and people in pain may enlist the support of bodily gestures in their attempt to communicate their inner experiences (Hydén & Peolsson 2002). Moreover, the terms in which patients express their pain may bear little similarity to those used in outcome assessment tools with which practitioners are familiar (De Souza & Frank 2002). Allied to this is the problem faced by people in pain of convincing others that their pain is real. Sometimes, as in the case of a fractured bone or a twisted ankle, the origin of pain is externally visible. Moreover, others can imagine – based on either their own or others' experience – the nature of the pain associated with such conditions. However, many painful conditions are not visible – especially those such as chronic fatigue syndrome or fibromyalgia that cannot be located to a single specific region of the body – and the absence of physical correlates of inner pain can make it hard to convince others of its reality (Fagerhaugh & Strauss 1977, Thomas 2000, Glenton 2003, Werner et al 2003). One of the informants interviewed by Thomas comments 'It's so hard for people to understand if I say I'm in pain because they don't see it; I'm not in a wheelchair or walking with a cane' (Thomas 2000: 691). In contrast, a scar provides clear evidence of the reality of symptoms, to the extent that a woman in Hilbert's (1984) study reported that she had contemplated having unnecessary surgery purely for the sake of a visible surgical scar. The problem of being believed can be compounded in situations in which pain fluctuates; others may find to hard to understand why somebody who is supposed to be in pain 'seems to be fine today'. Alternatively, physical actions consequent on pain may be misinterpreted; a painful gait may be construed as intoxication (Locker 1983). People with chronic pain may face a type of 'double jeopardy', whereby they are blamed both for being ill and for not getting well. Advice given by others may thus be perceived as a criticism of the individual's coping. A woman with chronic pain interviewed by Werner et al (2003: 500) comments: 'Poor people who're trying to give me advice! It'll make a large gap between us. First you're to blame because you have pain, and second you're to blame because you have chosen not to get well.'

Convincing others that one's pain is real is a necessary part of legitimating one's pain (Hilbert 1984, Kugelmann 1999, Werner & Malterud 2003). As the person in pain may have to withdraw from activities that others would normally expect them to perform, it is felt that this withdrawal needs to be justified. The person in pain needs to establish that the way in which he or she is behaving is morally justifiable. If people find that the authenticity of their symptoms is doubted, or their pain is considered by others to be 'just in the mind', they may interpret this as a threat to their moral character (Johansson et al 1999, Åsbring & Närvänen 2002). Work-related pain may raise morally discrediting suspicions of 'shirking' (Tarasuk & Eakin 2002). Some painful conditions may thus be stigmatizing, leading to a loss of social and moral worth that is perceived by both the person in pain and others (Sim 1990a). A woman with repetitive strain injury interviewed by Reid et al (1991) describes another type of 'double jeopardy' – being unable to fulfil social expectations in relation to work, but having a reason for this perceived failure that is stigmatizing: 'Some were very cynical. Others accepted it. I think one friend, though she hasn't said anything, her attitude is that you're going for the worker's comp … "compo bludger" or whatever you call it. But I never told anybody voluntarily that I had RSI because of the attitude toward it … You feel like a leper' (Reid et al 1991: 606).

This strong sense of moral legitimacy is central not only to individuals' experience of pain, but also to the way in which some types of pain are represented in medical discourse (May et al 2002). In addition, at the level of everyday clinical practice, the expectations of health professionals as to the credibility or appropriateness of the patient's pain are crucial to its legitimacy. If the nature of the patient's pain is readily explicable in terms of the presumed diagnosis, and if the degree of pain corresponds to that expected clinically, the patient achieves credibility in the professional's eyes (Baszanger 1989, Adamson 1997). Conversely, if this concordance between the pain presented and that deemed normal or appropriate is lacking, the patient may lose credibility and be subject to negative judgements. Kotarba & Seidel (1984) describe some of the ways in which patients with chronic pain are derogated and stigmatized in seminar discussions between practitioners. They report that 'the biggest and most vocal audience reaction seems to be laughter in response either to faculty jokes about pain patients or to demeaning statements about problem patients' (Kotarba & Seidel 1984: 1396).

The way in which pain is managed may also embody certain moral assumptions. The idea that one level of pain or discomfort is 'tolerable' and another 'intolerable' contains a clear expectation of what patients should or should not be expected to suffer. In this connection, Cassell (1978: 186) comments on the: 'almost moral sense to the way in which therapy for pain is given. First, as though a little suffering is good for the soul, and secondly, as though we must make sure the sick person is not taking narcotics for the pleasure they give rather than for pain relief'.

9.6.4 THE ROLE OF DIAGNOSIS

If a clear diagnosis can be obtained from a medical practitioner or a physiotherapist, this label may confer the necessary legitimacy to the experience of pain (Hilbert 1984, Reid et al 1991, Hydén & Sachs 1998, Raymond & Brown 2002, Lillrank 2003). Equally, if such a diagnosis is not forthcoming, the individual may feel that his or her pain behaviour has not been 'officially' sanctioned (Gerhardt 1989), and problems may arise in relation to work absence or disability benefit (Cooper 1997). However, in some conditions, such as chronic fatigue syndrome, there may be different views of the value of diagnosis; patients may value the diagnosis, but doctors may be reluctant to make it, fearing a self-fulfilling prophecy (Woodward et al 1995).

The nature of any diagnosis received may greatly influence the meaning of pain. If a clear, definitive diagnosis is provided, this may provide a meaning to the pain and dispel much of the ambiguity and uncertainty surrounding the symptoms experienced (Reid et al 1991, Henriksson 1995b, Hellström et al 1999, Greenhalgh 2001), and allow the pain to be explained by an objective cause – the pain becomes 'real'. One of Hilbert's informants commented:

> When the doctor called me and told me what I had, I remember I was so *delighted* to know that I had something that I didn't even hear what he said. I had to call him back and ask him what he said. I just knew I had something, and I was delighted. Even if they'd have told me I had *cancer*, I wouldn't have cared … I was desperate to be told that I had *some*thing. Cause *I knew there was something wrong*, but I didn't know *what* (Hilbert 1984: 368; original emphasis).

A diagnosis may also clear the way to specific forms of treatment, and very often carries with it a prognosis, giving the patient information on what is to come. A diagnosis also 'provides a sense that one is living in an orderly world, that one's condition can be located in medical indices and in libraries, that others share the condition, that one is sane' (Hilbert 1984: 368). Conversely, if no diagnosis can be given, the person has to look elsewhere for an explanation of the pain, and prognosis and therapeutic options are likely to be unclear. Indeed, in the absence of a formal medical diagnosis, patients may take steps to self-diagnose (Cooper 1997).

The message given by a physiotherapist regarding the nature and cause of a patient's pain may therefore have a marked effect on the person's understanding. Crucially, the terminology chosen may have different meanings for the patient from those intended by the practitioner. A study by Donovan & Blake (2000) has shown that words intended to reassure – such as 'mild' in relation to arthritis – may be interpreted by patients as ominous rather than comforting. One informant in the study remarked: 'The doctor tells me it is mild, not very much, but, you know, from mild it is going to be bad. I know that when my sister, when she got this illness, it was [mild], but now it is very bad' (Donovan & Blake 2000: 542–543).

9.6.5 COPING WITH PAIN

Pain, especially chronic pain, requires various coping mechanisms in order to minimize the disruption that it causes to an individual's sense of identity, social relationships and normal daily activities. As with chronic illness generally, the person with chronic pain can be described as having an illness 'career', marked by a number of successive stages (Price 1996). At different stages, different means of coping will be required. Kotarba (1983a) suggests that people with chronic pain may pass through three phases. In the first phase, 'onset of pain', pain is generally perceived as tractable and something that can potentially be eliminated from the person's life. Professional help may be sought at this stage. In due course, however, the pain may prove to be persistent, and professional treatments may be found ineffective. This marks the second stage, 'emergence of doubts'. If strategies to relieve the pain continue to be fruitless, the third stage, the 'chronic pain experience', is reached. Kotarba suggests that at this stage the patient may switch his or her allegiance from professional care to lay support and other non-medical resources. Although this model risks being rather deterministic – i.e. almost prescribing a series of phases through which people with pain are expected to pass – it emphasizes the fact that the pain experience should be seen as a longitudinal process. It also highlights the way in which professional intervention may be perceived and evaluated differently at different points in the person's pain career, and the way in which the balance between lay and professional sources of support may shift over time.

At a psychological level, there are a number of ways in which people deal cognitively and emotionally with their pain (see Ch. 8). In addition, those in pain may resort to sources of professional help, including physiotherapists, occupational therapists, and those providing various forms of psychological therapy (outlined in Ch. 18). However, an important way in which individuals cope with pain is in terms of the social meanings that they construct around their pain, and the way in which they adjust their social relationships.

The way in which people construct meaning around pain will depend upon a number of factors, such as: aspects of their personality (Section 8.4.1), the cultural resources they can draw upon (for example, notions of stoicism, traditional lay theories of health and illness), networks of social support that are available to them, and the relationship between their own understanding of their pain and that conveyed to them by health professionals. In general, the following aspects of the meaning of pain are likely to be influential on the person's ability to cope:

- The origin of the pain (for example, is it ascribed to a bodily dysfunction, or is it seen as a punishment for previous actions?)

- The extent to which the course and duration of the pain are thought to be predictable

- The relationship between pain and the individual's concept of health (e.g. is the pain a marker of ill health, or is it seen as part of normal life, perhaps as part of growing old?)

- Its perceived seriousness (e.g. does it reflect a benign or a serious underlying disorder?)

- Whether the pain is considered remediable

● The extent to which the individual perceives his or her pain to be understood and legitimated by significant others.

People with pain employ a range of psychological coping mechanisms (Skevington 1995; see Ch. 8). They may also draw upon cultural and religious beliefs (Kotarba 1983b). In their daily activities, people with pain use practical strategies, such as adopting schedules or routines that avoid or minimize pain (Henriksson 1995a, Schaefer 1997), and adjusting the nature and pace of their usual activities (Mannerkorpi et al 1999). People may also use distractions (Carson & Mitchell 1998, Ross et al 2001).

In conditions such as rheumatoid arthritis, daily uncertainty as to the nature, degree, duration and location of pain make it harder to manage and increase its disruptive effect on everyday life (Locker 1983). The individual finds it hard to plan activities in advance, and has to have available a wide range of coping strategies. Additionally, others have difficulty in forming reliable expectations as to the behaviour and capabilities of the person in pain, and such expectations are subject to ongoing and potentially troublesome negotiation.

Seeking professional help is an important means of coping with pain. It is important to remember, however, that professional input may be only a minor element in the way in which people deal with illness. Moreover, there is considerable evidence that aspects of the professional management of pain are unsatisfactory. Health professionals' knowledge of pain has been found to be poor (Wolff et al 1991, Sloman et al 2001, Visentin et al 2001), and in North America little time is devoted specifically to pain in the physiotherapy curriculum (Scudds et al 2001). Practitioners are apt to underestimate patients' pain (Solomon 2001), or construe it as unreal or unwarranted (Byrne et al 2001). There is also evidence that physicians' attitudes to pain and its management may lead to its undertreatment (Green et al 2002).

Aspects of pain management in clinics and hospitals have been shown to be deficient (Larue et al 1997, Schafheute et al 2001). Moreover, in an interview study of a pain relief clinic in the UK, Bendelow & Williams (1996) found ambivalent attitudes among staff to the role of the pain clinic. One nurse described it as 'where the real no-hopers go, you should see it, it's like a psychy [psychiatric] ward, they're all spaced out on tranks and anti-depressants, doing OT, making baskets, it's awful' (Bendelow & Williams 1996: 1130). The authors note that such attitudes tended to be picked up and reflected in patients' own responses. More generally, patients with pain may elicit negative attitudes from medical staff. One woman with back pain interviewed by Glenton (2002: 324) suggests that the lack of a definitive diagnosis and of clear therapeutic strategies may contribute to such attitudes:

> They're so sick of us ladies who come along with this sort of thing! There are so many of us and they don't know what to do with us, do they? And we complain and we hurt so much. One doctor has written about me 'her complaints are so massive …'. He could have written 'her problems' but it was the complaints that were the problem! Of course I was a pretty

hopeless case when they couldn't figure out what it was. I heard from a friend of mine that her daughter, who's a doctor, is training to be a radiologist now because she can't stand all these old women who hurt all over the place!

Mainstays of physiotherapy, such as exercise, may be found to be unsatisfactory by some elderly patients (Lansbury 2000). In general, the health care system may encourage passivity and chronicity in patients with pain, and may disempower rather than empower them (Walker et al 1999). Physiotherapists should therefore consider carefully whether the treatments they implement, or the advice that they give, is acceptable to patients and compatible with their usual or preferred lifestyle – if it is not, it is unlikely to be helpful.

It is also important to remember that people generally seek professional help for pain when their own resources have been exhausted. In other words, their symptoms are sufficiently troublesome that they have decided to cross the threshold of formal health care. What may seem to be a 'minor' pain is clearly not so to the individual, otherwise it would not have driven them to professional care. For therapy to be effective, patients must believe that they are believed, and that the practitioner is not trivializing their suffering.

The expression of pain in a clinical context is subject to a variety of psychological, social and cultural factors, and practitioners should be very cautious of the inferences they draw from overt behaviour or from the manifest, rather than the latent, meaning of what patients say. Cassell provides an illustration of the potential pitfalls: 'The patient often learns how bored others become by his pain. In the beginning, it is possible to say something hurts when asked, but after days and weeks the sufferer usually learns to be silent. It is a mistake to take that silence to mean acceptance of pain, when it is merely acceptance of the social rules' (Cassell 1978: 186).

9.7 CONCLUSION

This chapter has reviewed some central sociological aspects of pain, and has attempted to provide a complementary perspective to that of Chapter 8. Some of the issues explored will also link with Chapters 4 and 11.

An understanding of the social dimensions of pain should assist physiotherapists' awareness of the subjective experience of pain and the ways in which pain impacts upon the individual's life. It will also provide an insight into the assumptions that underlie practitioners' understanding of the nature of pain, and the way in which these may differ from the assumptions of patients themselves. As a result, the management of people with pain can potentially be more sensitive, appropriate and effective.

Chapter **10**

Recent perspectives on child development in relation to physiotherapy practice

Christopher A. Whittaker

10.1 AIMS AND SCOPE

In 1787, Tiedemann published what is generally regarded as the first scientific account of the behaviour of a young child (Tiedemann 1787). He carefully charted the ages at which specific behaviours occurred and emphasized the variability to be seen in development: 'I grant that what has here been observed cannot be taken as a general law, since children ... progress variously, the one with speed the other more slowly' (Tiedemann 1787: 206). In the last century, in particular, innumerable detailed attempts have been made to describe the behaviour of a wide range of children in naturalistic and experimental settings. Tiedemann (1787: 206) believed that when sufficient data had been collected, then 'it will be possible by means of comparison to strike an average for the common order of nature'.

Two centuries later his goal remains unrealized. There is no widely accepted notion of which invariant factors control child development. Part of the problem lies in the interface between theory, observation and interpretation – what we believe determines what we look for, what we see, and what we do about it. The particular theoretical orientation that we were trained to take, or which has emerged from our clinical practice, determines the sort of research questions we ask, the methodology we adopt, the instruments we use to record our observations, and the theories we apply to the interpretation of our findings about children. Broader cultural and sociopolitical issues related to gender, race, disability and power are also seen as influencing these processes of decision-making (Barton & Tomlinson 1984, Ribbens 1994).

Any overview of the psychology of child development, confined to a chapter, can only be highly selective. In my selectivity I have been guided by the need to provide a brief synopsis of some current major themes in the psychology of child development, with a focus on research relevant to the physiotherapist's clinical practice. Since the last edition of this chapter (Whittaker 1997), some issues have become more important in the literature other less so, while some have remained the same. The text has been modified accordingly. Quite extensive use will be made of references to key readings as a guide to in-depth treatment of the themes raised here.

10.2 DEVELOPMENTAL MILESTONES OR THEORETICAL ORIENTATIONS?

The concept of 'developmental milestones' is one familiar to physiotherapists, for many of the major traditional texts in this field have that orientation. More recent texts, for example Bedford (1993), while outlining Piagetian theory, also emphasize the developmental milestone approach. These accounts of childhood attempt to record, in more or less detail, what children actually do at different ages. Developmental milestones are key factors typically grouped under concepts such as language, motor development and play. Perhaps the most accessible text is Mary Sheridan's (1992) *Spontaneous Play in Early Childhood*, which has influenced a generation of professionals in the field of health and education. An equally seminal work, at a more complex and detailed level, is Holt's (1991) *Child Development: Diagnosis and Assessment*. The focus is on paediatric assessment but it gives an in-depth insight into the pattern of child development. A third key work, also in the paediatric literature, is Illingworth's (1987) *The Development of the Infant and the Young Child*.

Sheridan, Holt and Illingworth all give recognition to the pioneering work of Gesell (Gesell & Amatruda 1947). Four major fields are covered in Gesell's Scales: motor development, adaptive behaviour, language and personal–social behaviour. Gesell's developmental theory is essentially one of the uniform unfolding of biological mechanisms through the maturation of the nervous system: 'A behaviour pattern is simply a defined response of the neuro-motor system to a specific situation' (Gesell & Amatruda 1947: 4).

Such 'norm-referenced' scales have the advantages of: familiarity through long usage in clinical settings; ease of application without complex equipment; and intrinsic interest for many children. It might be thought that a detailed understanding of developmental milestones is a sufficient grounding for physiotherapists, given the other demands and constraints on their time during initial and postgraduate education and clinical practice. It will be argued that this is not the case. In particular, it is suggested that the differing theoretical positions outlined here can radically alter our perception of the relative importance of given aspects of the development of the child, and that these can lead to very different clinical outcomes.

Clarke & Clarke (1974) indicated that norm-referenced tests had their origins in the application of the concepts of normal distribution and correlation analysis to the field of intelligence at the turn of the century. An examination of scales such as the Gesell, or the Griffiths (1954), shows their empirical and observational foundation. They were devised to compare individual children with an identified pattern of development common to a supposedly representative population of children of the same age. Yet some were validated a generation or more ago, on cross-sectional, not longitudinal, samples. So different groups at each age band were tested, rather than the same group of children being monitored as they developed. Samples generally over-represented middle-class white populations from Western countries.

The empirical basis of test construction often leads to conceptually unrelated items being grouped together under broad headings as indicators of a particular developmental level. On the Cattell Scale (Cattell 1940) items such as patting a mirror and taking two cubes are seen as indicative of a 7-month level. Kiernan (1974) pointed out that this empirical orientation means that items are only included if they highlight differences between age levels, that is they occur at one age level not another. Yet a third item, excluded for spanning both ages, might be a vital conceptual link, which could be used in an intervention programme with a child with atypical development. In an important early study, Stott & Ball (1965) sought to explain the poor predictive validity of norm-referenced infant scales that show only low correlations with later intelligence test scores. They found inconsistent factor content at different levels indicating that the same abilities are not being measured at each stage. On the Gesell Scale the distribution of items by factor analysis, a powerful statistical technique for identifying underlying relationships in data (Kline 1994), is totally different from the format laid down by its authors: the items are measuring different abilities from those intended. Stott & Ball (1965) suggested that a Piagetian theory-based scale should prove of value with infants. Subsequent research, reviewed below, has supported this perception.

A recurring criticism of norm-referenced scales is that they concentrate on perceptual motor items while ostensibly measuring cognitive development (Jones 1972, Gaussen 1984). The Bayley Mental Scale (Bayley 1969), for instance, has six items which require the same cognitive object permanence skill of retrieving a totally hidden object, but some items demand significantly more complex motor skills. Such tests will clearly disadvantage motor-impaired children.

Practitioners need to examine the range of empirically based norm-referenced scales which they routinely employ and consider if these need to be supplemented by theory-based instruments in order to gain a more complete picture of the children they are assessing. To assist this process, theoretical issues in child development and the implications raised for clinical practice will be examined.

10.3 PIAGET AND VYGOTSKY

In 1896 two men were born who would dominate, in turn, the field of developmental psychology in the twentieth century. One, Jean Piaget, would live out his long life in tranquil Switzerland; the other, Lev Vygotsky, would die young in Stalinist Russia. Piaget's influence was greatest, particularly in the field of education, during the 1960s and early 1970s, while Vygotsky's impact has been most noticeable in the last two decades.

Developmental theory was significantly influenced, for much of the last century, by the work of Piaget, and a great deal of research which followed him was predicated on supporting or refuting his claims (Boden 1985). His output of research was prodigious and the depth and complexity of his argument, along with its uncompromising style, make reading Piaget hard, even for specialists in the field. These difficulties spawned a plethora of 'Guides to Piaget' of which Ruth Beard's (Beard 1969) is still one of the most accessible, and Flavell's (Flavell 1963) one of the most comprehensive. It is vital, however, to place Piaget's work in the context of more recent research and a very readable review is provided by Mitchell (1992). Ignorance of the subtle insights to be found in the original work may have blunted our perceptions of important aspects of Piaget's theory: however difficult, it rewards patient scrutiny. This is particularly true of his insights into the cognitive development of the infant leading up to the onset of mental representation.

10.4 RESEARCH INTO THE SENSORIMOTOR STAGE

Piaget believed that there are distinct stages in the child's development of understanding of the world, each qualitatively different from the preceding one. He did not mean by this the commonsense notion that older children had acquired more facts because they had lived longer. Rather, that a child's developing view of the world is radically different from an adult one. His stages are:

1. Sensorimotor stage – birth to 2 years
2. Pre-operational stage – 2 to 7 years
3. Concrete operations stage – 7 to 12 years
4. Formal operations stage – 12 years onwards.

Research of relevance to physiotherapists has mainly occurred in the first two of these stages, and it is these that will now be considered.

Piaget believed that babies develop by means of 'action schemas', which they generalize to different aspects of the environment: a process he called 'assimilation'. At the same time, the action schemas themselves become modified, so extending the range of behaviours the infant could employ. This process he called 'accommodation'. Optimal development comes when assimilation and accommodation work in unison. Piaget identified six hierarchical substages in the sensorimotor period, with gradual differentiation of action schemas into areas such as problem-solving, causality, imitation and object permanence. His sensorimotor theory (Piaget 1953, 1955) was developed by meticulous observation of only three children, his own – which by any reckoning is not a very representative sample.

Researchers were quick to see the potential of devising theory-based assessment procedures grounded in how infants think. By far the most widely used are the Ordinal Scales of Psychological Development (OSPD; Uzgiris & Hunt 1989). Standardized on a sample of approximately 200 infants in the USA, they generally confirmed the order and stages of concept development identified by Piaget. In 1980, Carl Dunst produced a useful clinical manual to supplement the OSPD (Dunst 1980), which contained an excellent profiling procedure, additional scale items, age norms and advice on educational programming. The OSPD have been used extensively with typically developing children (Uzgiris & Hunt 1987), people with severe and profound learning disabilities (see reviews by Kahn 1976, Hogg 1987), children with multiple impairment (Sharpe 1990) or cerebral palsy (Cioni et al 1993), and children with severe autism and minimal speech (Whittaker & Reynolds 2000, Potter & Whittaker 2001). Procedures that could be used to measure cognitive development using physiological rather than motor responses with both very young and motor-impaired children were reviewed by Gaussen (1984, 1985), although additional problems such as epilepsy may affect the reliability of such data. As costs fall, and techniques improve and become less intrusive, so brain imaging studies (see Gillespie & Jackson 2000) could prove to be a rich source of information on cognitive development in people with severe developmental disabilities. Stringent ethical guidelines would be needed to safeguard the rights and well-being of individuals in this situation.

The development of the use of 'mental imagery' or 'foresight' in solving problems marks the transition to pre-operational thinking. An example is searching for a causal mechanism to activate a novel wind-up toy without demonstration. Piaget (1951) and Werner & Kaplan (1963) contend that the child's idiosyncratic symbolic system – manifest, for example in deferred imitation and pretend play – is a precursor of the shared symbolic function of language. Normative data on the development of symbolic play in young children have been presented by Lowe & Costello (1988), McCune-Nicholich (1977), Rosenblatt (1977) and Largo & Howard (1979a, 1979b), and all of these authors give general support to Piaget's formulations. The pretend play of children with autism (Wing et al 1977, Jarrold et al 1993), severe learning difficulties (Jefree & McConkey 1976, McConkey & Martin 1980) and profound learning difficulties (Whittaker 1980) have all been reported to follow a broadly similar, although attenuated, sequence of development.

A serious and persistent criticism of Piaget is that he took too little account of the social dimension in development. This will be examined more closely when considering the work of Vygotsky and the social context of communication, below.

As well as underestimating the social dimension in his theory, Piaget stands accused of largely ignoring it as a researcher. His claim that the pre-operational child is egocentric has been seriously challenged in Donaldson's (1978) *Children's Minds*. Her thesis is that Piaget underestimated children's abilities because they did not understand what was required in the tasks that he set them. In a well-known experiment Piaget showed children a model of three mountains, each one of which had a distinctive feature at its summit. The child's task was to select a photograph of the scene representing the view of a doll that was sitting on the opposite side of the model. Children under seven tended to choose a view of the model from their own rather than the doll's perspective, and Piaget interpreted this as egocentric – a failure to perceive another's view of the world. Donaldson claimed that in fact, because the task was outside their experience and the questions were linguistically complex, the children had difficulty in working out what the experimenter wanted them to say. To illustrate this interpretation, Hughes (1975) devised a hide and seek game with toys in which the children had to hide a robber from a policeman in a model partitioned into four 'rooms'. Essentially, in the correct solution the robber could be seen by the child but not by the policeman. Ninety per cent of children between 3 and 5 years solved the problem, disproving, according to Hughes and Donaldson, that they were egocentric. They did this, so it was claimed, because the story was more within their compass of knowledge and made 'human sense'.

Mitchell (1992) challenged their interpretation. He suggested that the policeman scenario was a simpler problem than the mountain task and invoked Flavell's theory of Level One and Level Two perspective-taking (Flavell et al 1981) in explanation. This proposed that children as young as 3 can understand that someone does not share their perspective, but it is only 4-year-olds who can imagine what that person can see. Mitchell (1992) equated Level One perspective-taking to the policeman task and a Level Two perspective-taking to the mountain situation, providing a partial vindication of Piaget's position.

10.5 THEORY OF MIND

Another aspect of the perceived difference between 3- and 4-year-olds, which focuses on their developing social awareness, is 'theory of mind'. We talk and think not just about what people do, but also speculate on the motives behind their actions. This understanding that other people have needs, thoughts and beliefs seems a natural part of being a person; it is called a theory of mind, but when does it develop, and what would we be like if we did not possess it? Over almost two decades a burgeoning range of research has sought to answer these questions. The response to the first appears to be about 4 years of age. The answer to the second, some authorities (see Frith 1989) would have us believe, is that we would be labelled as having autism.

One aspect of theory of mind which has figured largely in this research is the attribution of a 'false belief' to someone else, where we have to suspend our own knowledge of a situation and imagine how someone else thinks about it. In a series of apparently simple experiments it has been claimed that many 4-year-olds can attribute a false belief to others while most 3-year-olds fail to do so (Perner et al 1987). In one version, 'the Sally-Anne experiment', a doll leaves her marble in one location then exits the room, and the second doll moves it. The child is asked where the first doll will look for the marble when she returns. Younger children are said to fail because they do not conceptualize that someone can have a false belief, when they (the children) know the truth. How far this finding will stand up to systematic variation in the language used, the use of multiple hiding places, or to non-verbal versions of the task still remains unclear. Astington (1994) provided an excellent introduction to theory of mind and its links with pretend play. More complex literature reviews are given in Astington et al (1988) and Baron-Cohen et al (1993).

10.5.1 AUTISM AND THEORY OF MIND

Autism is characterized by problems with reciprocal interaction, non-verbal/verbal communication and imaginative activity, as well as a markedly restricted repertoire of activities and interests (Frith 1989). People with Asperger's syndrome, a form of autism seen in more able individuals, show similar difficulties. Both groups have problems in understanding the subtleties of social interaction, and taking language on a literal level is very common. Jones (1995) outlined the difficulties faced by someone without a theory of mind: difficulty predicting what others will do; failing to understand what people will find interesting; difficulty in appreciating hidden meanings as in teasing or sarcasm; an inability to realize that a factual statement of truth can be hurtful. Comprehension of the reasons behind these difficulties could aid tolerance and help professionals develop more effective social skills programmes.

Inconsistencies underlying theory of mind experiments were examined in Whittaker (1997). In order to demonstrate that theory of mind problems are specific to autism, careful 'mental age matching' needs to take place between the experimental group of children with autism and control groups of typically developing children and youngsters with learning disabilities (Frith 1989). Many of the studies in this area, reviewed by Happé (1995), use a simple vocabulary measure, the British Picture Vocabulary Scale (BPVS; Dunn et al 1982), to compute the verbal mental age of the participants in order to match groups. Given the well-reported language difficulties in semantics and pragmatics that people with autism have, and the verbal bias of the theory of mind tests, the use of BPVS seems somewhat surprising. When a much more robust measure of verbal mental age, the Wechsler Intelligence Scale for Children – Revised (WISC-R) (Wechsler 1974), was used by Yirmiya & Shulman (1995), no significant differences were found between individuals with autism and those with severe learning disabilities on the false belief task, thus calling into question the view that failure in theory of mind tasks is specific to autism, and not a function of learning disability. Yirmiya & Schulman (1995) argue persuasively for studies which examine a broad spectrum of cognitive, linguistic and social–emotional factors alongside a wider range of theory of mind tasks.

In the period since 1996 the influence of theory of mind has continued to wane in autism research. This may be partly because of methodological concerns and also because the symptoms characterizing autism tend to emerge in the second year of life, well before the cognitive structures tapped by theory of mind research. Baron-Cohen & Swettenham (1997) have claimed, in defence of theory of mind, that developmentally earlier behaviours, such as lack of joint attention, are precursors of theory of mind, but so far this link has not been convincingly demonstrated.

10.6 PIAGET'S INFLUENCE

Piaget's greatest impact was on education, particularly in the 1960s and 1970s when his followers were influential in the child-centred approach to primary education (Plowden 1967). Criticisms of his stage theory, and the lack of control of the social dimensions in his experiments, meant that his influence waned considerably after his death. Indirectly, however, the influence of both Bruner (Bruner et al 1976) and Piaget can be seen in the play-orientated curriculum in nursery schools and in cognitive approaches to learning, such as that of Floyd (1979).

Physiotherapists are primarily concerned with the motor system and movement, yet much of their treatment with children is through play, so an understanding of recent advances in cognitive psychology is essential in appreciating the child's perspective. Children under 7 years are clearly more capable of logical thought than was believed a generation ago, and the 3–4-year-olds are less egocentric. But there is perhaps more evidence that they struggle to make sense of the complex social encounters that adults draw them into. Clinicians, as well as cognitive researchers, would do well to think carefully about the context of their social encounters with children – to be wary of the language employed, and the level of comprehension assumed, in these often unnatural settings. Aspects of Vygotsky's theory are helpful in relation to these issues.

10.7 VYGOTSKY: A SOCIAL CULTURAL PERSPECTIVE

Interest in Vygotsky increased after Piaget's death in 1981 and accelerated after the demise of the USSR in 1989, since when there has been greater access to Vygotsky's original writings. His emphasis on the social dimension of learning also accorded well with other contemporary evidence. Vygotsky's writing is generally more accessible than Piaget's, for he has an open, more fluid style. A modern readership may have greater difficulty with aspects of the content; his references, for example, to now obscure

1920s' debates with contemporaries such as Karl Buhler and, more importantly, with understanding the cultural setting of Stalinist Russia.

In the last decade there have been a number of commentaries placing Vygotsky's work into the context of education (Daniels 1993), cognitive science (Frawley 1997) and educational psychology (Das & Gindis 1995), while Smith et al (1997) compared the work of Vygotsky & Piaget in relation to educational theory and practice. A useful introduction to many of the key features of Vygotsky's thought is given in Daniels (1996).

Fundamental to Vygotskian psychology is his claim that higher mental functions in children emerge from the prevailing social and cultural setting rather than from the individual child. This is in direct contrast with Piaget who sees them being constructed through the child's sensorimotor actions on the environment. Vygotsky's 'general genetic law of cultural development' summarized his position on this issue: 'Any function in the child's cultural development appears twice ... first it appears between people as an interpsychological category, and then within the child as an intrapsychological category' (Vygotsky 1981: 163). He then extends this principle to processes such as concept formation, voluntary attention and logical memory, concluding: 'Relations among people genetically underlie all higher functions and their relationships'.

This perspective explicitly rejects the individualistic view of psychological phenomena by stressing the social origins of mental functioning. Two key concepts follow from this general law: the zone of proximal development (ZPD) and inner/egocentric speech (Vygotsky 1978). The ZPD is the difference between children's actual developmental level seen in independent problem-solving and the level of their potential development under adult guidance, or in collaboration with more capable peers. Vygotsky draws some important implications from this both for assessment of intelligence and for the processes of teaching. The ZPD is the aspect of Vygotsky's theories that has been most influential in the West in relation to both the dynamic assessment of children's abilities and to educational theory (see Daniels 1993). Egocentric speech, which emerges around the age of 3 years, is observed in children talking aloud to themselves about their actions. Vygotsky interpreted this as a new self-regulatory mechanism, being a transition phase between external and inner speech. This is seen as evidence for his view that all higher mental processes are derived from social and cultural contexts and only then internalized.

Vygotsky interpreted culture as the product of human social activity and emphasized that all human mental function is inherently sociocultural, because it is undertaken with socially organized cultural tools, the foremost of which is language (Wertsch & Tulviste 1996). The sociocultural setting can also impose constraints on the conceptual framework used to scaffold these higher mental functions: some of these manifest limitations are now discernible in Vygotsky's own position.

10.7.1 LIMITATIONS OF VYGOTSKY'S THEORY

Wertsch & Tulviste (1996) point out that Vygotsky had a restricted view of culture, even by the standards of his day, seeing it largely in terms of the mediating effects of signs, especially language. Particularly uncomfortable for us today is his evolutionist view of the development of culture, which was specifically Eurocentric: he believed that some cultures were inferior to others, although all were capable of development, and that through education Soviet Russia could turn all children into 'supermen'. These views, of course, preceded the emergence of Nazi Germany and the major Stalinist purges in Soviet Russia; we cannot even speculate how these events may have changed Vygotsky's perspectives.

Another significant limitation of Vygotsky's theories is his insistence that the process of development is solely a function of the environment: 'the environment here plays the role not of the situation of development, but of its source' (Vygotsky 1934: 113). This view gives little credence to the role of the active individual in the process of development. Research, some of which is reviewed here, has shown that far from being a passive recipient, the child is an active participant in a complex dialogue with his or her socially mediated environment.

Our sociocultural experience since his death makes it easier for us to see these limitations in Vygotsky's position, but more difficult to apprehend the world in which he wrote them. He probably would have appreciated this scenario, as an apt example of the importance of historical–cultural perspectives on ways of thinking.

Vygotsky's most significant contribution to current theory may prove to be his analysis of the complex social exchange that takes place between child and teacher, in the process of learning in educational settings. But the social interchange between child and adult begins in earliest infancy, as we shall see in the next section.

10.8 THE SOCIAL CONTEXT OF COMMUNICATION

Many of the children referred to physiotherapists have language and communication difficulties in addition to motor impairments, and it is important to keep informed about developments in this complex area. Until the 1960s the intriguing question of how children acquired language was dominated by the 'operant conditioning' theory of B. F. Skinner (Skinner 1957). He believed that caregivers unknowingly 'shaped' the infant's production of sounds, reacting very positively to new ones that the child made. Words would be shaped and vocabulary extended in the same way. It is important to note that 'external reinforcement', in this case the caregiver's positive response, was seen as the controlling process, with the child having a largely 'passive' role.

Where Skinner's theory collapsed as an overall explanation of language acquisition was in its inability to explain the 'grammatical' development of the child. When children come to put words together they do so grammatically, so that by the age of 6 years they have mastered most of the syntactical rules. This rapid expansion of ability could not be accounted for by external reinforcement, but it was seen by many to be explained by the psycholinguistic theories of Noam Chomsky. In 1959, Chomsky published his famous rebuttal of Skinner (Chomsky 1959) and his own theory followed shortly thereafter (Chomsky 1965). Chomsky came to believe that we are born with an inherited 'language acquisition device' (LAD), which is able to identify the particular 'surface structure' of the grammar of the language we are brought up in, and convert this into an innate 'deep structure'. This deep structure has a universal grammar, which he claimed was possessed by all human beings. In this way he sought to explain the rapid growth in the child's understanding of the rules by which words can be linked to make acceptable utterances. His theories dominated language research for well over a decade.

Those working with children with no speech and with complex learning disabilities during the 1970s did not find Chomsky's theories particularly helpful in practice. What did help were views that emphasized the reciprocity of the communication process within an understanding of the child's cognitive development (Schaffer 1971, 1977, Whittaker 1984). Donaldson (1978: 38), reviewing the Chomskian revolution of the previous decade, placed importance not on grammatical structure but on the child's development of meaning: 'it is the child's ability to interpret situations which makes it possible for him through active processes of hypothesis testing and inference, to arrive at a knowledge of language'. The search to determine how this process of 'construction of meaning' works, and how it affects children's thinking, is an ongoing one. Aspects of it were examined when considering Donaldson's work and theory of mind earlier in the chapter. Mitchell (1992) gives an important review of more recent research. This suggests that young children's comprehension of the distinction between what is said and what is meant emerges gradually between the ages of 3 and 6 years. It has significant ramifications for the way professionals interact with children in this age group, the nature of the settings in which this takes place, and our appreciation of the child's actual understanding.

The child's construction of meaning, then, is a long-drawn-out process, but when does it begin? The answer seems unequivocally to be in infancy, perhaps in the neonatal period itself. This research has its theoretical foundations in concepts of 'attachment' (Ainsworth 1964, Bowlby 1971), 'joint reference' (Bruner 1975), and 'reciprocity' (Schaffer 1977), all of which relate to the interactive nature of the child–caregiver relationship. Meltzoff & Moore (1985) outlined a series of sophisticated and apparently well-controlled experiments in which neonates appeared to be capable of facial imitation, indulging in tongue/lip protrusion and mouth opening following the presentation of these gestures by an adult. Given that neonates produce these movements anyway, Meltzoff & Moore's task was to demonstrate that they occurred at a greater than chance level, which they do report. It would be interesting to see these results replicated in another laboratory, and to compare the neonates' 'imitation' responses to other face-like objects as in the early smiling experiments (see Schaffer 1971).

Research has examined the interactional patterns between mothers and their premature babies in neonatal units. Henriksen (1994) described the 'helplessness response' of these infants and the dangers in mothers modelling their behaviour on the professionally detached 'efficient' pattern of care seen as necessary by staff in these high dependency units. The extremely specialized role of the physiotherapist within the neonatal intensive care unit is covered in an informative overview by Sheahan & Brockway (1992).

A wide range of prelinguistic communication with infants has been investigated, including: modified adult facial/vocal behaviour; gaze; the use of motherese (the speech of adults to young children); touch; variation in rhythm and pace of the interaction and turn-taking (see Schaffer 1977, Nind & Hewett 1994). The baby is not the passive organism envisaged by Skinner, but an active partner engaging in a reciprocal relationship. At the core of these interactions is the adult's belief in the infant's 'intentionality', for early interactions 'are sustained only through the mother's initiative in replying to the infant's responses as if they had communicative significance' (Schaffer 1977: 10). An acceptance of intentionality, the use of non-verbal approaches along with an understanding of the child's mental representational abilities, are at the core of work with children having complex learning disabilities. Whittaker (1980: 259) suggested that children seen as having profound learning disabilities 'have tended to be identified in terms of what they could not do'. A generation later this negative labelling persists, particularly in relation to children with severe autism and minimal speech. Whittaker (1996) argued that the triad of impairment, which is the basis of the prevailing diagnosis of autism (American Psychiatric Association 1994), in seeking to identify how people with autism differ from others, inherently focuses on what they cannot do. It is a *deficit model*, and the deficit is located in the individual. The majority of psychological research in autism follows this deficit paradigm, is experimental laboratory-based, and focuses on those with mild autism, who form a small minority of those with the diagnosis.

In contrast, Potter & Whittaker (2001) examined in detail the quality of the communication environment experienced by 18 children with severe autism and minimal speech in the natural setting of school classrooms. They also developed an intervention programme with five of these children over a 2-year period. They found that the rate and quality of the children's spontaneous communication were not dependent on their age, degree of autism, adaptive behaviour levels or on staffing ratios. It was directly related to the quality of their communication environment, with some environments having a negative effect on the children's social engagement. The communication environments which were most enabling were those in which adults used minimal speech, reduced verbal prompts, provided pauses at critical points to allow time for the children to respond, and taught the children a non-verbal communication system such as multipointing (Potter & Whittaker 1997). The use of non-verbal proximal communication (Whittaker 1996a) in rough-and-tumble play led to immediate and significant improvements in social responsiveness. From a theoretical perspective, Potter & Whittaker (2001) concluded that the role of language impairment in autism should be carefully re-evaluated. Subsequent preliminary analysis of results from their longitudinal intervention study suggested that some children with severe autism and minimum speech may have a form of auditory verbal agnosia, or word-deafness, which could be a fundamental element underlying their autism.

Physiotherapists need to be aware that very young babies appear to have a greater awareness of their social and material environment than was thought a generation ago. Similarly, the non-verbal aspects of the social communication of disabled children need careful consideration.

10.9 WORKING MOTHERS, INFANT DEVELOPMENT AND POVERTY

According to official statistics, there has been an increasing trend over the last two decades, in both the UK and the USA, for mothers of infants under 1 year of age to return to full-time employment. By 1999, 49% of British and 55% of American mothers in this category were in employment (Office for National Statistics 2000). The assumption that the mother is also the child's primary caregiver is difficult to ratify although increased maternal employment is undoubtedly related to the greater provision of non-maternal day care arrangements external to the home. The effects on children of these day care arrangements have been widely and acrimoniously debated. A fierce controversy began with Belsky's (1986) review of research that concluded that more than 20 hours per week of non-maternal child care in the infant's first year posed risks to both the subsequent behavioural adjustment of the child and the mother–child relationship. Clarke-Stewart (1989) and others attacked Belsky's analysis on methodological and substantive grounds. Belsky (2001), although one of the main protagonists, gives a reasonably balanced overview of the key issues involved in this complex and long-drawn-out debate.

In an attempt to clarify the effects of day care provision, the National Institute of Child Health and Human Development (NICHD) supported a major longitudinal study – 'NICHD Early Child Care' – in the USA. This was a large, well-designed collaborative study, involving many of the protagonists in the day care argument. It followed, from birth, 1300 children and their families living in 10 different American communities. Possible confounding variables that had marred earlier research, such as methodological problems, family economic status, maternal educational level, and ethnic origin, were carefully controlled. Detailed intensive observations of children's day-to-day experiences in their usual non-maternal day care arrangements were made at 6, 15, 24, 36, and 54 months of age in order to examine the quality of that care. Early findings indicated that enhanced language and cognitive development during the first 3 years, and again at 4½ years, was associated with high-quality non-maternal care (NICHD Early Child Care Research Network 2000). The quality of mother–child interactions was also systematically monitored in this study during the child's first 3 years of life. More time in day care during this period was shown to be associated with less sensitive interactions between mother and child (NICHD Early Child Care Research Network 1999). Insecure attachment of the infant to the mother was related to the poor quality of non-maternal care and more than one care-giving arrangement. Children who had over 10 hours per week of non-maternal care in the first year of life, and whose mothers were insensitive in their interactions, were also at risk of showing insecure attachment at 15 and 36 months (NICHD Early Child Care Research Network 1997).

The NICHD study provided general support for Belsky's (1986) position, indicating a direct relationship between an increased quantity of care from an early age and later problem behaviour. Item analysis showed that the children's problems included aggressive and destructive behaviour rather than, as Clarke-Stewart (1989) had theorized, assertiveness resulting from the independence supposedly fostered in child care settings. Belsky (2001) pointed out that the NICHD findings are not restricted to any particular racial, ethnic or demographic group. The results do not support the view that infants from economically disadvantaged families might benefit from high-quality early day care rather than staying with their mothers. Belsky (2001) concluded that extensive paid parental leave, tax incentives, strategies such as part-time employment and the expansion of good-quality child care could be justified by the NICHD's findings on economic, as well as humanitarian, grounds. This would enable more parents to follow their reported option of choice and have a full-time parental presence at home with very young children (Farkas et al 2000).

The NICHD's findings and Belsky's (2001) conclusions do not accord easily with the current British government policy to encourage mothers of young children to return early to the workplace. Young unemployed single mothers have been identified as one target group for government initiatives in this area because of the link with child poverty. For it is clear from official statistics that childhood poverty in Britain increased dramatically during the 1980s. In 1979 less than one in ten children was living in a household whose income was below half the national average, but by 1993 this had increased to one child in three, while over three-quarters of children living in one-parent families were living in poverty (National Children's Homes Action for Children 1998). The issues surrounding child poverty are complex but a detailed review is provided by Kumar (1993). The link between poverty and poor health has long been recognized, with the most recent examination (Department of Health 1998a) indicating that the gap in health between those in social classes 1 and 5 has widened in the last two decades. The Acheson Report was positive, however, that: 'Provided an appropriate agenda of policies can be defined and given priority, many of these inequalities are remediable' (Department of Health 1998a: v).

The British government has the laudable and ambitious aim to eradicate child poverty in Britain by 2020. A major cornerstone of this policy is the Sure-Start programme (www.surestart.gov.uk) which also aims to prevent learning difficulties from developing in children by supporting parents, in identified regions of greatest need, to promote the physical, intellectual and social development of their children between birth and 4 years of age. This support is provided by integrated health care, family support, child care, and play facilities. Programmes are locally based, differ in emphasis from each other, and are evaluated individually by independent agencies appointed by each programme. While encouraging responsiveness to local circumstances, such a structure may be very difficult to evaluate overall against the expressed national objectives, although a large-scale national evaluation is also planned.

10.10 CONTROVERSY AND EVOLUTIONARY PSYCHOLOGY

Professional disputes among academics are nothing new; indeed, argument and counter-argument are the very stuff of the scientific method. Usually these dialogues take place in arcane journals where wary editors dutifully expunge any diversion into personalizing criticism. The debate over what has come to be called 'evolutionary psychology' (EP) has, by contrast, been conducted in part through 'popular science' books, where few constraints on personal criticism seem to apply. This is a field in which barbed invective abounds, dressed, of course, in suitably sophisticated prose.

Evolutionary psychologists seek to explain human behaviour, and our past and current societal and cultural systems, on the basis of universal features of human nature that, they claim, have not evolved since the dawn of mankind in the Pleistocene age 100 000–600 000 years ago. They believe that this explains many of the problems we face in coping with our complex social and cultural milieu: Stone Age minds coping with a postmodern society. The claims of EP are disarmingly wide, covering the disciplines of philosophy, sociology, anthropology, as well as biology, psychology and social policy. An introduction to important aspects of the EP perspective is given by Pinker (1997). Rose & Rose (2001) present a powerful multidisciplinary critique of EP, which is seen as a 'dangerous ideology'. They liken the adherents of EP to religious fundamentalists, point out that its basic precepts cannot be falsified and are therefore not scientific, and outline a range of political programmes its adherents have espoused, including the dismantling of the welfare state. Rose & Rose (2001: 3) believe that the claims of EP 'are for the most part not merely mistaken but culturally pernicious'.

Of direct relevance to this chapter is Karmiloff-Smith's (2001) important critique of the 'modular view of the mind' (Fodor 1983). This is the idea that the brain is genetically pre-specified for higher-order cognitive, language and perceptual abilities and that these domains function independently of each other. The analogy here is with a Swiss army knife, where each blade has a specific and completely separate function, although there appear to be varying perspectives in the EP camp as to whether these modules are mental constructs, or map on to specific anatomical brain structures. Karmiloff-Smith examines the evidence of *double dissociation* – damage to one area of the brain causing one type of loss while sparing another function. If the damage is to another region the outcomes are reversed. These phenomena seem, on the surface, to be strong evidence for a modularized brain with functionally specific areas. But Karmiloff-Smith pointed out that this evidence, from adult brains, does not mean that the brain started out with this level of specialization: 'it could be that specialisation builds up gradually and is actually the *product* of child development, not its starting point' (Karmiloff-Smith 2001: 147).

Karmiloff-Smith then goes on to review evidence of the plasticity of brain structures in childhood. For example, recent brain imaging studies have demonstrated that the localization of language is a process of gradual specialization, not something fixed at birth. Grammar is processed by both hemispheres in typical children until they are around 6 years of age and only then does the left hemisphere become more specialized and localized for grammar in right-handed individuals (Johnson 1997). This explains the finding that if the left hemisphere is removed early, in cases of severe epilepsy, then the prognosis for language development in the remaining right hemisphere is much better than if the child is older when this operation takes place (Mills 1994). This empirical evidence from recent brain imaging studies suggests a greater degree of plasticity in brain specialization than was generally accepted, rather than less, and suggests that the modular view of the brain needs at least some modification. These data also reinforce the importance of intensive and well-resourced early intervention.

10.11 ASSESSMENT OF MOTOR DEVELOPMENT

Eckersley (1993) gives a comprehensive overview of the field of paediatric physiotherapy, emphasizing a 'whole child' approach. Here some current protocols and tests related to the process of motor development in typically progressing children and disabled children will be examined. A useful summary of gross motor development in infancy with suggestions for further reading is provided by Van Sant (1994). Erhardt (1992) gave an extensive overview of eye–hand coordination in infancy, while Exner (1992) examines in-hand manipulation skills, and the Erhardt Developmental Prehension Assessment (Erhardt 1982) outlines in detail manipulative activity from the neonatal period until 6 years of age.

Physiotherapists often need a method of rapidly screening the motor behaviour of a young child to decide if formal treatment procedures are required. The Milani-Comparetti Screening Test, first described by Milani-Comparetti & Gidoni (1967), has undergone extensive revision. In its current form (Stuberg 1992) it can be administered in less than 10 minutes by an experienced observer. The test allows the recording of both spontaneous and evoked responses from the child, with an emphasis on functional motor behaviour and the reflexes underlying it. Results are presented graphically on an accessible and well-designed scoring chart, which provides a useful overview of the normative timescale expected for the reflexes of early childhood.

The Bruininks–Oseretsky Test of Motor Proficiency (Bruininks 1978) can be used to give separate and combined scores for fine and gross motor skills with typically progressing, and developmentally disabled children from the age of 4½ to 14½ years. Although it has excellent test–retest reliability, the standardization is based upon US norms from the 1970s.

The Pediatric Evaluation of Disability Inventory (Haley 1992) has a different premise from the Bruininks–Oseretsky, based instead upon an assessment of functional skill in children from 6 months to 7½ years. The areas covered are self-care, mobility and social function. An important distinction is made between capability and functional performance.

10.11.1 SENSORY INTEGRATION AND PSYCHOMOTOR APPROACHES

In the USA in particular, there is a long history of psychomotor work with children with varying degrees of learning difficulties. Building on the theories of Strauss in the 1940s (Strauss & Lehtinen 1947), Frostig (1966), Cruickshank (1967), Kephart (1971) and Cratty (1974) all produced detailed programmes for working with children labelled as brain-injured, attention-deficit disordered, or having learning disabilities. British approaches of the same era are summarized by Haskell et al (1977). The most enduring body of work in this field is the neurobehavioural approaches to Sensory

Integrative Therapy (SIT) of Jean Ayres. Her Southern California Sensory Integration tests included scales that examine space visualization, figure-ground perception, position in space, kinaesthesia, manual form perception, finger identification, graphaesthesia, localization of tactile stimuli and double tactile stimuli perception (Ayres 1978, 1989). Highly detailed therapy programmes are presented based upon the tests, language measures and clinical observations (Ayres 1973). In an exhaustive review, however, Hoehn & Baumeister (1994: 348) declared unequivocally that SIT was 'not merely an unproven, but a demonstrably ineffective' remedial treatment for its target populations.

Smyth (1992) provided an important review of the literature on so-called 'clumsy' children and stressed that secondary emotional problems are common in the mildly and moderately affected members of this group. Clumsiness has also been associated with Asperger's syndrome, a form of autism (American Psychiatric Association 1994), and with dyslexia in some children (Tansley & Panckhurst 1981). There is an important and largely unfilled role for physiotherapists in the identification and remediation of these subtle difficulties, in conjunction with other members of the interdisciplinary team.

10.12 CONCLUSION

The nature of physiotherapists' work means that they are often in close and prolonged contact with children and their families. They need a broad grasp of changing perceptions of development, and to be able to communicate these easily and effectively to parents and caregivers. Useful guides to the professional skills of working with parents are McConkey (1985), Cunningham & Davis (1985) and Hartley (1993).

The importance of subtle prelinguistic communication in the social interaction between children and adults has been stressed in this chapter. This is particularly true when the child is operating at a sensorimotor level, whether as a baby or as an older child with learning disabilities. Touch and movement are subtle and powerful communicators, and it may be precisely because of the intimacy of contact that some physiotherapists believe that a brisk professional detachment is best adopted. The child is the likely loser in such an exchange. Obviously professionals who wish to use a more intensive interactional approach need to do so within clearly defined and agreed ethical parameters (Nind & Hewett 1994, Potter & Whittaker 2001). Therapists need to be aware also of the context of social encounters when working with older children who have language – and to monitor carefully their own style of communication.

The child develops within the primary ecosystem of the family, and the secondary ecosystem of the culture. For it is now generally recognized that social cognition is an essentially reciprocal process that takes place between the child and the socially mediated environment. The parents' role has long been acknowledged, but the part played by siblings and culture in this process remains relatively unexplored (Bornstein et al 1992, Azmitia & Hesser 1993, Farver & Wimbarti 1995). Yet, despite a growing acceptance of the reciprocal nature of development, concepts of disability and typicality are still often located 'within the child'. It is particularly difficult for professionals to accept that they may be involved, however unwittingly, in the construction of the very disability that their vocation has drawn them to ameliorate.

Almost invariably, physiotherapists practise in interdisciplinary teams drawn from professions with different training, cultures and power structures. In this situation efficient communication, always a crucial element in any workgroup, is vital. A key element has to be that members strive to understand and appreciate the professional orientation of colleagues. A sharing of knowledge on different perspectives of child development is not an undermining of professional expertise, but a way of strengthening bonds, and a recognition of the rich complexity and fascination of children.

Chapter 11

The subjective experience of illness

Frances Reynolds

11.1 INTRODUCTION

The purpose of this chapter is to examine the subjective experiences that are frequently associated with illness. Medical and therapy students spend much of their courses studying the objective, physical aspects of disease in the form of anatomy, physiology and pathology. Patients, however, have argued that health professionals know a lot about disease but little about illness (Iezzoni 1998, Frank 2001). The 'subjective' aspects of illness are the personal, experiential or psychological aspects – the lived experience. This chapter introduces some relevant concepts and research that will help practitioners to work with patients in a more empathic manner, and thereby achieve better working partnerships. First of all, consider some ways in which disease is affecting the lives of two people in the following case examples.

Case study

Sue is 48 years old. She is married, with a grown-up daughter. Sue has had multiple sclerosis for 15 years, and has mobility, fatigue and incontinence problems. She uses a wheelchair. In order to improve her strength and stamina, she attends weekly physiotherapy at a local multiple sclerosis therapy centre. Since retiring from her social work job on health grounds 3 years ago, she spends much of her time painting, and has had her work accepted at local exhibitions. She also participates in charity fund-raising. She describes her husband as hugely supportive in every area of her life.

Case study

Robert is 21 years old. He has cystic fibrosis, a genetically inherited condition which results in mucus building up in the lungs and digestive system. Robert lives at home with his parents and works in a part-time clerical position for the local authority. He has regular physiotherapy treatment, at home and in hospital, to manage his breathing problems. His parents have been very proactive to secure the physiotherapy that he needs to maintain his functioning. Robert writes and sends out a newsletter to local youngsters with cystic fibrosis every 2 months, when his health allows. He spends much of his spare time on the internet searching for information about new research into treatments for cystic fibrosis.

11.1.1 THE BIOMEDICAL APPROACH TO DISEASE AND IMPAIRMENT: WHAT IS MISSING?

The traditional biomedical approach to disease and impairment focuses on the objective, disrupted workings of the physical body. 'Disease is the problem from the practitioner's perspective' (Kleinman 1988: 5). The aim of medical treatment is to cure or modify the disease process through a range of physical interventions, such as medication, radiotherapy and surgery. Although proven to be effective with many acute conditions, the biomedical perspective offers rather little beyond assessment and a biological explanation for patients with incurable conditions, such as Sue and Robert above.

With the rise of biomedicine, the patient's own subjective experience of illness has been ignored by health practitioners because considered irrelevant to treatment and recovery. However, in the last 20 years or so, this assumption has been disputed. A biopsychosocial perspective gives due weight to the psychological and social as well as the biological aspects of ill health and health care (Ader 1980). This perspective helps us to understand why individuals differ markedly in their responses to 'similar' health conditions. For each patient, being ill is a unique challenge. Each person confronts a particular set of stressors associated with illness, and each brings different coping resources. For example, some people respond with optimism and high levels of perceived control whereas others are pessimistic, their thoughts filled with worst-case scenarios (Sullivan & D'Eon 1990, Scharloo & Kaptein 1997). In order to adopt a more client-centred approach, health professionals need to develop empathy for the patient's own personal experience. This enables the health professional not only to appreciate the many ways in which illness affects a person's life, but also to make better use of the patient's motivation and various coping resources. A more effective partnership with the patient can then be established, optimizing treatment outcomes.

In common with many other patients with chronic conditions, both Sue and Robert encounter unpleasant, sometimes distressing symptoms on a daily basis, such as breathlessness, coughing, spasms, and profound fatigue. They both experience restrictions in their daily lives and are confronted with limited choices about work, and leisure activities. Sue has had to retire from work on health grounds, because of her increasing mobility, fatigue and incontinence problems. Robert's health and daily treatment regime only leave him with sufficient energy for a part-time sedentary job, in a career that would probably not have been his first choice if he had been completely well. Although both seem likely to encounter daily frustration at not being able to carry out preferred activities, it seems from the brief information given that both are committed to personally meaningful occupations (painting, charity work, paid work, writing newsletters, computer use). Both Sue and Robert seem to experience their family as highly supportive, in both practical and emotional terms, and regard this support as helpful for coping with illness. At a deeper level, it is quite possible that both Robert and Sue have worries about their future prognosis. They both experience a deteriorating condition, which is likely to shorten their life-span, and they may be concerned about their access to suitable care. Their immediate family may no longer be able to provide this if and when their condition worsens.

Sue and Robert have had differing experiences of health in previous years. From the information given, Sue appears to have had no major health problems until her early thirties, whereas Robert has lived with cystic fibrosis all of his life. This may affect the adaptation process, because Sue has more clearly experienced loss of her former health. For Robert, ill health is a normal part of life. Although they both have regular physiotherapy, for Robert the treatment penetrates into daily life at home, and may therefore seem more intrusive. Each person seems to have somewhat distinctive coping strategies. Robert appears to adopt a more problem-solving approach, searching for information about his disease and continuing to seek medical solutions. Perhaps he hopes for an ultimate cure. Sue appears to be immersing herself in creative and social pursuits, making the most of her existing abilities. Their ages and life stage may affect their illness experiences. Sue has achieved a successful marriage and has a daughter. She had a rewarding career as a social worker until recent years. These achievements may not only provide self-esteem but ongoing social support during her illness. On the other hand, Robert may be finding that his illness is making it harder for him to leave the parental home and achieve an independent adult lifestyle. He has not yet found a partner and may have some concerns about whether he will find one who is accepting of his health problems. He is engaged in paid work, but not the career that he would have chosen. Sue has found that she possesses creative talent and enjoys painting. Her work has received some recognition locally and has been accepted in exhibitions. These aspects of her lifestyle would seem to offer high levels of satisfaction and a sense of continuity with her pre-illness self. Robert may not receive such public acclaim but nevertheless, he is proud of providing a useful service to others via his newsletter, which serves an educational and support purpose for young people in a similar situation. Sue has functional problems, including incontinence. This could be a source of considerable embarrassment, and may lead to shame and social difficulties unless effective self-management strategies are developed. Mobility problems create further barriers to her full and active participation in the community, as local facilities and transport services are rarely designed with wheelchair users in mind. This can lead to a loss of independence. Robert enjoys much easier access to community facilities.

These speculations may have made it easier to reflect about the variety of experiences that people have when living with illness. Such experiences include much more than disease symptomatology. A useful approach to understanding the illness experience is to consider illness as comprising a range of stressors, encompassing physical, emotional, social and practical difficulties. The person's interpretations of these various difficulties will both influence, and be influenced by, their emotional state, belief system, coping strategies and support resources.

11.1.2 ACUTE AND CHRONIC ILLNESS

Before looking further at the illness experience, a distinction needs to be drawn between acute (or short-term) illness and injury, and chronic (or long-term) conditions. Both acute and chronic health problems present a range of stressors – anxiety, discomfort and activity restrictions, for example. The distinction is not always clear-cut. For example, some short-term conditions, such as injuries sustained during sports, may have far-reaching consequences. A knee injury that is a nuisance for an amateur sportsperson may lead to the curtailment of a professional footballer's career. Nevertheless, for most people, acute illness and injury follow a limited, fairly predictable time-course. The person expects medical and therapeutic treatments to be effective, and assumes that a good recovery will take place. These expectations and assumptions are challenged by chronic illness, although the person usually starts out by hoping that recovery will be possible (Charmaz 1999a). Chronic illness sets in train a long process of adaptation. A range of trial and experimental treatments may be embarked upon, and the person may feel quite alienated from a body that can no longer be trusted (Ellis-Hill et al 2000). Chronic illness may pose considerable challenges to the person's identity, lifestyle and relationships. The remainder of this chapter will focus on the experience of chronic illness. Nevertheless, acute conditions sometimes present similar issues.

Since the late 1980s, a variety of research and writing has been carried out to illuminate the experience of illness (see, for example, Kleinman 1988). Some of the research has been based on quantitative assessment of patients' psychological responses such as depression and anxiety, but more recently, qualitative studies have suggested several recurring themes. Let us now turn to some of the research that has been carried out in this area.

11.2 THE ILLNESS EXPERIENCE PRIOR TO DIAGNOSIS

In the early stages of disease, before medical help is sought, the appearance of unusual symptoms may or may not create concern. Some people appear to be perceptive monitors of their internal state, and note changes in health quickly. If they interpret the health change as substantially affecting their valued activities, or as heralding possibly serious disease, they may readily seek medical opinion and advice (Levine & Reicher 1996). Others seem to suppress information about their bodily state and may fail to notice (or fail to report concern about) health changes. For some, this response may reflect a way of coping with fear, but for others, it may be grounded in undue optimism and a sense of invulnerability (Leventhal et al 1997). In such cases, medical help-seeking may be delayed – sometimes with fatal consequences. Even at the outset, cognitive interpretations and emotional responses to changes in health play a part in determining the person's experience of illness.

Receipt of a diagnosis can have very different emotional consequences for different people. Reactions are partly determined by the patient's perceptions of the seriousness of the disease, and the established effectiveness of available medical treatment. Clearly the diagnosis of a life-threatening condition is likely to generate very high levels of anxiety. Additionally, responses to diagnosis vary according to the person's belief system. People with high levels of perceived control, an optimistic outlook and a belief in the curability of their disease may respond to symptoms with more equanimity (Scharloo & Kaptein 1997, Williams & Barlow 1998, Leventhal et al 1999). The person's social and cultural milieu also influences responses to illness and diagnosis. For example, a socially stigmatized illness may be particularly feared within a particular culture because it leads to ostracism, disgust from others and/or family shame (see, for example, MacDonald 1988, Santana & Dancy 2000).

A diagnosis may be too threatening emotionally for some patients to accept immediately. They may instead respond with denial or disbelief, possibly seeking second opinions. Others may experience powerlessness, which may be expressed as depression or anger towards others (including health professionals). Yet for some people, a formal diagnosis – even of a serious disease – can provide considerable emotional relief, because the medical recognition reassures the person that his/her health problems are not imaginary, and also serves to inform others that the person is not 'malingering'. For such reasons, many people with multiple sclerosis, or chronic fatigue syndrome, report relief at receiving an eventual diagnosis (Charmaz 1999a; see Section 9.4).

11.3 LIVING WITH A CHRONIC ILLNESS

Living long-term with illness can entail a variety of negative experiences. According to Moos & Schaefer (1984) and Charmaz (1999b), these include:

- Ongoing bodily symptoms such as pain, dizziness, fatigue, incontinence
- Psychological distress, such as depression, anxiety

- Challenge to the self-concept
- Disrupted activities and lifestyle
- Altered roles and social relationships
- Reduced expectations about the future.

Obviously, the illness experience is very much shaped by the symptoms of the disease itself, including the degree to which they fluctuate over time, and their intrusiveness into everyday life. 'Discomfort can be a constant companion. It grows at the edges of one's life and sometimes devours it' (Charmaz 1999b: 364). While pain is a central feature of many chronic illnesses (for example, rheumatoid arthritis), it is not present in all chronic conditions. Nevertheless, regardless of discomfort, almost all chronic conditions appear to challenge the person's sense of self. Illnesses which create very visible outward signs (such as disfigurement or difficulties in walking) readily communicate the person's health problems to others, and may therefore be experienced as a 'master status', overwhelming the person's identity (Charmaz 1999a). Less visible health problems (such as profound fatigue) may be easier to live with in some ways as the person has more choice about whether to 'pass' as healthy. However, less understanding and support may be forthcoming if other people forget about the person's illness, or doubt its veracity (see Section 9.6.3). Many facets of the illness experience are shaped by the person's own interpretations, beliefs, values and emotional response, together with the acceptance and support of others. Some illnesses and impairments attract social stereotypes and stigmatization (Charmaz 1991). Such reactions are likely to diminish the person's sense of control over their illness status and their self-esteem.

11.4 NEGATIVE FEELINGS AND GRIEF

The appearance of a chronic illness, particularly in adulthood, may lead to a period of grieving for the former healthy self, for the future that had been previously planned, and for prior cherished assumptions that the world is fair and orderly. The person may wrestle for a long time with the question 'Why me?' The symptoms and ensuing sense of uncontrollability may leave the person feeling completely directionless (Hafsteindottir & Grypdonck 1997). A participant with HIV in Crossley's study (2000: 141) expressed such reactions in these terms: 'Absolutely everything, everything that you have had in life just breaks down, becomes dust, powder, you know, and you become completely naked and utterly lost, you do not know what to do.' Loss of physical function is likely to affect daily occupations, leading to further experiences of loss and bereavement. For example, the majority of people with multiple sclerosis become unemployed within a few years of diagnosis (Jackson & Quaal 1991). With loss of employment comes financial insecurity, loss of professional status and reduction in social contacts. Loss of function also affects daily leisure and self-care pursuits (Wikstrom et al 2001). Indeed, difficulties in managing leisure and personal care may have a more detrimental effect on quality of life than physical symptoms per se (Lundmark & Branholm 1996).

Grieving may take a variety of forms, including anger and sadness. Everyday activities may lose their meaning. Depression is highly associated with experience of loss and powerlessness. Unsurprisingly, substantial numbers of people become depressed following the onset of stroke and other serious conditions (Hafsteindottir & Grypdonck 1997). Such responses do not necessarily resolve quickly. Several studies have shown that people's experience of struggle and despair can continue for many years. For example, Mannerkorpi et al (1999) noted that negative experiences predominated interview reports given by people who had experienced fibromyalgia for more than 3 years.

Some people with life-threatening conditions such as cancer describe additional emotional pressures – to appear brave, to show oneself to be 'fighting' the illness, and to shield others from seeing one's distress. These social 'obligations' add to the emotional burden of chronic illness (Diamond 1999, Sutherland & Jensen 2000).

Grieving is generally accepted as progressing through a number of phases. These should not be considered as strictly sequential. There are likely to be periods of emotional turmoil interspersed with plateaux of relative calm and possibly – but not necessarily – acceptance. Several studies have shown that emotional distress is most marked in the first year or so of illness (see, for example, Ellis-Hill et al 2000).

11.4.1 CHANGES IN SELF-IMAGE AND SELF-ESTEEM

Although health professionals in the past have tended to focus treatment on physical dysfunction, there is increasing awareness that chronic illness often brings about profound changes in personal identity (Ellis-Hill & Horn 2000). The person is likely to experience a marked disjunction between their current and former selves, or a 'biographical discontinuity' (Bury 1982). Frank (2001: 354) provides a profound illustration of this when describing his own experience of cancer as: 'being disconnected from my life as I had been living it and from the lives of others around me. Suddenly, they (including my recently healthy self) were standing on shore and I was in a small skiff being carried toward an opposite shore.'

Not only are individual characteristics and abilities affected (such as the ability to walk without effort), but the illness may also impede 'normal', 'taken-for-granted' and self-defining social and occupational roles. For example, some mothers with arthritis report guilt at not being able to play physical games with their small children (Barlow et al 1999). A person who has taken early retirement from work on health grounds may mourn not only the loss of professional status but also the disappearance of his/her role as provider to the family (Charmaz 1994). Also, because self-esteem is fostered by the praise and recognition of others, it can become progressively eroded if the person becomes increasingly confined to quite isolated activities within the home and family environment (Day 1991).

Both the individual's value system and also wider cultural values influence the extent to which self-image and self-esteem are undermined by the lifestyle changes induced by illness challenge. For example, the Western Protestant work ethic is said to make it harder for people to accept reduced autonomy and independence when they become frail through illness or old age (Day 1991). Such transitions appear to be easier for people living in cultures that value obligations of care towards the extended family. However, the family context may also reinforce helplessness and passivity, infantilizing the person and reducing his/her role and status to that of 'sick person'. Both overprotective and critical family contexts can undermine the person's independence and sense of self (Schwartz & Kraft 1999).

There may also be gender differences in the illness experience, because of the different social roles that women and men occupy. For example, women tend to value their role as home-maker, even when also engaged in paid work. Many women retain aspects of their home-making role, even when in poor health, and this possibly contributes to their sense of continuity, coherence and well-being (Day 1991). With fewer alternative roles available, premature retirement from work on health grounds may have a more devastating impact on the self-esteem of men, through challenging their masculinity (Charmaz 1994, 1999a).

On the other hand, women may experience greater distress from disfiguring illnesses, given the cultural emphasis on female appearance (Williams & Barlow 1998). Health professionals do not always appreciate that altered appearance – as well as altered function – can be an upsetting aspect of long-term health problems. For example, some of the people with spinal cord injury interviewed by Seymour (1998) commented on how self-image was undermined by the 'enforced' use of clothing that was easy to put on, as well as changes in body shape brought about through the injury itself (such as slackening of abdominal muscles). Stenstrom et al (1993) and Williams & Barlow (1998) also found that women with rheumatoid arthritis often described concern not only about pain, but also about their appearance. Swollen joints on the hands and restrictions on clothing and footwear made many self-conscious and lacking in social confidence.

Self-image may also be diminished through the responses of others to illness. Although other people may initially be quite sympathetic to a crisis of illness and hospitalization, care and concern can rather quickly evaporate, particularly among colleagues in the workplace. Rather than being attributed to illness, the person's ongoing difficulties with tasks (for example, when fatigued or in pain) may be misinterpreted as a moral defect – a problem of 'character and competence, of will and worth' (Charmaz 1999a: 221). Such 'moral' judgements are also all too commonly applied to those whose symptoms can be confused with drunkenness or mental confusion (for example, a stumbling gait in multiple sclerosis). Not surprisingly, such social responses add considerable stress to the illness experience.

Jensen & Allen (1994: 353) summarize these issues by arguing that illness can prompt 'the recognition and redefinition of one's self, roles and goals. Considerable energy is expended in re-framing one's place in the world … in learning to live again with a "new me".'

11.4.2 LOSS OF PREFERRED ACTIVITIES AND LIFESTYLE

The effects of ill health on social roles and occupations have already been partially examined in connection with self and identity changes. Changes in lifestyle due to illness create additional sources of stress. For example, loss of paid employment brings about financial uncertainties, and can plunge the person into an unfamiliar world of unemployment and disability benefit, which some regard as operating according to arcane, even punishing, rules. Reductions in income are likely to reduce choice – over care arrangements, transport options and leisure pursuits. To maximize quality of life with a chronic illness, the person requires supportive contact with community resources, including adult education, leisure facilities, and libraries, as well as medical services. However, financial difficulties may create barriers to access, resulting in increased isolation.

Chronic illness may also disrupt previous lifestyle in ways that increase health risks. Pain and functional limitations may make physical activity more onerous. With reductions in physical activity, loss of fitness may ensue, with negative effects on physical and mental health (Reynolds 2001).

Isolation and lack of stimulation can have the unfortunate effect of focusing attention on illness symptoms and medical treatments, and decreasing the person's sense of control and self-efficacy (which is a belief that desired goals can be accomplished; see Section 8.5.3). Low levels of perceived control have been shown to predict future decreases in functional performance in some chronic conditions (Thompson & Kyle 2000). Negative beliefs can indeed act as 'self-fulfilling prophecies'.

11.4.3 ALTERED SOCIAL RELATIONSHIPS

Illness often raises issues about how others will respond. Over-sympathetic reactions may be as unwelcome as rejecting ones. Hence, many people with chronic conditions wrestle with the dilemma of telling – or not telling – others about their health problems. Not telling is a way of keeping control over the situation and the relationship, avoiding stigmatization and preserving 'normality' (Charmaz 1991, Admi 1996). However, non-disclosure may also result in strained relationships and lack of support.

For some people, illness is associated with a contraction of social networks. In part this is because reductions in work and leisure activities lead to loss of acquaintances and colleagues. After the initial period, friends, too, may not respond well to the changing health status and needs of a chronically ill person. Some people describe the changing role of their partner, from intimate lover to 'carer', as the most painful aspect of their illness (Seymour 1998). Changes in sexual functioning, resulting from neurological damage and/or chronic pain, may also be a difficult – even unspeakable – aspect of the illness experience. Health professionals all too rarely help chronically ill patients and their partners to manage their sexual needs (Seymour 1998).

11.4.4 AN UNCERTAIN FUTURE

Moos & Schaefer (1984) regard living with an uncertain future as a major challenge of chronic illness. Crossley (2000) examined the narratives of people with HIV infection and discovered that the unpredictability of the illness trajectory, and an awareness of short-ened life, led some to experience the future as meaningless. This could be expressed as a reluctance to engage in major projects – such as taking an educational course, having and caring for children or embarking on a new job. However, once a sense of future is lost, the person can easily become locked into 'an empty present'. Futile thoughts about 'what could have been' may preoccupy the person, and depression becomes more likely (Crossley 2000). The person may find that everyday experience is tinged with anticipatory grief, thinking about death and leaving their loved ones. Alternatively, others commit themselves to long-term projects as a way of maintaining belief in the future and perhaps with the aim of leaving others a reminder or legacy (Reynolds 1997).

11.5 NORMALIZING THE ILLNESS EXPERIENCE

Some patients do not seem to encounter the negative experiences outlined above. In interviews at least, they 'normalize' their experience. Rather than allowing the illness to occupy a central place in their lives, they refuse to let it disrupt current roles and future plans, and tend to minimize the effects that it has had on self-image. Crossley (2000) noted that some of her interviewees with HIV infection described their illness experience in this way. A study of adolescents with cystic fibrosis found that most viewed their illness as a normal part of life, not as a catastrophe (Admi 1996). Despite statistical evidence showing that many people with cystic fibrosis die before the age of 40, the young people in this study did not appear to be preoccupied with anxiety about their own futures, and were making plans like others of their age.

Some people seem to defend themselves against experiencing the anxiety-provoking aspects of illness. Denial as a defence mechanism can serve a positive function in maintaining hope and well-being, although it may give way to a painful period of adjustment later on if and when symptoms worsen. Crossley (2000) also suggests that some people's roles and obligations (for example, as breadwinner or father in the family) are so powerfully self-defining that the illness is not 'allowed' to intrude. However, it is only possible to normalize some illnesses in this way. The person is unlikely to be able to ignore the functional impact of increasing muscle weakness that may occur in a neurological condition such as multiple sclerosis. Familiarity with illness may also lead to the person regarding their health problem as 'normal'. Those who have lived with a condition for many years – indeed a lifetime for those with inherited diseases such as cystic fibrosis – are less likely to focus on loss. Some people do not regard disease or impairment as a barrier to achieving positive life goals, but instead endeavour to raise awareness of the many barriers created by environmental design and societal attitudes. They explicitly reject 'tragic' or 'heroic' interpretations of illness/impairment (Morris 1993; see Section 17.4).

11.6 EXPERIENCING ILLNESS IN POSITIVE TERMS

Although, understandably, many healthy people anticipate that long-term illness would be a wholly negative and stressful experience, some with direct experience of chronic health problems come to view their illness as having at least some positive aspects. There are some people – even with extremely debilitating conditions – who argue that illness has for them been 'a blessing' (Young & McNicoll 1998, Mohr et al 1999, Petrie et al 1999, Reeves et al 1999).

Looking back at the case examples, we would need to ask Robert & Sue directly to understand their personal interpretations of the meanings of long-term illness. Yet it seems from the two brief accounts that illness has not been a wholly negative experience. For both, it has been a stimulus to contribute to others' well-being. Sue is actively engaged in charity fund-raising, and Robert creates newsletters to inform and provide support to others in a similar situation. Sue appears to be using her early retirement from work to explore her artistic talents and interests, and enjoys public acclamation for her work. Robert is gaining expertise in the research literature on cystic fibrosis, and in desk-top publishing skills. It seems that both appreciate the deep concern and care shown by family members. Some of the research evidence relating to the positive framing of illness will be considered further.

11.6.1 ILLNESS CAN PROVIDE OPPORTUNITIES FOR DEEP FRIENDSHIP/ FAMILY CLOSENESS

Although for some people chronic illness brings about distressing changes in family relationships, such as transforming intimate partners into 'carers', for others it deepens closeness and affection (Petrie et al 1999). Where family members and friends show unconditional support and acceptance, the person's sense of belonging is enhanced and his or her sense of identity is more likely to withstand assault by the illness.

Illness may not only deepen ties within the family, but may lead to the development of meaningful *new* relationships. Because illness so often contracts social networks, research has rarely examined the *expansion* of social networks during illness. However, some people with long-term illnesses use their leisure opportunities to meet others with similar interests, for example, on adult education courses (Reynolds 1997). Others gain new relationships through involvement with self-help organizations (such as multiple sclerosis therapy centres) or volunteering. These new contacts can improve stimulation and quality of life (Day 1991). Social involvement increases the availability of social support, and is likely to strengthen the person's sense of self. It also provides opportunities for the person with a chronic illness to contribute to others (Kleinman 1988).

11.6.2 ILLNESS MAY PRESENT WAYS OF CONTRIBUTING TO OTHERS

Health professionals are so used to regarding the ill person as in need of support that the human need to care for others is often overlooked (Erikson 1982). Yet some people with long-term health problems report much satisfaction from using the opportunities that illness affords to contribute to others, particularly those in similar circumstances. For example, in a study by Reeves et al (1999: 353), a participant with HIV described herself as having a 'mission' to 'get out and get involved'. Participation in self-help organizations (for example, the Multiple Sclerosis Society), advocacy, disability equality training, user involvement in research, charity fund-raising and counselling are diverse examples of ways in which people with long-term health problems are enhancing the lives of others, through bringing their insights, expertise and enthusiasm to 'make a difference'. Nevertheless, it is important to recognize that not all contributions are illness-related. Many people with long-term health problems continue to be active in wider society, teaching skills, doing research, reciprocating care, being neighbourly, and so on.

11.6.3 ILLNESS STIMULATES PHILOSOPHICAL THINKING ABOUT THE MEANING OF LIFE, AND LEADS TO A REVISION OF PRIORITIES

For some people, illness brings about the impetus to think deeply about philosophical issues and life itself. While a heightened sense of mortality can be highly anxiety-provoking, some people find that it encourages transcendence – a focus on the global community and environment – rather than self. The person may reject what they discover to have been a shallow style of living, and endeavour to live authentically. Some argue that without the experience of serious illness, life would almost certainly have continued on its previous unreflective, unsatisfying path.

Crossley (2000) reported that some people in her study described their illness in conversion/personal growth terms, that is, they interpreted their illness as a stimulus for personal growth and self-actualization. The illness experience had resulted in shifted priorities so that remaining energy and time were as a consequence devoted to the things in life that matter most, including relationships, creativity and making a lasting contribution to others. Charmaz (1991) wrote about people with chronic conditions living in the 'intense present', making the most of their opportunities. 'With the intense present comes a sense of urgency – urgency to act, to experience, and to bond with other people' (Charmaz 1991: 246).

Some also argue that shifting one's priorities is protective of psychological well-being (Weitzenkamp et al 2000). By selectively valuing roles and activities that can still be accomplished despite illness or impairment, the person focuses less on the experience of loss and more on the possibilities of personal achievement, thereby enhancing self-esteem.

11.7 THE ILLNESS EXPERIENCE AS PROCESS

Although this chapter has focused upon a variety of responses to chronic illness, both negative and positive, it is important to recognize that the illness experience is not static, and is not 'simply' a matter of symptoms being refracted through the lenses of personal and social values. It is more accurate to portray the illness as a culmination of a lengthy process of meaning-making. In the early stages, the person may be overwhelmed by grief and anxiety. The capriciousness of disease and misfortune may call up questions such as 'Why me?' The person may find it very difficu to adjust to inhabiting an unfamiliar body in an unpredictable world – in other words, wrestling with 'biographical discontinuity' (Bury 1982).

Some people appear gradually able to work through these grieving responses, over months and years. Positive reframing of illness and its implications for life may be one outcome. However, others are unable to find meaning or opportunity in the illness experience and are more likely to become depressed and defeated. Some go through cyclical patterns of response. Where the health condition fluctuates (as in relapsing–remitting forms of multiple sclerosis), an exacerbation of symptoms may bring increased worry and anger. Fresh adaptations need to be made. During periods of relative symptom quiescence, the person may feel more positive about their degree of control, identity and future.

The social context appears to play a part in influencing the process of coming to terms with illness. Highly supportive contexts offer emotional and practical resources for coping, whereas people who live in relative isolation or with critical partners or families may continue to experience illness as highly stressful. Highly visible health problems can attract unwelcome social responses, including prejudice and stigmatization. These add to the burden of illness.

11.8 CONCLUSION

Illness involves more than physical disease or impairment. Although disease processes often result in pain/discomfort, mobility limitations and other physical difficulties, the illness experience is also shaped by much more than the disease itself. Both individual and social–cultural factors influence the meanings of chronic illness. Influenced by personality, values and social context, some individuals respond to long-term conditions with considerable emotional distress, and experience the illness as threatening their core identity. They may doubt their ability to influence the progress of the illness and are highly disturbed by changes that ensue in roles and relationships. Others tend to deny the emotional impact of illness and seek to carry on as normally as possible. Some, perhaps paradoxically, come to regard their illness as life-enhancing, because it has motivated deep reflection, revision of priorities, closer relationships and a more authentic way of living. These various experiences and interpretations have profound influences on the person's coping strategies, and may have long-term effects on physical health and well-being. These issues are examined in Chapter 4.

Chapter 12

Loss, bereavement and grief

Mary F. McAteer

12.1   INTRODUCTION

The emphasis in this chapter is on bereavement by the death of a loved one, which is the ultimate loss. Bereavement is the conceptual basis for understanding many of the losses that confront the physiotherapist (McAteer 1989).

Grief is a universal phenomenon that affects people of every age and culture. Loss of one sort or another permeates almost every aspect of life. It is self-evident that loss and grief are the concern of everyone, yet throughout most of the twentieth century these topics were largely the preserve of psychoanalysts, psychiatrists and sociologists, but were neglected in the curricula of other health professionals. The general public took loss and grief into public ownership, as it were, with the advent of confessional-type television and radio shows along with a myriad of self-development courses. Subjects of such fundamental importance as loss, bereavement and grief should be placed at the very core of a health professional's understanding of human nature. Thanatology, the study of death and its related phenomena and rituals, is a vast resource for physiotherapists who encounter death and dying on an almost daily basis. In the past 30 or so years there has been considerable knowledge acquired in the vast subject of loss and there is a much greater understanding of the nature of grief in the context of the societies in which people live.

Medical literature on death and dying is relatively inaccessible to the public but the increasing use of information technology enables more widespread dissemination of information. There is a paucity of information on death and dying for physiotherapists. Miller et al (1996), using MEDLINE and CINAHL searching for 'physical therapy', 'rehabilitation' and 'grief' from 1982 to 1996, identified only four articles, two of which are attributed to this author (McAteer 1989, 1992). The situation has not changed since Miller's time of writing.

It may be useful at this point to attempt some definition of terms used in this chapter. Walter (1999) provides a concise formulation:

- *Bereavement* is the objective state of having lost someone or something
- *Grief* refers to the emotions that accompany bereavement
- *Mourning* is the behaviour that social groups expect following bereavement.

The exploration of loss and grief first came to global prominence with the work of Sigmund Freud in the early days of the twentieth century. Freud viewed grief and mourning from a psychiatric viewpoint, giving credence to the notion that grief was a disease rather than a response to loss. As a consequence, people were expected to deal with a loss, come to terms with it and generally put it out of their lives quite quickly and neatly. From the 1960s onwards, John Bowlby in particular worked extensively to counter the Freudian approach. Bowlby (1980) published widely on the nature of attachment and loss, chronicling the nature of the extreme distress and disability of bereavement along with a deep understanding of the difficulties of adjustment to permanent loss.

Losses occur in ways other than by death or separation (Olders 1989). Losses in the material world include loss of personal possessions such as money, jewellery, loss of a home due to fire or storm damage, theft of a car. Losses in the physical sense with which physiotherapists are familiar include loss of limb, loss of breast, loss of hair, eyesight, hearing, mobility, independence, and, ultimately, loss of life itself. In the spiritual world, the inner self, people endure loss of self-esteem, loss of faith and trust, to name but a few aspects. Losses may also straddle the categories suggested here when the loss involves home or homeland due to enforced emigration and compulsory or elective rehousing. Miller et al (1996) refer to two categories of loss encountered in physiotherapy: physical, such as in hemiparesis, and symbolic, such as loss of mobility.

It is virtually impossible in one chapter to explore the vast range of losses that affect people. The large number of refugees in the world must cope with multiple losses: those of bereavement, family ties and country of origin. Eisenbruch (1990) proposes a type of cultural bereavement where losses are not only personal but embrace loss of social systems and cultural meanings.

12.2 ATTACHMENT AND LOSS

The underlying feelings around all losses, whether physical or otherwise, are essentially the same but the intensity of the grief is related to the degree of attachment. There are conflicting views on the nature of attachment. Bowlby's (1982) thesis is that attachments come from the need for security and safety. Attachments are formed early in life, are usually directed towards a few specific individuals, and tend to endure throughout a large part of the life cycle. Forming attachments is considered normal for children and adults alike. If it is considered that the aim of attachment behaviour is to maintain bonds of affection, then it is reasonable to expect that situations that endanger these bonds give rise to certain specific reactions. The greater the loss, the more intense and varied the reactions are likely to be. Olders (1989) contends that relationships are so essential for human growth that evolution has provided for pain on separation to ensure that we work on relationships. Giving up childhood attachments is part of normal growth. Bowlby's (1980) view of loss and grief is conceptualized as a form of separation anxiety, the motivation for which is to restore proximity to the lost object. Theories of attachment and loss are fundamental to understanding bereavement and grief yet they frequently neglect the extent to which their subject is historically and culturally defined. The Romanticist ethos of the nineteenth century viewed the breaking of bonds of attachment as a type of destruction of one's identity and a denial of the meaning of life. Twentieth-century modernism, with its emphasis on goals and rationality, would see the breaking of bonds or ties as a good outcome and adjustment and this would be the prevailing view in the professional literature (Stroebe et al 1992). Appreciation of the importance of attachment is fundamental to the understanding and management of all losses. The loss of an attachment to a loved person or of any other significant attachment leads to a prolonged period of distress and disability. The disability following the loss of an attachment is the product of three interlocking factors:

- The pain of the rupture in the bond and the agony of coming to terms with this reality

- The handicapping privation of the missing assets previously derived from the lost person or resource

- The cognitive erosion and reduction in problem-solving capacities and of the will to persevere (Caplan 1990).

12.3 BEREAVEMENT

The British royal family was the focus of many studies of grief, at each end of the twentieth century. The death of Queen Victoria in January 1901 was an event that unsettled Britain and the Empire to an extent that few today could comprehend (Rennell 2000). Although Victoria had reigned for 63 years and was in her ninth decade, her death seemed virtually impossible, such was her strength and stability. The development of telegraphic services and the popularity of the national press ensured that her death was public knowledge throughout Britain within minutes of the announcement. The sense of loss resulted in a massive outpouring of grief that impelled people into the streets and villages, not only to express their grief but also to voice concern for the uncertainty of the future without the guiding hand of the monarch to whom they had a loyal attachment. In 1997, the premature death of Diana, Princess of Wales, was perhaps less about the institution of the royal family than about her youth and beauty and the fact that she was very much loved by ordinary people the world over. While much has been written about Diana, her life and work, the name of Queen Victoria has been evident in bereavement literature since shortly after her death, not only in terms of Victorian culture, but also because of the publicity attendant on her particular grief and mourning practices after the death of her husband, Albert.

Many of the practices and rituals around bereavement in modern society are relics from the Victorian age when infant mortality was commonplace (Walter 1999). In the twenty-first century few children in Western cultures die in infancy and most people go on to live into old age. Death rituals and customs are shaped by the secularist and consumerist society of increasingly greater numbers of older people. Responses to a death will be related to the nature and duration of the attachment, whether the death was sudden or expected, natural, accidental, suicidal or homicidal. The concept of anticipatory grief as described by Worden (1991) suggests that in cases where death is expected due to a protracted illness, there may be time to prepare for the death of a significant person. In such circumstances, the loosening of the emotional ties with the dying person to some extent modifies the great outpouring of grief often experienced at the time of death.

Grief as a subject for research received considerable attention in the twentieth century. Connotations of psychopathology attached to the expression of grief in much of the literature. Ramchandani (1996) points to more than 75 years of investigation in the controversy around the concept of pathological grief and finds the notion rather tenuous. By mid-century, the notion of grief being 'normal' began to emerge.

One of the key researchers in this area was Eric Lindemann, often described as the father of the modern study of grief. His article 'Symptomatology and management of acute grief' (1944) is regarded as a seminal work of such importance that 50 years after its publication the *American Journal of Psychiatry* saw fit to republish the article. Lindemann studied a significant sample of people who were bereaved as a result of a fire in the Coconut Grove Nightclub, Massachusetts, in the autumn of 1942.

12.4 DESCRIPTIONS OF GRIEF

The fire was responsible for the deaths of 500 people, and Lindemann studied 101 bereaved people prospectively in the immediate aftermath.

One of the novel aspects of Lindemann's work was that it described not only the feelings of the survivors but also the physical sensations of their acute grief. His findings point to the principal manifestations of acute grief as being:

1. Somatic distress
2. Preoccupation with the image of the deceased
3. Guilt
4. Hostile reactions
5. Loss of patterns of conduct, manifested by restlessness, lack of daily routine and an inability to sit still
6. Appearance of traits of the deceased in the bereaved.

In almost all descriptions of grief, authors will caution against any neat and ordered progression. Various phases or stages will overlap since emotions are wide-ranging and constantly changing. This caveat is particularly important to health professionals who may, in a mechanistic way, look for a linear progression through the grief process in their clients.

Shock, disbelief and denial may be experienced even when a death is expected but these emotions are likely to last longer and be more intense when the death is unexpected (Sheldon 1998). Typical responses in cases such as the deaths of young people in traffic or drowning accidents are likely to be 'there must be some mistake' or, 'there must be another person of the same name' or 'I don't believe it.' This incredulity echoes the initial response to the diagnosis of a terminal illness as described by Kubler-Ross (1969).

Anger is a common and confusing emotion experienced by bereaved people and is frequently vented on accident and emergency professionals. Murray-Parkes (1975) found in his important study of widows in the first year of bereavement that anger is prevalent around issues such as insurance, lack of funds and other less tangible assets. Later work by Worden (1983) suggested that anger was at the root of many problems associated with the grieving process. Frequently anger is directed at friends and family but when it is directed at the medical profession it may be rationalized by blaming the doctor in charge for the death and in such circumstances complaints may proceed to litigation.

When the shock and anger abate, the reality of the loss makes its impact. Sadness fills the bereaved person's waking hours, and crying and tearfulness are common. The bereaved person goes about their daily business but with despair, in what Karl (1987) calls a coping phase. Aimlessness, apathy, confusion, lack of confidence and indecision take their toll. Crying is a variable feature since tears do not always manifest sadness. Many subjective accounts of bereavement report waking in the morning and for a moment feeling that the death of the loved one was a dream, only to be shattered quickly by the reality of the day to come. During this 'feelings' phase of grief, the physical signs as described by Lindemann (1944) include transient visual and auditory hallucinations of the dead person, restlessness and searching behaviour (Sheldon 1998).

Guilt is widely reported in the literature (Lindemann 1944, Worden 1983, Walsh 1995, Sheldon 1998). Families may feel guilty that they did not get a second opinion, a special nurse, or that they should have dissuaded the patient from having surgery. Others feel guilty at their expression of relief when a loved one has died, even though they may have cared for the person over many years. Parents whose children die are particularly vulnerable to feelings of guilt around the fact that they were unable to ease the child's pain or discomfort (Worden 1983).

Anxiety ranges from a mild sense of insecurity to a more persistent and intense, almost pathological, response. The bereaved person may feel that they will not be able to survive alone, or they may have fears for their own health. Anxiety relates to an awareness of one's own mortality, heightened by the death of a loved one (Worden 1976). The anxiety over the death of his wife prompted C.S. Lewis to write one of the most accessible and powerful descriptions of this phase of bereavement: 'No one ever told me that grief felt so like fear. I am not afraid, but the sensation is like being afraid. The same fluttering in the stomach, the same restlessness, the yawning. I keep on swallowing' (Lewis 1961: 5).

A phase of despair or depression occurs when the bereaved person finds loss of meaning and direction in life (Sheldon 1998). It is at this time when the bereaved person possibly feels the loss in its fullest sense. Apathy makes it difficult for the person to make decisions and this may encourage some dependency (Hegge & Fischer 2000). This depressive aspect of bereavement has been the subject of much research among widows. Close to 50% of American women are widowed by the age of 65 and it seems that the situation is similar elsewhere. For many, the loss of a spouse leads to depression, yet there is variability in responses to widowhood. There are suggestions that where a spouse has been seriously ill for a long time before death, the surviving partner feels relief that their loved one's distress is over, whereas in cases of sudden death there is more distress and greater vulnerability to depression (Carnelly et al 1999).

Acceptance or adjustment comes to the bereaved, in most cases, after time and the person enters the mainstream of daily life. Lay people often speak of 'recovery', which in itself is impossible since the dead person cannot be recovered.

12.5   MOURNING

Mourning a loss is considered an essential part of the restoration process (Imara 1983). There is little doubt that a normal mourning process is necessary after a bereavement in order to promote healing and to enable psychological growth to continue. Olders (1989) suggests indeed that all losses can be considered developmental phases. All societies throughout history have had their own particular funeral and mourning practices. Some cultures banish their dead, burying them quickly and not speaking of them in public, while others retain the bond and honour the memory. An excellent source for this topic, from a sociological perspective, is Walter (1999).

Much of the English-speaking Christian world has been influenced by the Victorian model in which the dead person is buried in a coffin and laid to rest in a graveyard, in many cases either in or adjoining a church-yard. In the twenty-first century, urban sprawl dictates that cremation is the only real option for many funerals. Jews and Muslims bury their dead before sundown on the day of death while Christians may not be buried for several days. Burial may be a very public or an entirely private occasion, depending on the wishes of the dead person, if known, or on the prevailing wishes of the survivors. At any rate, the funeral celebrates a rite of passage for the deceased and is also a rite of passage for the living. Many contemporary authors agree that Western affluent societies are unable to look upon death and its rituals as a rite of passage to be compared with birth, coming of age, marriage and retirement (O'Gorman 1998).

The funeral is a set of psychologically healthy mourning practices for the bereaved, allowing the mourners to act out their grief in the presence of a strong support group. Walter (1999) makes an interesting observation when he refers to the luxury of time and solitude available to middle-class Victorian women to indulge themselves in their sorrow – a facility the poorer classes could not have. In contrast with Western cultures where health professionals view the breaking of bonds with the deceased as the desirable goal, in the Orient, and in Japan in particular, the maintenance of ties with the deceased is not only accepted, but also sustained and nurtured by society through religious ritual. The Shinto and Buddhist religions believe that contact should be maintained with the deceased. In both of these religions the dead person joins the ranks of one's ancestors, remains accessible so the mourner can talk to him or her at the family altar which most Oriental homes have, and in this way the deceased remains with the bereaved (Stroebe et al 1992). This notion resonates with the ancient Celtic beliefs of pre-Christian Ireland where there was a sense of the dead not being absent but being all around the living, minding them and generally looking out for them (O'Donohoe 1997). These practices contrast with modern Western culture where a person offering prayers or gifts at a dedicated altar in their home would most likely be regarded as being in need of treatment for a pathological fixation, since this would not be deemed to be culturally appropriate.

Grief and mourning are inevitably closely linked. In the chaos caused by the death of a loved one, culture becomes the means whereby there is some control over the inevitable and unpredictable: 'The two functions of culture are the integrative, those beliefs and values that give individuals a sense of identity and a sense of security, and the functional, those prescriptions for a behaviour that teach its members the right way to do things, to behave, and to express emotions' (Kagawa-Singer 1998: 1753). Mourning practices have been in place in all societies in order to facilitate the expression of grief. To this end, all the literature refers to the 'tasks' of mourning in order to achieve the grief 'work'. However, Copp (1998) cites Stroebe (1992) in challenging the necessity for any grief work, arguing that there may be potential benefits in not confronting a loss.

The concept of tasks for the bereaved is not entirely new. Most pre-industrial and modern societies recognized that the dying also had tasks such as the desire to make provision for their families and generally to put their affairs in order (Copp 1998).

The influence of developmental theories led Worden (1983, 1991) to identify the tasks of mourning as being to:

1. Accept the reality of the loss
2. Experience the pain of grief
3. Adjust to an environment in which the deceased is missing
4. Withdraw emotional energy from the deceased person and invest it in other relationships (Worden 1983) but revised (Worden 1991) to emotionally relocate the deceased and to move on with life.

12.5.1 TASKS OF MOURNING

Task 1

To accept the reality of a loss by death is not an easy task. The manner of death and the age of the deceased are important factors. With older people, especially if their death has been preceded by a long illness, there is not the same difficulty of realization as when the death is sudden and involves a child or young adult. The sight of the body is the first recognition of what has happened. Even though the survivor may feel quite numb at the time, this image may be recalled in the days and weeks ahead when numbness fades and reality emerges.

The absence of a body leads to prolonged and perhaps complicated grief (Van der Hart 1988). Searches for suspected victims of drowning accidents, earthquakes, avalanches, air crashes and other disasters are constantly portrayed on television news programmes. When hope of finding a person alive has vanished, the intent to find the body and restore it to the relatives is of equal urgency as the search, such is the recognition of the importance of this task. Parents who have been dissuaded from seeing the body of their child killed in a mutilating accident are likely to experience difficulty and regret at a later stage (Jones 1988).

Accepting the reality of death is likely to be facilitated when loved ones play a part in preparing the body for burial. In some societies and religions there are clear directives as to who performs this task. In Western cultures and in the USA in particular, death has become sanitized to such an extent that when the mortician's art has been employed, the dead person looks not only alive, but also better groomed than they were in life. This deception, along with euphemistic language such as 'gone to sleep' or 'resting with the angels' helps to deny reality. The challenge lies in deciding which coping strategy suits the individual who has been bereaved; in not succumbing to any dogma. Rituals at time of burial or cremation further help to confirm the reality of the death, especially if they take place after an interval of several days. Keeping the bedroom or study of a dead person exactly as they left it creates a type of shrine, and in Western thought, this is considered denial of the death. However, Queen Victoria kept a symbolic shrine to Prince Albert by having his former valet lay out his clothes each day as though her husband were still alive. Since mourning is about coping with reality, this author suggests that if the queen derived comfort from this practice, a more enlightened view should be taken than to consign her behaviour to maladaptation.

Task 2

To experience the pain of grief is to give expression to the range of emotions which includes, among others, sadness, pining, anger, guilt and regret. How people manifest these responses is as variable as are the people themselves. Expressions of grief, like funeral practices, are to a considerable extent culturally determined. There are also gender differences to be considered. There are perceptions among lay people and bereavement workers that women find it easier than men to express the pain of grief. Yet, hospice researchers in the state of Colorado who studied men and women and their responses to spousal bereavement using the Grief Experience Inventory found no significant differences between the two groups (Quigley & Schatz 1999). But the unequivocal view of Clare (2000) is that men find it difficult to express their feelings, to reach out and ask for help. Men are more isolated, psychologically and socially, and they have fewer close personal supports than women do. Feelings of helplessness are difficult for most men and women to acknowledge and express.

Many people today actively seek counselling services, both professional and voluntary, because there is considerable recognition of the need for release or catharsis. It is now considered the norm that after large-scale accidents or other disasters helping and counselling agencies are put in place. One of the main reasons for this type of intervention is to facilitate the expression of feelings and to give legitimacy to them, whatever form they take. Examples of disasters where the bereaved received counselling intervention along with the rescue and health workers are the Lockerbie bombing in 1988 and the Oklahoma City bombing in 1995. One of the terrible tragedies of the twentieth century occurred in the village of Aberfan in Wales in 1966. The collapse of a colliery spoil heap resulted in the deaths of 116 children and 28 adults. A case study of the management of this disaster suggests that many of the inadequacies of the government responses of the time are still extant in the current UK methods of dealing with man-made disasters (Johnes 2000).

To experience the pain of grief is an intensely private and individual experience, even where there is open and public expression of the feelings. It would be unwise to assume because a bereaved person does not show feelings that feelings are not dealt with. Many people deal with the gamut of emotions while containing them. Others may express their grief through music, art, writing or visiting the cinema. A substantial minority does not show any significant distress after a major loss (Exline et al 1996).

Task 3

The task of adjusting to life without the deceased may necessitate practical adjustments depending on the relationship with the person who has died. Almost all the research in this area concerns spousal bereavement, which, in turn, depends on the nature of the marital bond. Loss of a loved one has many connotations. It may mean loss of breadwinner, loss of best friend, sexual partner, banker, cook, gardener and so on. Sheldon (1998) found that a dependent or ambivalent relationship with the deceased made the adjustment more difficult. Bereaved people have the self-imposed task of searching for meaning in what has happened to them and to look for meaning in the death of a loved one is a painful process (Sheldon 1998). Aristotle, in ancient Greece, recognized that the least bearable of losses was the death of a child before its parents. It may be that when any bereaved person is searching for meaning, they are trying to reclaim order and control of their own life.

Task 4

When Worden wrote the fourth task of mourning in 1983, it was as 'withdrawing emotional energy from the deceased and reinvesting it in another relationship'. He revised the task in 1991 to read 'to emotionally relocate the deceased and move on with life'. His rationale in the rewording was that the original task sounded too mechanical, almost like pulling a plug and reattaching it somewhere else. The concept of relocation facilitates an ongoing relationship with the deceased, but one that allows people to continue their lives in a meaningful way. It is when this task is embraced that widows and widowers would feel happy and willing to enter into a new partnership or marriage, not leaving their dead partner behind but rather taking them with them in a less prominent place.

The processes of mourning will take varying periods of time, ranging from months to years. Society supports the bereaved in many ways but some mourners are denied societal affirmation when the loss is either covert or secretive. Situations of this nature might include those who grieve for:

- Unborn babies lost through miscarriage, stillbirth or abortion
- Small babies or very young children
- A pet which has died
- A homosexual partner or lover
- A divorced or separated partner
- A dead person with whom they had a secret relationship (Walsh 1995).

12.6 DETERMINANTS OF GRIEF

As mentioned earlier, loss and grief are directly related to the nature of the attachment. Nevertheless there are a number of factors that may help to predict the emotional and cognitive responses to any loss, and to bereavement in particular:

1. Who the person was. It is almost axiomatic that the intensity of grief is determined by the intensity of love. Grief for the death of a spouse or a child is vastly different to the grief over the death of a grandparent, for example.

2. The nature of the attachment, as to its strength and security. For some people the greater attachment is to friends as distinct from family members. For health professionals working with children, for example, Pfefferbaum et al (2000) cautioned that loss of a friend or acquaintance as opposed to a relative was significant as a cause of post-traumatic stress symptoms.

3. The ambivalence of the relationship. In any close relationship where the person is loved there are almost inevitably some negative feelings as well. Usually the positive feelings far exceed the negative ones, but in a highly ambivalent relationship where the negative feelings coexist in almost equal proportion, there is likely to be a more difficult grief reaction due to feelings of guilt and possibly anger at being left alone (Worden 1991).

4. The nature of the death will have an important influence on how the survivor grieves. Of the traditional categories of natural, accidental, suicidal and homicidal, there is considerable evidence that suicide brings unique problems for the bereaved (Exline et al 1996). Any death involving a perceived 'stigma' may be problematic.

5. The bereaved person's mental health and history of dealing with other losses are relevant. There is a perception that people with a history of depressive illness and those with anxious and insecure temperaments fare worse in coping with bereavement (Exline et al 1996), but research by Carnelly et al (1999) suggests that prior depression does not make a woman more vulnerable to depressed mood following the loss of her spouse.

6. Cultural factors. Ethnic and religious subcultures provide rituals for most life events including death, burial and mourning. Much is written in bereavement literature about the funeral rites of Irish Catholics and Orthodox Jews in determining a healthy grief process but the evidence is largely anecdotal. Sheldon (1998) claims that people from minority cultural or ethnic groups may experience problems if, at the time of death, they are unable to follow the rituals and customs they feel to be appropriate.

7. The bereaved person's ability to cope without a significant person. If a person masters his or her problems by working out effective means of coping, he or she may emerge from the experience with increased competence and resilience. Eventual mastery of the burdensome experience involves reorganization of the individual's 'assumptive world', namely of the individual's intrapsychic maps of external reality and internal system for guiding and motivating behaviour (Caplan 1990).

12.7 HEALTH FOLLOWING BEREAVEMENT

Physiotherapists are concerned largely but not solely with the physical health of the patient, and physiotherapists use largely but not exclusively physical means to treat the patient. There are a myriad of health implications following bereavement and any other significant loss. Lindemann's (1944) major contribution to the understanding of grief was the recognition of the somatic as well as the psychological signs. The pain of grief has been a rich resource for poets, musicians and artists through the ages. The classic 'broken heart' was given credibility by Murray-Parkes (1985) on the basis of his extensive research into the death of a spouse, which is followed in many cases by the death of the surviving partner from heart disease. There is a significant increase in death rates from heart disease in men in the year following their wife's death. The death of a spouse has long been recognized as one of life's most stressful experiences (Schleifer et al 1983). Few survivors of conjugal loss can be healthy in the first year of bereavement, given the range of physical symptoms such as tightness in the throat, shortness of breath, nausea (Lindemann 1944); headaches, dry mouth, lump in the throat, aching limbs (Murray-Parkes 1975); hollowness in the stomach, sleep and appetite disturbances (Worden 1991). American health care cost analyses show that harmonious marriages have a protective effect on health while widowhood costs twice as much (Prigerson et al 2000).

Bartrop et al (1977) provided the first laboratory confirmation of the link between bereavement and the immune system. Schleifer et al (1983) demonstrated a significant suppression of lymphocyte response in the first 2 months after the death of a spouse. It is possible that this suppression of the immune system is, in turn, affected by the changes in sleep patterns, food and drink consumption and levels of exercise. In the acute distress that follows many bereavements, physical symptoms surface which are often a facsimile of the symptoms of the deceased (Sheldon 1998). It has been known for some time that grief and mourning exert direct effects on neurotransmitters or neurohormones such as cortisol, ACTH, or noradrenaline (norepinephrine) (Olders 1989).

12.8 OTHER LOSSES

Failure to mourn any loss can result in psychopathology or psychosomatic illness and appropriate mourning equates with healing (Olders 1989). Losses other than by death have long been recognized as predictors of change in health status. The Holmes-Rahe Scale of Stress ratings list various losses such as divorce, jail term, son or daughter leaving home, and retirement. The rapidly developing science of psychoneuroimmunology will probably offer more enlightenment on the many connections between mind and body that will contribute to existing knowledge on loss and grief.

12.8.1 AMPUTATION

An important study by Murray-Parkes (1972) identified the loss of a limb as one of the most stressful losses outside of bereavement. He identified the components of the reaction to loss of a limb and loss of a spouse. With the help of a study by Marc Fried, he compared his results with Fried's analysis of the loss of a home due to compulsory rehousing. A brief consideration of his findings indicates the similarities in reaction to bereavement and amputation: both widows and amputees reported shock and numbness in the first hours or days after the loss. During this time, there was a strong sense of denial. In the widow it was expressed as a sense of incredulity while in the amputee it was one of puzzlement – he saw that his leg was gone but he felt that he should still be able to move it. In the amputee, there is a known physiological basis for the phenomenon of the phantom limb. In the widow, the strong sense of the presence of the dead husband demonstrates the similarity of the two phenomena. The shock or numbness was followed by a period of distress, the so-called 'pangs of grief'. This period was common to both widows and amputees and was characterized by crying and extreme sadness. When sadness abated, the grieving widow and the amputee each expressed apathy and depression. Amputees experienced a sense of mutilation that served to accent their separation anxiety. Murray-Parkes suggested that grief is the means by which amputees began to come to terms with the loss of limb. Just as the manner of death influences grieving, so also must the nature of the amputation. Traumatic amputation associated with accidents may be compared to the shock of a sudden death. Elective amputation may have been preceded by years of pain and, possibly, anticipatory grief so that when the decision to amputate is reached, patients may be somewhat prepared for it and may even view it as a life-enhancing procedure since it may provide complete pain relief after years of suffering.

The emotional sequelae to amputation are similar to those of bereavement and should be recognized by the physiotherapist as deserving the same attention as other aspects of impairment and disability (McAteer 1989). Murray-Parkes (1972) outlined the elements for a successful outcome to spousal bereavement and loss of a limb:

1. Realization of the loss
2. Preservation and protection of the damaged self
3. Old models of the world relinquished, new models developed
4. Relationship to new external objects in a satisfying manner.

Murray-Parkes's work on this topic predates Worden's tasks but the similarities are evident.

12.8.2 SPINAL CORD INJURIES

The sudden and often dramatic onset of paraplegia or tetraplegia is one of the most traumatic of all experiences, bringing with it the fear of total dependence on others, helplessness and sexual dysfunction. People thus devastated are in the unique position of grieving for themselves insofar as life as it previously was is gone but the body and mind live on. There are no mourning rituals to help people traumatized in this way, but the role of the physiotherapist, along with other members of the care team, is to facilitate the patient's passage from an able-bodied person to a disabled but functioning one. Friedman-Campbell & Hart (1984) stated that spinal-injured people or others suffering chronic illnesses could be understood and cared for when bereavement was the conceptual model.

Using the 'tasks of mourning' concept, the first task is for the patient to accept the reality of the loss of function. This is difficult to accept when the patient is in a state of shock, even if he or she has had a full explanation as to the extent of the injuries. Intensive care aimed at preventing further deficit may create in the patient's mind a sense of false expectation of recovery. Only as acceptance begins to surface can the patient begin to cope with denial and despair. Some patients may begin the process of realization based on their own deductions. When, in time, the person begins to feel the pain of grief, anxiety, anger, guilt, sadness, hopelessness and crying, these affective aspects of loss may compound the extreme physiological changes that are due to the spinal lesion. Sooner or later, the patient will start to adapt to the changed environment and relationships with people and places. This task involves not only physical adaptations but emotional, financial and vocational adjustments also. The final stage of coping is in withdrawing emotional energy from the bodily losses and investing it in new models of the world. This may be the most difficult task of all, involving as it does being able to contemplate the loss without undue pain but accepting that the loss is permanent. Christopher Reeve believes that spinal cord injuries will, in time, be cured but despite the momentum in research he is more subdued than he was when first he became a powerful fundraiser and advocate for the cause. He poignantly articulates the sense that in physical losses, just as in bereavement, there is not recovery, but adaptation:

> I have to admit that I wake up every morning and have to get over the shock of not being able to move. I am still jealous when I watch others merely stand up and stretch or walk down a hallway. Every time I think about all I took for granted in the past – making love, sailing, acting on stage, or simply giving a friend a hug – I am conflicted between the desire to revisit these memories and to keep them alive, or to try to let them go now that they are receding further into the distance (Reeve 1999: 299).

Not all disabled people, however, feel that their situation is tragic or undesirable (see Chs 4 and 17).

12.9 DEALING WITH LOSS

It has not been this author's intention to suggest any particular way of dealing with loss in the context of physiotherapy practice. It is hoped that the knowledge presented in this chapter will enhance the interactions between physiotherapists and their patients. A therapeutic, empathic milieu will encourage the re-emergence of personal worth and dignity when rehabilitation programmes are based on appropriate knowledge, skills and attitudes. There are some suggestions from the literature:

1. The patient's coping and ego mechanisms must be given time to work. He or she must be allowed to express anger, sadness, guilt, inadequacy, unusual humour, and even hatred.

2. Should the patient manifest non-destructive mechanisms such as shouting, it is important that he or she knows he or she is still accepted, even if the behaviour is not acceptable.

3. The physiotherapy programme should contain realistic challenges to encourage self-motivation and, consequently, self-worth.

4. There must be no delay in responding to the patient's problems. Prompt attention affirms the patient that he or she is a cherished human being.

Each individual has a personal timeframe for healing and rehabilitation. Professionals must let the process run its course (Stewart & Shields 1985).

Physiotherapists working in the area of women's health will be likely to have preparation for dealing with loss by stillbirth, spontaneous abortion and infant mortality. Central to an understanding of these particular losses is the understanding of attachment, coupled with the age-old fantasy of a perfect child, which starts in early pregnancy. The birth of a disabled child may mean the loss of the dream that was anticipated during the pregnancy (Worthington 1989). The unwilling separation from this bond of affection may result in distress, anxiety, anger, depression and emotional detachment. Parents experiencing losses such as this may need particular understanding on the part of health professionals.

It should be borne in mind that women are more accustomed than men to making transitions in their lives. Health professionals can make an important contribution by increasing their understanding of men's needs. Early pregnancy loss occurs in one in four pregnancies. The role of men, as they share their feelings and try to support their partners, has received little attention. Miscarriage is a painful and difficult situation for men. Their own feelings may not be acknowledged and yet they have to cope with the feelings of grief in their partner (Murphy & Hunt 1997).

Older men and women who have been bereaved may have deteriorating physical and mental health and may need alternative living arrangements for proper care. Referrals to social services or other agencies may relieve daily stresses. Home care or other home support services may be needed to keep widows and widowers in their own homes for as long as possible. Their readiness for institutional life should be ascertained before decisions are made to effect major changes. Sensitivity to the person's cumulative losses and their fear of dependence must be maintained (Hegge & Fischer 2000).

12.10 CONCLUSION

An attempt has been made to explore the nature of grief and mourning with specific reference to the physical and psychological manifestations that are likely following the death of a loved one. Most of the literature has dealt with spousal bereavement. The incidents and states that evoke a grief reaction are myriad. The diagnosis of a terminal illness has not been discussed here as was done in the second edition of this book. Bereavement forms the basis for understanding a wide range of losses, both physical and symbolic or conveyed losses. The degree of loss and grief is determined by the nature of the attachment. Miller et al (1996) urge physiotherapists to recognize their active role in supporting a grieving client. In providing client-centred care, physiotherapists must consider the client's grief and incorporate emotional goals along with physical ones when formulating a plan of treatment and management. Central to most treatment plans is physiotherapeutic intervention for pain. Physiotherapists have long departed from simplistic views of pain as always having a mechanical or readily identifiable cause. It is difficult to accept that physiotherapists working with patients with chronic illnesses, in extended care or in palliative care, would not have an understanding of the emotional and spiritual dimensions of pain. The helplessness of many people seems to make their pain worse. Wall (1999) contends that pain is merely one fact of the sensory world in which we live and that it is 'inherently ridiculous' to consider pain as an isolated entity.

Linguistically, pain and suffering are often intertwined, but Clarke (2000) contends that many patients experience suffering rather than pain. Physiotherapists frequently encounter patients whose distress and discomfort appear disproportionate to the underlying pathology or impairment and Clarke's view of suffering is distinct from pain and more about the process whereby people lose an acceptable idea of themselves, through disease or life events. Physiotherapists seeing newly referred patients will recognize the anxieties and threat to self-image that accompany illness and disability (McAteer 1993). It may be reasonable to assume that in everyday physiotherapeutic interventions there may be more covert grief than one would immediately estimate.

Understanding loss and grief requires a receptive and sensitive approach. Boundaries should not be drawn around a body of knowledge that is finitely physiotherapeutic when it comes to something as ubiquitous as loss.

SECTION 3

Patients and practitioners

Chapter **13**

Professions and professional work

Jackie Waterfield

13.1 INTRODUCTION

For many, physiotherapy has been, and always will be, referred to as a profession (Richardson 1992). However, by definition it would appear to fall into the category of a 'semi-profession' (Etzioni 1969). One way of trying to address the professional status of physiotherapy has been through education (Chartered Society of Physiotherapy 1979a), on the assumption that changes in education will enhance other attributes associated with professionalism, such as autonomy and social status.

Professionalization is considered a process, rather than an event or an ascribed status (Johnson 1972, Houle 1980). Note that achievement of professional status implies the attributes of professionalism, and if these attributes are lacking, a claim to professional status is likely to fail. However, it is possible for those who have not formally achieved professional status to exhibit the same attributes, that is to say attitudes and values (such as altruistic concern, an ethical orientation to practice), as those who have (Sim 1985). Accordingly, physiotherapy has tried to mould its own professional development in fields such as postgraduate education, research and titled roles, to achieve professional recognition and possibly to achieve a similar status to that of medicine. However, the question remains: what value is the label 'profession' to an occupational body such as physiotherapy?

This chapter will initially discuss the general area of professionalism and then focus on the issues of education, autonomy and altruism in relation to physiotherapy, and the professional work that its members carry out.

13.2 PROFESSIONALISM

13.2.1 CHARACTERISTICS

Bottery (1998) suggests that there are several key characteristics held by professions: *expertise*, the notion that the occupational group have exclusive knowledge and practice; *altruism*, or an ethical concern for others; and *autonomy*, in relation to control of both entry to the profession and the nature of practice carried out within it. Physiotherapy is categorized as a 'semi-profession' by defining characteristics such as its membership being predominantly female (Short 1986) and working in large institutions. The terms 'profession' and 'occupation' are in many cases used interchangeably, which perhaps reflects the way in which the language relating to professionalism and professionalization is culturally based. This has not helped in giving a clear picture of the global development of professions and professionalization, as a substantial amount of archival evidence comes from the USA or the UK and not from non-English-speaking communities (Burrage 1990). Many of the emerging professions, among which occupational therapy classes itself (Barclay 1994), or the semi-professions, are measured against the traditional professions such as law, medicine and the church. However, society has changed since these traditional professions were established, and they too have evolved over time; the church, for example, may no longer even be considered a profession. Therefore, is this established model of a profession just an abstract concept (Selander 1990) or of any value in defining issues relevant to practice?

13.2.2 SOCIETY AND STATUS

Professions have to practise in an economic and social context, characterized by increasing market forces (Bottery 1998), which may place boundaries around their practice. The concept of a profession should therefore be seen as socially constructed, and subject to change in relation to the social situations in which people live. Purtilo (1986) suggests that physiotherapists as professionals should develop a sense of responsibility to both their own professional life and the protection of the society within which their profession functions. Thereby, an occupational niche is found which is normally based around widely agreed societal concerns; for physiotherapy this niche is health care (Jackson 1970). Society gives status to the professions by valuing their skills and knowledge, and there is therefore an onus on professionals not to abuse this position. This also places a responsibility on professionals to reflect on the ever-changing domain in which they work and reassess their role in society.

Medicine, an established profession, has been used to a high-status profile, based on the knowledge and skills that it has acquired (Coburn & Willis 2000, Harrison & Ahmad 2000), and to which the general public has had little or no access. This position has been achieved sometimes to the detriment of other occupations that historically delivered health care, particularly before a National Health Service (NHS) was formed in the UK (Witz 1992). Thus, through both academic and legislative control, medicine has forced many occupations into subservient roles (for example, midwives, physiotherapists), consequently excluding them from the category of profession and the accompanying benefits. Note that this societal status often brings not only financial rewards but also power and control to professional bodies and individual members (Wilensky 1964, Burrage 1990, Witz 1992). However, the traditional view of these characteristics on which professions have been based may no longer be of value in negotiating a place in today's society, and with the political bodies that influence and determine the work agenda.

13.2.3 PROFESSIONALIZATION

Professionalization is a diverse and variable process with both social and historical links, and while some professions share similar processes of professionalization, others may be quite unique (Wilensky 1964, Siegrist 1990, Evetts 1999). This process includes the internalization of professional values and practices through education. It determines such things as what a novice professional will pay attention to, how knowledge and theory influence practice, how individuals perceive the purpose of the profession as a whole, and how professional goals can be achieved. Hence, a professional paradigm is developed and while, as Parsons (1968) suggested, there might be ambiguity at the fringes, the central occupational characteristics are strong.

For physiotherapy in the UK, professionalization through formal education began in 1956 when degree education was sought, initially only for those involved in teaching or occupying positions of professional leadership. By 1992, physiotherapy in the UK had become an all-graduate profession, but its professional status still seemed unconfirmed. A first (bachelors) degree was the educational goal of UK physiotherapy, but in the USA the profession has for several years had entry by masters degree only, and is now considering doctorate-level entry (Simmonds 2000). Australia and the UK now have masters programmes that give licence to practise, but that are not called physiotherapy degrees. It is interesting to consider how this diversity in professional education affects the understanding of what a physiotherapist is – for the individual professional, for the profession itself and for the public. With increased globalization it is also interesting to consider this diversity internationally.

13.2.4 PROFESSIONAL EDUCATION

Higgs et al (2001) suggest that physiotherapy education is about graduating competent practitioners. Formalizing education was initially based on a belief that this education must be seen by other professionals to be of adequate standing in order that the evaluative judgement of physiotherapists would be respected. Hence, it became imperative for physiotherapy to be recognized as a suitable subject for inclusion in higher education (Chartered Society of Physiotherapy 1979a). A degree, it was suggested, would not only improve quality of care for patients but would also offer a better career structure and status for the practitioner (Piercy 1979). These latter issues have become an increasing concern with regard to staff retention and recruitment within the UK health system (Newman 1997, 2001). So education – both its length and level – has become more central in both establishing professional status and suggesting a specialized and superior knowledge base for professions. A degree has made the practitioner much more marketable and opportunities for employment are no longer confined to the government-provided health care system; increasingly, the private sector, industry and overseas posts offer greater financial rewards, often with better working conditions. So while graduate level education may be a means of advancing the status of the profession, this now presents a problem for the service the profession was primarily created to serve, and which in the UK currently funds the qualifying education of the professional.

13.2.5 APPRENTICESHIP OR FORMAL EDUCATION

The 'true' professions of medicine, law and theology were founding subjects for many universities and it is suggested that the increase in the number of professions may be linked with the rise in the number of universities (Johnson 1972) and greater access to higher education. This form of education moves away from apprenticeship or experiential learning, with its emphasis on craft knowledge, towards a more 'intellectual' education, or knowledge for knowledge's sake (Teichler 1999). The UK nurse education Project 2000 is an example of where the *apprentice* has become a *student*, illustrating a move from a service-led training to an education-led training (Grindle & Dallat 2000). Teichler (1999) suggests that the opportunity to explore 'knowledge about knowledge' may be beneficial in becoming aware of the norms, values and assumptions underpinning one's own scope of practice. Education, rather than training, also offers the opportunity to develop new knowledge and practice, rather than possibly just operating within the traditional boundaries of practice. For physiotherapy, it was argued that a degree course would offer a more systematic intellectual stimulus, producing evaluative students and more research or evidence (Onuoha 1981). Hence, physiotherapy's unique body of knowledge, autonomy and professional status would increase.

It would appear that a certain amount of discordance exists between the two approaches to education – 'intellectual' and 'practical' – to which universities contribute, as they have developed the role of legitimizing expertise through intellectual knowledge. For physiotherapy, skills and knowledge are equally important and the 'art or science' debate within physiotherapy (Peat 1981) continues. Gesser (1985, cited in Selandar 1990) describes a concept of 'scientification of the occupations' where specific research, language and a university education can be important to both professions and occupations, but Selander (1990) suggests that scientification and professionalization are not synonymous. Interestingly, in establishing itself as a profession, physiotherapy has initially tried to emulate the scientific methods of medicine (Ritchie 1999), yet this suggests a reductionist approach – the kind from which many health professions allied to medicine have tried to break free as a means of defining themselves as equal to, but 'different' from, medicine.

Ludmerer (1999) reflects what many practising therapists doubtless feel: that formal courses alone are insufficient to develop professionalism, and that interaction with peers, role models, other disciplines and clients, both within the academic field and in the real world of work, is important (Becher 1996). However, this integrated form of socialization can have its own problems. For example, not all mentors of new professionals will necessarily have similar attitudes to those advocated by the professional body (Ludmerer 1999, Richardson 1999b); nor do they necessarily have the skills to mentor (Williams & Webb 1994). Some would argue that it may be in the best interests of the profession to keep newer recruits away from established members (Chartered Society of Physiotherapy 1979b). There also remain the questions: how long is needed to develop appropriate professional attitudes, and who is to be the judge of this?

How education is structured will perpetuate the debate between skills and knowledge. Managers perceive competence through the ability to complete tasks safely, efficiently and effectively (Clouder 2000a), so they appear to be very *product*-orientated. Educationalists, meanwhile, want students to be reflective and evaluative and hope to develop practitioners who will continue to learn throughout their professional life; here the emphasis is on the *process*. Another balance must be struck between increasing one's self-knowledge and the professional knowledge base (Clouder 2000b). Professionalism should incorporate all these things, but again external pressures may come from the social and institutional context in which the professional practises.

13.3 KNOWLEDGE

Currier (1984) and Higgs & Titchen (2000) suggest that a profession possesses a unique body of knowledge that is different from that of other professions, such that it defines and delineates professional boundaries. However, it is becoming more difficult to define this uniqueness as knowledge increasingly crosses boundaries. For example, the use of qualitative research in health care in determining policy and practice demonstrates the impact of social science upon an area traditionally governed by the tenets of science (Taylor 1911). Perhaps more important in distinguishing one profession from another is the context in which the knowledge is utilized, and physiotherapy considers this in its search for professional status. Therefore, education must allow for specialist knowledge to be developed, and encourage research and practice that preserve the uniqueness of the different professions (Richardson 1999a).

For professions, it is suggested that this knowledge should be acquired through a substantial period of education and professional socialization; so education can be seen as a form of initiation to a profession. If socialization is important then a form of occupational control is exercised over recruitment – that is, a process of training and licensing through formal awards and professional standards of practice to ensure that only certain types of members are allowed into the profession from the beginning (Jackson 1970). While physiotherapy is a popular educational course in the UK (Green & Waterfield 1997), access is still limited; for example, men and minority groups are still underrepresented. This is an important issue, if it is felt that a profession should represent the society it serves.

The relationship between professional governing bodies – such as the Chartered Society of Physiotherapy, the American Physical Therapy Association and the Canadian Physiotherapy Association – and external factors – such as the state (Johnson 1972) – will influence professionalization and the control of educational processes. This balance of control is related to another attribute of a profession to be considered in the next section: autonomous action.

A negative consequence of having strong demarcations in the skills and knowledge between occupations (Witz 1992) is that accessibility to areas of work is reduced (a form of occupational control), as is the mobility of the workforce (Francis & Humphreys 2000). Also, if education is too narrow in its scope and focuses only on immediate practice needs, there is a concern that it will inhibit the development of innovation and preparation for indeterminate tasks. This ability to adapt and apply both craft and knowledge to complex, novel problems is a key aspect of professionalism (Southon & Braithwaite 1998, Teichler 1999). Clearly, a balance is needed.

13.4 PROFESSIONAL AUTONOMY

13.4.1 AUTONOMY

Autonomy for physiotherapy is about providing high-quality practice (Higgs et al 2001) and a responsibility or duty of care to the recipient of such practice. Health practitioners are increasingly being asked to demonstrate this accountability (Evetts 1999, Grimmer et al 2000), as well as consider the issues of cost-effectiveness, more than they ever used to. The consumers of health care, both patients and purchasers, want to be part of the decision-making process and are no longer content to take the professional's word as truth, often seeking independent opinion (Dauphinee & Norcini 1999). There is an assumption, particularly in medicine (Mirvis 1993), that these consumers cannot evaluate practice, because of the technical nature of the profession's knowledge and skills. Thus, if evaluation is attempted by an outside body, this is deemed to be an infringement on the autonomous function of professions to regulate themselves. However, Irvine (1997) suggests that if the public is involved in the process of standardization of practice and education, then trust is more likely to be developed between public and profession. This trust can then be interpolated from the profession as a whole down to the individual practitioner, thereby enhancing rather than reducing autonomy, and reinforcing societal status. Thus, just as professionalism is a social construct, so professionals must accept that policy formation is also a social action and should not be seen as an imposition on practitioners, threatening their autonomy. Bottery (1998) recommends that professionals should participate in the process of making and evaluating policy. Professionals need to acknowledge that they can only give what they have the right to give, that is their specialist knowledge and skills, and only then in the context of what has been determined by public policy to be available to the consumer (Mirvis 1993). This suggests that it would be 'unprofessional' not to be part of the policy process and that contributing to policy formation actually strengthens and broadens the altruistic role of a profession.

So autonomy can exist at several levels. Clinical decision-making is still an autonomous practice for the health professional (Harrison & Ahmad 2000), but this cannot be exercised without due regard to cost. Professions therefore need to be 'managed'; however this management may mean increasing legislation, both about practice and about the context of practice. Some practitioners may consider the introduction of, for example, guidelines and protocols a positive means of standardizing practice, offering equity and parity to all recipients of health care, while others may feel it reduces professional autonomy and constrains practice (Garfield & Garfield 2000). Any changes through standardization, either at an institutional or at a societal level, need to be evidence-based and negotiated by professionals and the policy makers. Sometimes, these changes may also produce a feeling that 'management' is being devolved downwards, such that those directly involved in patient care have less time to do the 'real' job. Clearly, professions and their practice need to be both transparent and accountable to consumers and commissioners, but this will mean their autonomy will come under pressure. A more negative view of this phenomenon is that this transparency may give the state information that might actually be used to legislate against professions (Bottery 1998).

13.4.2 EVIDENCE–BASED PRACTICE

Other possible threats to autonomy are perhaps linked with the advent of evidence-based practice (EBP) (though this is not a new concept, and has been around since the eighteenth century). Sackett et al (2000) and other proponents suggest it is about balancing the use of best external evidence, such as that derived from empirical research, the practitioner's expertise, and the rights and preferences of the individual patient. It should encompass financial resources as well as other physical resources, and should be about addressing the greater good. This has met with mixed responses from professions and from individual practitioners within professions (Armstrong 2002). As discussed earlier, some see the development of EBP standards and guidelines as a means of restricting practitioners' autonomy and rationing services, whereas others have welcomed it as a means of defining the skills and knowledge base of their profession. Physiotherapy, as a relatively young semi-profession, has found its empirical evidence lacking in many areas of practice and it has relied on experiential evidence to justify its practice. Some therapy research has been done under the auspices of doctors, with therapists being essentially the research technician; the evidence may, therefore, not be truly applicable to physiotherapy practice. All these factors also impact on the physiotherapist's ability to be truly autonomous and imply that the profession does not have its own knowledge base – again firmly placing it in the category of a semi-profession. Physiotherapy has tried to address this by having graduate entry into its practice, and by increasing the profile of research within the professional body. Interestingly, even though medicine was one of the founding professions, it is suggested that only 20% of its practice is evidence-based (Imrie & Ramey 2000). Ideally, practitioners should share research or evidence for the greater good, but this practice may be inhibited by competition between professions and businesses (Bottery 1998).

13.4.3 CONTINUING PROFESSIONAL DEVELOPMENT (CPD)

All practitioners are encouraged by the profession and their employers to be lifelong learners. Lifelong learning can be defined as 'those novel forms of teaching and learning that equip students (learners, individuals) to encounter with competence and confidence the full range of working, learning and life experiences' (Kogan 2000: 341). However, the process of learning for a role or job may be better described as continuing professional development (CPD); while being part of lifelong learning, it is more circumscribed. It is defined in *A First Class Service* (Department of Health 1998b) as: 'a process of lifelong learning for all individuals and teams that meets the needs of patients and delivers the health outcomes and health care priorities of the NHS and that enables professionals to expand and fulfil their potential'.

CPD includes both formal and informal learning, such as experiential learning. Interestingly, Alsop (2000), Jordan (2000) and Dowswell et al (1997) suggest there is little evidence that improved health outcomes are directly associated with CPD. Moreover, while much of one's professional knowledge could be said to be developed through experiential learning in the workplace, a study by Turner & Whitfield (1997) showed that physiotherapists in Australia and England relied on information gained from formal pre- and post-registration courses to influence their choice of treatment techniques, rather than informal CPD. Increasing concern is also raised, by authors such as Fieldhouse et al (1996) and Marks (1999), that education may be more about 'training' workers for a job, thereby devaluing the other benefits of learning for its own sake (see Section 13.2.5). As a result, competent practitioners may fulfil the needs of both clients and employers and the public face of the profession, but they may not be developing their own knowledge base (Chartered Society of Physiotherapy 2000), or contributing to the knowledge base of the profession. Hicks (1988) feels quite strongly that members of a profession should take responsibility for adding to the professional body of knowledge, as it is how practice is rationalized. Globalization and technology are moving so rapidly that this limited vision of education may restrict innovative development of new knowledge (Wringe 1991, Teichler 1999), such that professions may be unable to compete in future markets.

Increasing technology may also change the current conventional work patterns (Heinz 1999) and health care practice. Therefore, lifelong learning, as earlier defined by Kogan (2000), could also be seen as about equipping workers to deal with this change. CPD is also related to issues of registration to practice, particularly with state health care providers.

Continuing professional registration

It is easier to control the entrance into a profession by admission requirements than to control the continued practice of its members. Policies and initiatives around lifelong learning, standards and EBP may be ways of continuing control post-qualification in the future. Part of the process of professionalization is the development of a profession's codes of conduct (Sim 1985), and professionalism is about individual responsibility to maintain competence to practice. Professional bodies characteristically have rules of professional conduct (Purtilo 1977, Hewison & Sim 1998; see also Section 15.5). If professional autonomy involves working within professional guidelines/codes of practice, where there is a personal commitment to ensure that one remains competent, professions may question the amount of control any further external body, such as (in the UK) the Health Professions Council (HPC), needs to exert. If self-regulation is an attribute of a profession then physiotherapy has achieved this, but in future this may be governed much more by the state. The public's trust in the professions may or may not be increased by this form of state intervention and doubt could be cast on other areas of professionalism.

The consequences of external influences, such as the HPC, identified in the two previous sections may be that practitioners are pressurized to learn primarily to fulfil the requirements of employment and registration. Additionally, the boundaries of professional practice may also be externally defined, resulting in only certain practices being acceptable to those who control employment. As a result, new or evolving aspects of the profession may be reduced and controlled, resulting in a loss of the profession's autonomy and a return to technical status (Wilensky 1964).

Control of practice

Professionalization, if seen as a form of occupational control (Freidson 1994), brings with it educational endorsement and closure of a market, controlling both knowledge and service delivery. Wilensky (1964) suggests that where competence is not exclusive, occupations will look for legal protection of title; this has occurred recently in the UK. This 'closure' suggests that the public may be protected from those who may have little or no relevant knowledge and skills, although Totton (1999) feels that this is not guaranteed. However, it may also be seen to restrict the practice of those already in the occupation, as to gain closure one must define what one does that is distinct from what others do. Parry (1995) and others believe that physiotherapy still cannot define itself. Closure may be beneficial, to a degree, but may also have the negative effect of producing both dissent within the membership and increasing competition in a limited market.

13.5 INTERDISCIPLINARY BOUNDARIES AND WORKING

There has always been a certain rivalry between physiotherapy and other practitioners such as osteopaths, nurses and occupational therapists (Lloyd 1999). Interestingly, a practitioner writing to an internet mailbase for physiotherapists expressed the view that there was more difference within the professions of chiropractic, osteopathy and physiotherapy than between them, and most professions do indeed appear to have factions and an internal hierarchy. Skills and knowledge of different occupational groups may overlap in some areas – for example, intensive care, stroke rehabilitation, low back pain – and this may be seen as a challenge to the uniqueness of physiotherapy as a profession.

Evetts (1999) argues that professionalism is about being able to work interprofessionally, while Kumar (2000) feels that specialization has caused a decrease in communication between disciplines and that to achieve a goal of rehabilitation, that is the greater good, professionals should work multidisciplinarily (Capilouto 2000).

Client-centred professional philosophies identify collaboration between professions as essential (Lloyd 1999). But the mechanisms for such collaboration are as varied as the terminology for this activity, utilizing words such as multidisciplinary, interdisciplinary and transdisciplinary team working which, though often used interchangeably (McCallin 2001), mean different things. In an attempt to clarify issues, Sorrels-Jones (1997) suggests multidisciplinarity is about a collaborative process where professions act independently in managing the client but share information; in contrast, interdisciplinarity is much more about evaluation and planning that is done collaboratively, with a pooling of knowledge to problem-solve. It appears, therefore, that multidisciplinarity is more professional task-orientated and interdisciplinarity is orientated to a client-centred process.

One approach to increasing understanding across professions is through shared teaching and learning, which has been advocated by many, including the World Health Organization (WHO 1988, Finch 2000, Lavin et al 2001). This must be underpinned with sound educational reasons, and should not be just an economic imperative, in the way that fiscal management in health care systems may be a major driver for collaboration (Perkins et al 2000). Interprofessional education has been seen as a way forward to addressing the understanding of other professions, and yet there is little evidence that it achieves this or that it is benefiting client care (Zwarenstein et al 2002). Its strength seems to lie in providing activities that allow professions to interact in decision-making, and not in gaining an in-depth understanding of individual professions' boundaries of practice. For collaboration to be useful in practice, professional stereotyping must be addressed in education, as well as the skills of working within a team (Hilton 1995). Identifying the means of achieving greater collaboration in both universities and the workplace, and measuring the outcomes, is an ongoing task (Barr 2002).

Professional boundaries, and therefore autonomous practice, are constantly being redefined (Smith et al 2000), but this needs careful evaluation.

Professional practice within health has historically been seen on a 'care–cure' continuum, with 'cure' being of higher profile and in the medical domain and 'care' being associated with the allied health professionals and nurses (Baumann et al 1998). Currently some nurse practitioners and physiotherapists are carrying out activities that junior doctors used to do. There appears to be a need for these tasks and for them to be done effectively and economically, and nurses and therapists, both of whom are looking for increased professional status, appear willing and able to include these tasks in their roles. Is this a welcome expansion of professional boundaries or further subordination under medicine's auspices (Shepherd et al 1996)? Also, while these boundaries are still in flux these practices challenge the definition of the profession and professional and civic accountability (Dowling et al 1996). It could be argued that these changes in scope of practice do satisfy an economic, a societal and an occupational need and as such market forces, as illustrated here, may play a part in developing a profession and professional identity. Therefore, who delivers a service could become driven on an economic basis (Armstrong 2002) and not on the basis of traditional professional boundaries.

13.6 ALTRUISM

Professions 'profess' a calling to promote the general good and justice, as well as an ethical commitment to carry out the work needed to achieve this good (Dyer 1985). Competent health practitioners should demonstrate this highly valued characteristic of engaging with others to relieve their suffering (McGaghie et al 2002). However, Jackson (1970) suggests that there is no reason to believe that professionals are more charitable or more interested in others than non-professionals. If education is part of professional development, then the promotion of the greater good must begin here and must involve attention to how professional knowledge produces benefits, and to whom these benefits flow (Goodlad 1984). Illich (1977) and Wilding (1982) suggest that although professions aim to 'enable' individuals by acting in their best interests, that action itself may 'disable' the individual, but benefit the professional emotionally, financially and occupationally.

Historically, doctors were paid for their services, many seeking patronage from wealthier clients. Those in society who could not afford doctors sought out cheaper lay practitioners. In today's culture, both private and public health services continue, with doctors having key roles in both. In private practice, the conduct of professional activities may be determined, at least partially, by monetary considerations (for example, increased patient throughput will augment income). In government health schemes, on the other hand, the way in which practice is carried out rarely affects the remuneration of the practitioner, and financial considerations are therefore unlikely to influence professional practice (except, perhaps, in terms of any promotion that may result from higher levels of professional skill). The suggestion here is that a prime function of the private practitioner is contributing to the wealth and success of a private business, whereas in the public health arena the prime function is about working for the greater good in society. The existence of *pro bono publico* work in US medical and legal practice (where fee-for-service is the principal basis of the practitioner–client relationship) points to a certain tension between personal remuneration and public service (Scott 1993). Whereas personal gain from fulfilling people's *desires* raises few qualms, there would seem to be an unease at the idea of personal gain from fulfilling basic *needs*. An argument of the last UK Conservative government (1979–97) against more than minimal pay rises for public sector workers, such as nurses, was that it is important not to attract the wrong sort of people into the profession (presumably those who would be driven by financial gain rather than by an altruistic drive to help others). However, increasingly public health can also be considered to be operating in a competitive and business market place (Bottery 1998) and in light of this, professionals should re-evaluate their roles in this market place. Historical practices and the power of one of the oldest professions (medicine) can be difficult to break. Possibly, some practitioners may mourn the loss of 'a sense of vocation' that the semi-professions had early on in their history which appears to be being replaced by a more career-oriented practitioner. Positively this could be viewed as about looking for optimum working conditions that allow the practitioner to function autonomously and for the greater good, or more negatively it could be related to gaining optimum financial reward and prestige. For the majority it may not be an either/or situation, but represent two ends of a spectrum. If professionalization is a process governed by changes in society, this may influence where along this continuum one practises at any one time.

13.7 CONCLUSION

Professional education and practice have a social responsibility and a wider benefit beyond immediate professional and economic utility (Teichler 1999). Attributes such as lifelong learning and codes of conduct may be important for an 'ecological' approach to occupations: one which 'ensures that they as individuals and as a profession are aware of developments within their society and are able to locate their practice within a wider picture of social and political issues' (Bottery 1998: 170). However, education and the socialization process must be considered carefully to avoid producing an inflexible 'profession', which may bring only rivalry and exclusion and which ultimately will not enhance the development of either society in general or health care in particular.

Physiotherapy has largely achieved the attributes of the 'established professions'. However, as in all the existing established professions, these attributes are being challenged and redefined by greater public access to previously closed areas of knowledge and practice and continuing state control. Part of being a profession means participating in the processes that contribute to this redefinition. Thereby, policies impacting on health practice are not only implemented by practitioners but also shaped by them. In addition the recipients of that practice, the public, must understand the limitations of practice (Mirvis 1993). This should enhance satisfaction with physiotherapy and health care on the part of both practitioners and public, as expectations are not unnecessarily raised or left unfulfilled. Perhaps it is the characteristics attributed to professions that are worth pursuing in their own right and not the label 'profession' (Sim 1985). These characteristics may help to define the future boundaries of practice and engender interprofessional collaboration.

Chapter **14**

Interpersonal communication

John Swain

CHAPTER CONTENTS

14.1   INTRODUCTION

A chapter is a small contribution to the literature about communication generally, and more specifically the body of literature aimed at medical and health practitioners. This is a huge and complex arena and it is of central importance to physiotherapists. Indeed, physiotherapy can be thought of as a form of communication; the whole process is one of communication between the client and the physiotherapist, between the physiotherapist and colleagues, including other physiotherapists, doctors and so on, and also between the physiotherapist and members of the client's family. The purpose of this chapter, then, is to examine interpersonal communication in the particular context of physiotherapy practice.

The first section contrasts two models of interpersonal communication: the linear or skills-based approach and the social or dynamic model. The following two sections engage with two central themes: that is, understandings of 'self' and 'power', in the context of the practitioner's relationship with the client. Both are actively produced, or brought into practice, through processes of interpersonal communication within particular social and historical contexts. It is in this context that barriers to effective communication are considered, including situations in which clients might be thought to have a communication difficulty. The following section explores the notion of reflective practice, a theme throughout the chapter, as a process of engaging with the challenges of interpersonal communication.

14.2 ONE ANOTHER

Communication is one of those terms that seem to have an intuitive and obvious meaning but are hard, if not impossible, to define precisely. Interpersonal communication is part of our social existence as human beings, as much as the air we breathe is a part of our physical existence. It is inevitable in encounters between people. Everything about us communicates, including hairstyle, clothes and posture. However, interpersonal communication is much more than how and what is communicated in individual encounters; it is the cement that holds us as people together and characterizes the society and culture in which we live. Cherry encapsulated this some years ago:

> The very word 'communicate' means 'share', and inasmuch as you and I are communicating at the moment, we are one. Not so much a union as a unity. Inasmuch as we agree, we say that we *are of one mind*, or, again, that we understand *one another*. This one another is the unity. A group of people, a society, a culture, I would define as 'people in communication' (Cherry 1957: 3).

Given the complexity of communication, it is hardly surprising that there are numerous definitions and ways of understanding the processes – almost as many as there are people who provide definitions. It is possible, however, to identify two models or ways of thinking about communication and, in doing so, draw out some key issues. These are linear and social (sometimes referred to as dynamic or social constructionist) models (Pearce 1994). The former seems to be a dominant way of looking at communication that also seems to accord with common sense; communication as a process of sending and receiving messages. Rungapadiachy (1999) adopts such a model, suggesting that most social and behavioural theorists would agree on the same basic model. A popular communication model that is used in the literature is as follows:

1. Sender (self)
2. Encoder (converting thought into message)
3. Channel (verbal, non-verbal, both verbal and non-verbal)
4. Decoder (interpretation of message)
5. Receiver (other/others) (Rungapadiachy 1999: 195).

Though this is the basic template of the linear model, it has been developed in various ways. Northouse & Northouse (1998: 17), for instance, have developed a 'health communication model which specifically focuses on transactions between participants in health care about health related issues'. This takes a broader systems view of communication, to take account of major factors in the health communication process: relationships, transactions and contexts.

The linear model of communication can underpin skills-based approaches to communication (Minardi & Riley 1997). Such skills-based approaches involve identifying small discernible elements or units of interpersonal communication, such as eye contact or use of questions, which can be analysed in terms of the effectiveness of communication and incorporated into training packages. There are times when it seems useful to consider what we intend to achieve through communication, for example when preparing a report. Indeed, intentional communication tends to be given priority in education and literature aimed at health care professionals. In physiotherapy practice such instrumental communication can be found, for instance, in assessment procedures used for gaining information to: formulate aims and goals for therapy; select means by which aims and goals are to be achieved; and devise a detailed programme of treatment. For example, in 'eliciting information from the client' within the context of clinical interviews, Williams (1997) covers topics of: listening; the structure of the interview; questions; keeping control of the interview; and checking on accuracy.

Nevertheless, linear models of communication, conceived as the sending and receiving, or transmission, of information, have been increasingly challenged. From a social model of communication, improving communication is not a simple matter of improving physiotherapists' skills of expressing and listening to information. Communication is 'meaning making' rather than 'information processing' and meanings are constructed between people. Communication is both based on and generates our perceptions, descriptions and understandings of the world or, more specifically, physiotherapy.

A social view of communication posits a dynamic model in the sense that communication is seen as a *trans–action* constructed between people. Social models concentrate more on the communication process itself, rather than the notion of message sending. Hartley (1999), for instance, bases his approach on Clampitt's (1990) model of communication as dance: 'This uses the analogy of a dance where partners have to co-ordinate their movements and arrive at a mutual understanding of where they are going. There are rules and skills but there are also flexibilities – dancers can inject their own style into the movements' (Hartley 1999: 18). Hartley broadens the basic model in terms of different contexts: the nature of the audience; relationship between the participants; and medium or channel of communication (for example, written or spoken). As to the last of these, in more recent years the rapid uptake of mobile phones has been something of a revolution in channels of communication, not just verbally but texting has even developed something of a new language of symbols. Information technology, particularly e mail and the internet, have opened the gates for what can be thought of as the information era.

There are a number of important aspects to a social model of communication. Interpersonal communication is viewed as an interplay between people, in which participants are both active agents, affecting the interplay, and reactive agents, affected by the interplay. There is no simple one-to-one correspondence between acts of communication and the meaning expressed. The context is all-important, giving and given meaning. Silence, for example, can 'say' more than words, but has no meaning outside the particular interpersonal and social context. It could be taken to mean the person is experiencing boredom, fear, respect, deep mutual understanding, passion, hatred – the list is potentially endless. Even signals that usually have a well-defined meaning, such as raising the hand to signal 'stop', depend on the context of the two-way flow. If accompanied by a smile, for instance, the raising of the hand could be meant as, and understood to be, a joke. Furthermore, there are differences between cultures in the actual behaviours used and their possible meanings (Bimrose 1998). Unlike British children, for instance, black American, Puerto Rican and Japanese children tend to avert their eyes when listening to another person. This can be understood by British adults to be a sign that the child is not listening or, even worse, is purposefully showing that he is not listening. Similarly, white British and Americans require a much larger personal space and they also touch less than people from some other cultures. Such generalizations are difficult, however, particularly in cosmopolitan societies, and there is variability within as well as between cultures. Furthermore, this model is holistic rather than being concerned with isolated 'atomistic units' (Pearce 1994). Meaning-making is constituted through the organization and system of a conversation and the whole is greater than the sum of the parts.

Within a social model, acts of communication do things. Communication always has an action orientation (Wetherell & Maybin 1996: 244). Speech, and indeed writing, is a form of social action. In particular, social relationships are achieved through and enmeshed within interpersonal communication. Relationships between physiotherapist and client are defined or maintained through all the communication between them. To illustrate this, consider the following statement: 'Please do these exercises at least twice a day, though stop if it gets too painful' (assuming that the statement is made by the physiotherapist to the client). In this example, the intention is to establish the treatment regimen as planned by the physiotherapist. The action, in terms of the professional–client relationship, will obviously depend on the existing relationship between the physiotherapist and the client and their history of communication as to whether it is being defined, maintained or redefined. The crucial point is that the relationship dimension provides the context for the meaning of the content dimension. The content can be interpreted in many ways by the client. If, for instance there is a trusting relationship, the client may interpret this as a useful suggestion to which he or she should comply. If, on the other hand, their relationship is distant and the client feels the physiotherapist has no real knowledge of him or her as a person, this might be seen as a rigid directive more to do with the physiotherapist complying with the expectations of the professional role. Furthermore, not only does the social context give meaning, it is also given meaning. Pearce (1994: 75) explains:

> The social world is in a process of continual creation. The actions you perform in this moment add to the sum of human experience; the future of the human race is not fixed, it is still being developed through our actions … When we communicate, we are not just talking *about* the world, we are literally participating in the creation of the social universe.

Physiotherapy–client communication is not just a means for undertaking physiotherapy practice; the participants are creating physiotherapy practice.

The next section moves on to consider the self in relation to communication, developing, in particular, a social model of communication. At this point, physiotherapist readers could usefully think about themselves and what they bring to communication in physiotherapy practice. How did they decide to become physiotherapists? What do they understand to be the relationship between therapist–client interpersonal communication and physiotherapy practice? What are the main values, opinions and beliefs that they bring to interpersonal communication in practice? What unique abilities, aspirations, expectations and personal concerns do they have that might influence the communication process generally and also in more specific situations (for example, with disabled clients and clients from ethnic minority communities)? In reflecting on such questions it can be useful to compare answers with other people's – both other therapists' answers and also, if possible, clients' answers to similar questions.

14.3 COMMUNICATING SELVES

An examination of processes of communication usually involves consideration of the concept of self. As with the concept of 'communication', we need first to stand back and consider the notion of self or identity (in this context, the two terms are used interchangeably). Within a social model, the whole notion of self is embedded within communication. This can be thought of in at least two ways.

- You bring yourself into the communication within physiotherapy practice. You are being you. You bring your own personal stamp to the identity of 'physiotherapist', though within available social resources and choices.

- You are you through communication within physiotherapy practice. Who you are is through being with others. To use Cherry's words again, 'We are one' (Cherry 1957: 3).

Let us look, then, at the concept of self and what it means. The concept of self and the transformation of its meaning in different societies and at different times has provoked debate within philosophy and the social sciences for two millennia (Bruner 1995: 25). The common-sense view, or dominant understanding in contemporary Western societies, is that each of us is an entity, a 'self' or 'I', irrespective of the context or the society in which we live. In more recent years, however, this way of understanding the self has been challenged. In the local context of our daily lives we can be seen as moving between and within many selves, including, in my case, father, husband, lecturer, friend, researcher, man, white, middle-aged, disabled and the list continues seemingly endlessly. This 'self-pluralistic approach' denies the subjective 'reality' of *my self*: 'Rather, it postulates an individual who encounters his or her world from a plurality of positions, through a plurality of voices, in relation to a plurality of self-concepts, yet who still retains a meaningful coherence, both at the level of the constituent pluralities and at the level of the total system' (Cooper & Rowan 1999: 2).

Even the understanding of self as 'independent being' and 'coherent being' has a particular social and historic context. Changing understandings of self or social identity have been associated with broad social change. As Jenkins (1996: 9) suggests, the centrality of 'social identity' as 'one of the unifying frameworks of intellectual debate in the 1990s' is possibly a sign of the times. Echoing the widely held belief that 'the times' are themselves rapidly changing, Jenkins (1996: 9) writes: 'Popular concern about identity is, in large part perhaps, a reflection of the uncertainty produced by rapid change and cultural contact: our social maps no longer fit our social landscapes'.

In the changing social maps there has been the emergence of the notion of 'relational selves'. This could perhaps be crystallized by rewriting the well known phrase, 'I think, therefore I am', as 'I relate, therefore I am'. Gergen is more expansive: 'the conception of relational being reduces the debilitating gap between self and other, the sense of oneself as alone and the other as alien and untrustworthy. Whatever we are, from the present standpoint, is either directly or indirectly with others ... We are made up of each other ... we are mutually constituting' (Gergen 1999: 137–138).

From a social model viewpoint, then, the person is not understood simply as a sender and receiver of messages. A person's identity as a physiotherapist is established through and within his or her work as a physiotherapist. Harré (1998: 68) writes: 'What people have called "selves" are, by and large, produced discursively, that is in dialogue and other forms of joint action with real and imagined others. Selves are not entities, but evanescent properties of the flow of public and private action.' The notion of narrative, that is a continuing account of ourselves and the series of occurrences in our lives, to ourselves and others, is important in the social model or social construction of selves. Anderson (1997) says we understand and give meaning and intelligibility to our experiences through narrative or storytelling.

Selves, then, are socially constructed through language and maintained in narrative. A self is not a thing inside an individual, but a process or activity that occurs in the dynamic space of communication between people (Freedman & Combs 1996). In this understanding of human beings, the focus of interest is moved from the inside of an individual to the person as part and parcel of the social world. Writing of the link between identity and narrative life history, Widdershoven states:

> What then is narrative identity? It is the unity of a person's life as it is experienced and articulated in stories that express this experience ... the unity of a person's life is dependent on being a character in an enacted narrative. We live our lives according to a script, which secures that our actions are part of a meaningful totality. Our actions are organized in such a way that we can give account of them, justify them by telling an intelligible story about them (Widdershoven 1993: 7).

This accounting of actions can project existing stories into a presumed future: 'I'm overburdened with my work and suppose I always will be', or 'Physiotherapists are undervalued in multiprofessional contexts and I can't see there'll ever be any way out of that'. Stories, however, can also narrate into a preferred future, for example 'I'm overburdened by work at the moment but I expect I'll be able to sort it out and I'll see light at the end of the tunnel'. Somers (1994: 613–614) states that 'people are guided to act in certain ways and not others, on the basis of the projections, expectations, and memories derived from a multiple but ultimately limited repertoire of available social, public, and cultural narratives'.

Mattingly has investigated the complex interconnections between narrative and experience in clinical work through the 'therapeutic narratives' of occupational therapists. She states that therapists 'operate with multiple storylines, multiple possible plots which point towards different possible selves, and they experiment with a variety of self understandings through the actions they take and the experiences they try to create for themselves and others' (Mattingly 1998: 119). Narratives are constructed by professionals, stories of themselves, their roles, their practice. Mattingly suggests that professionals are particularly likely to tell stories to make sense of difficult relationships and interrelations with others, managers, colleagues and clients. She emphasizes the dramas that underlie encounters in therapy when there are collisions between expectations and intentions, and unfolding events with others, particularly when desires run high, creating significant experiences.

A study by McKay & Ryan (1995) is an example of a narrative approach in therapy research. It is based on the idea that narrative reasoning is a means of enabling therapists to explain their practice. A student and an experienced therapist were asked to tell their story about one particular client with whom they were working. The experienced therapist 'presented a future or conditional image of the person which guided the intervention: "it's up to us to get her home"' (McKay & Ryan 1995: 236). The student's story, however, kept strictly to the formal therapy process. It was a story about means, or strategies of intervention, rather than ends in terms of the implications from the viewpoint of the client. There are inherent self-stories here in terms of how therapists see themselves in relation to clients and in communication with clients. Ryan & McKay (1999) extend this to argue that, by using narratives, individual learning and theorizing are enriched. Practice includes the individual's feelings, the way they perceive their situation, their reactions to that particular situation, the interactions between the therapist and the client and 'many other highly personal facets' (Ryan 1999: 7).

Physiotherapist readers might find it useful, at this point, to write a narrative from their own practice. This could involve the following steps:

1. Focus on work with a client that you consider involved collisions between your expectations and intentions and those of the client.

2. Write your story of the encounters with the client. You might, for instance, cover how you perceived the situation, your actions, reactions and feelings, though it is important to tell your story in your own way.

3. Stand back from the narrative and reflect on how you saw yourself as a therapist and what you were communicating about yourself in these encounters.

4. It is useful to compare your narrative with other people's, if possible, particularly the client's.

14.4   COMMUNICATING RELATIONSHIPS

We turn next to the construction of relationships through interpersonal communication, with a particular focus on power in therapist–client relations. Social divisions, class, race, gender, age and disability inequalities are manifested and experienced in everyday interpersonal communication, including physiotherapy practice. Notions of power have underpinned analyses of professional–client relations and their social and historical context. Hugman (1991: 1) states: 'Social power is an integral aspect of the daily working lives of professionals. The centrality of power in professional work has been increasingly recognized' (see Ch. 13).

As Thompson (1998: 43) argues, 'an understanding of the workings of power is an essential part of challenging inequality, discrimination and oppression'. He suggests that power in relations between professionals and clients manifests itself in a number of ways including: control over the allocation of resources; the legitimization of knowledge, expertise and skills; and statutory powers. In physiotherapy practice, power relations can be communicated, for instance, in assessment procedures which gain information to: formulate aims and goals for therapy; select means by which aims and goals are to be achieved; and devise a detailed programme of treatment.

Some areas of professional practice are often assumed to come under the authority of the professional rather than the client (Winslade et al 1996):

1. Diagnosis of client's concerns according to external definition criteria

2. The asking of questions in order to interpret the answers

3. Knowledge of what the client needs to do to overcome the problem he or she is concerned about and the development of a treatment plan

4. The writing of reports in which the professional is the first-person author and the central character in the story is relegated to third-person object status

5. The conveying of information about the client to other people or agencies in referral situations

6. Discussions with other professionals about the client and his or her life

7. Note-taking at the clinical interview, decisions on what is appropriate to include in the notes, and the maintenance of such notes for professional purposes.

These authors suggest that these areas of professional practice are conducted without reference to the object of such practices, that is without any real inclusion of the 'voice' (beliefs, opinions, aspirations, expectations and so on) of the client. To take an example from the area of learning difficulties, drawing on stories told by people with learning difficulties, key workers and care staff, Gillman et al (1997: 676–677) found that:

> Many respondents looked to the case records of professionals to provide background information and personal history material, but they frequently found that the kind of information they were seeking was not contained in 'official' records. For many people with learning difficulties who have been in long-term institutional care and who have lost contact with relatives, official files are the only record of their lived experience. Yet such records are often inaccessible (both literally and conceptually) to those who are the subjects of their deliberations. White and Epston (1990) argue that the case file has a narrow readership of professional experts and is a vehicle for the presentation of the worth and expertise of the author, namely the professional.

We shall return to the above list of professional practice areas at the end of this section.

Such unequal power relations can be constructed throughout every aspect of communication processes, and the complex, delicate and subtle processes of communication can be distorted and blocked in many ways. The remainder of this section, then, reflects on the barriers and difficulties that can be encountered in interpersonal communication. We shall concentrate first on the role of the professional in the construction of such barriers and difficulties. One focus for analysis is the control of listening by the professional, and the barriers to listening that block and divert two-way mutuality in communication. First, there is the control of the context, time and space, dominated by the professional. Lack of time is often quoted as a barrier, by professionals at least. The professional's attention can be focused on another pressing appointment and his or her own need to limit the encounter. When time is felt to be pressing, for instance, it is quicker to offer a word or two of reassurance than to allow the client to talk through his or her feelings, experiences or needs. Communication, however, is not limited by time alone. In general terms, the amount and kind of attention a person receives in social interaction is shaped by gender, social class and other factors believed to determine the person's social worth (Derber & Magrass 2001). It can be argued, then, that it is the quality of the interaction that is important, irrespective of time constraints.

Second, power relations can be constructed through distortion, devaluing and the drowning out of the client's voice. The barriers to listening include criticizing, labelling and diagnosing. The terms 'labelling' and 'diagnosis' can have more formal, technical meanings in therapy, but they can also be seen as general processes within communication. Each of the barriers is a violation of the voice of the other person that can channel the flow of conversation towards the judgements of the professional.

Criticizing is the inner judgmental voice of approval or disapproval. It can begin before a word is spoken. Judgements can begin from the way a person is dressed – from make-up, hairstyle, gait, jewellery and so on. Deep-seated values, beliefs and prejudices can be a screen to listening to the individual. Preconceptions and feelings can be so strong that criticism is an impenetrable barrier to listening. Labelling and diagnosing are ways of categorizing people that can devalue them and what they are saying. Labelling can be seen as the making of presumptions, pre-judgements and prejudices about a supposed type or stereotype of person. There are, of course, many such labels: aggressive, chauvinist, disabled, deaf, and derogatory name-calling labels. It is not that labels are wrong in themselves. Indeed, they can be used to affirm positive identity ('Black is beautiful') and bring people together to challenge the discrimination and abuse they experience. In the context of these discussions, however, labelling can be a barrier to listening to another person as a unique individual. Diagnosis does involve listening, but a form of technical listening to pick up clues about conclusions being drawn. It might be concluded, for instance, that the other person is under stress or deceiving him- or herself. Everything the other person says and does is sifted for signs to confirm the diagnosis. Labelling and diagnosing are part of the processes of physiotherapy. The dilemma for physiotherapists is that the techniques involved can themselves play a role in constructing unequal power relations.

Third, unequal power relations can be constructed through ways of responding that block, divert, distort and re-channel the track the client is on, or the client's narrative. Interpreting, for instance, can direct the flow of conversation in accordance with the professional's judgements and diagnosis about the client. Changing the subject is simply switching the conversation from the other person's to the professional's concerns. This might involve, for instance, avoidance of emotionally difficult concerns, such as death, sickness and personal conflicts. Reassurance can also be a denial of the strength of the client's feelings. The rushed few words of support may be an attempt to show caring, but can be a means of closing down conversation. Clichés are a form of reassurance: 'time's a great healer' or 'you've got to take the rough with the smooth'. Such stock platitudes avoid rather than reflect the client's particular concerns.

Finally, professional power can be constructed through taking over and dominating the flow of conversation, deciding needs and solutions for the other person. This can involve advising, excessive questioning, ordering, and defensiveness. Advising certainly has its place in physiotherapy practice as, for instance, in health education. Stock advice, however, can pre-empt listening to the client. It is easy to provide solutions without really knowing the problem as perceived by the client. Ordering is a form of advising backed with authority: 'you'll have to live with the consequences if you don't'. Such threats do not have to be explicit, but can be inherent in people's perceptions of physiotherapy. Professional defensiveness can be a barrier to listening to the client. Excessive questioning, advising and ordering can all be expressions of defensiveness. They can be ways of putting up a screen of expertise that promotes the credentials of the professional. All the baggage of professional education, accountability, appraisal, and professional responsibility can help cement the wall between physiotherapist and client with defensiveness.

Within a dynamic model of interpersonal communication, barriers and difficulties are constructed between the client and the professional. Thus, a role is played by expectations from both sides. Sometimes, for example, clients expect physiotherapists to be 'all-knowing' and may lose confidence if the professional's knowledge is seen to be incomplete. Furthermore clients are not necessarily passive in client–professional power relations. Miell & Croghan found evidence of client resistance in the literature:

> There is ample evidence of resistance in clients' responses to professional intervention ... The self-advocacy groups set up amongst young people who have been in care, people with disabilities, and women dissatisfied with medical intervention show that those on the receiving end of professional intervention can not only define their own needs but they can also actively resist attempts to impose definitions upon them (Miell & Croghan 1996: 298–299).

Many physiotherapists might also cite non-adherence to treatment and advice as a common expression of resistance. Furthermore, other power relations can play a part in physiotherapy encounters, particularly age and gender. Some female physiotherapists, for instance, have experienced sexual harassment from male clients (McComas et al 1993, DeMayo 1997).

The barriers to communication in physiotherapy practice can be compounded in situations where the 'mechanics' of communication are problematic, again from both sides. A variety of speech, language and communication problems can be encountered:

1. The client's possible difficulties in expression, including a range of impairments such as stuttering, lack of speech, lack of control over movements of the body and so on, sometimes associated with medical conditions such as Parkinson's disease or cerebral palsy and sometimes with mental health problems, e.g. depression, where the client may not want to communicate

2. The client's difficulties in comprehension, including learning difficulties, hearing impairment, visual impairment or general anxiety (e.g. before major surgery), where the client may not listen

3. The physiotherapist's difficulties in expression, including use of jargon, patriarchal attitudes and so on

4. The physiotherapist's difficulties in comprehension, including lack of time to listen, preconceptions and so on.

At this point you might find it useful to reflect on the barriers to interpersonal communication that you face in your own practice. Return to the list of seven areas of professional practice that can be assumed to come under the authority of the professional (Winslade et al 1996). Take each in turn and give examples from your practice in which you, rather than the client, have been in control – making decisions that will have real implications for the client's life. Work through the list again and identify strategies that increase the control and authority of the clients you work with.

14.5   REFLECTING ON PRACTICE

In this final section, I shall draw together and focus on a theme that has been developed throughout the chapter, that is, reflecting on physiotherapy practice. In doing so, I shall draw on one particular perspective that can provide a foundation for reflective practice, that is, social constructionism. The term 'social constructionism' is an umbrella term for a broad-based perspective in philosophy, the humanities and the social sciences. The idea that a perspective or theory from the social sciences has relevance in considering the effectiveness of their practice can be problematic for physiotherapists. However, within a social model, addressing interpersonal communication involves consideration of physiotherapy from a broad viewpoint. The effectiveness of physiotherapy practice is not just dependent on the technical skills of a physiotherapist but on the whole complex process of interpersonal communication through which physiotherapy practice is realized. We looked above at reflection through narrative and you have also been asked to reflect on power relations in your practice. Here, we explore the general process of reflection in theory and practice. Perspectives, or theories, are an integral part of the basic values, assumptions, beliefs and feelings that therapists bring to their work. Therapy cannot be detached from the therapist, his or her views not only of physiotherapy but also of what we are as human beings and of the society we live in. Being a reflective practitioner involves exploring deep-seated beliefs and taken-for-granted assumptions. The social constructionist perspective does not offer direct and substantial implications for the practice of physiotherapy. Nor does it offer physiotherapists a pertinent field of study as an academic abstract discipline in its own right. It is one way of viewing personal and social worlds that can inform the standpoint of physiotherapists seeking to reflect critically on their practice as socially constructed encounters through and within interpersonal communication.

Social constructionism is founded on the notion that every aspect of our existence is fundamentally social and actively produced in the relationships and interrelations between people. Experience and meaning are not merely actively created by an individual, they are created in social encounters that are embedded in and shaped by culture and the wider social world. Nightingale & Cromby (1999: 229) state: 'Basically, social constructionists are concerned with the ways in which social and psychological reality are actively constructed (rather than pre-existing) phenomena'.

As Burr (1995) points out, however, there is no single definition of social constructionism. Indeed, it can be argued that social constructionism, as with other perspectives such as humanistic psychology, is a 'broad church' and is also ever-developing (Gergen 1999). Burr (1995: 3–5), however, summarizes key assumptions that would be widely accepted as the foundation for social constructionism, and which can also provide a foundation for reflective practice. First, social constuctionism takes a critical stance towards taken-for-granted knowledge. There is no single way of defining 'truth' or 'reality', and each construction has its potentials and limits. Assumptions, taken-for-granted knowledges and, ostensibly, unquestionable truths should therefore be challenged and alternative framings of reality considered. Thus, from a social construc- tionist perspective the world of 'hard facts' becomes less tangible and more provisional. 'Facts of life' are actively constructed meanings in the daily social life of communication between people. Thus, for instance, the 'fact of life' that disability is an abnormality of the individual is ques- tioned with the recognition that disability has different meanings in dif- ferent societies and at different times through history (see Section 17.4).

Another assumption, according to Burr (1995), is that knowledge is sustained by social processes. Knowledge and power are inextricably intertwined and, as Dallos (1997: 149) points out, 'a prime aspect of this is the rise in influence of scientific thought, medicine, technology, economic analyses, and so on'. Social constructionism emphasizes the role of lan- guage as the essential feature of human societies (Clarke & Cochrane 1998). A particular emphasis is given to the use of discourse; that is, ways of speaking, the words we use, and the rules regulating what it is possible to say, who can say things, under what conditions and with what con- sequences. The concept of discourse, then, addresses power relations between people within interpersonal communication. Hugman explains:

> Discourse is about more than language. Discourse is about the interplay between language and social relationships, in which some groups are able to achieve dominance for their interests in the way in which the world is defined and acted upon. Such groups include not only dominant economic classes, but also men within patriarchy, and white people within the racism of colonial and post-colonial societies, as well as pro- fessionals in relation to service users. Language is a central aspect of discourse through which power is reproduced and communicated (Hugman 1991: 37).

Foucault (1980) argues that there is an inseparable link between know- ledge and power: the discourses of a society determine what knowledge is held to be true, right, or proper in that society, so those who control the discourse control knowledge. Power cannot be simply seen as the prop- erty of individuals or groups but is produced within interpersonal com- munication and emerges through interactions.

The social constructionist view of knowledge and power can underpin reflective practice, that is the capacity of a therapist to think, talk or write about a piece of practice with the intention to review or research a piece of practice with clients for new meanings or perspectives on the situ- ation. At a personal level, it can help therapists to examine the beliefs and values they bring to their practice for signs of stereotypical thinking or prejudice. At a professional level, it can provide a framework for evalu- ating theories and models of practice in terms of their potential to oppress or marginalize people. Such reflection can help therapists to con- struct models of practice informed by notions of social justice and based on collaboration and partnership with clients. The process of reflecting is traditionally seen as something that professionals do, either alone or together. However, Anderson (1992) has developed an approach in which professionals reflect in the presence of those who consult them and then invite the clients to reflect upon their reflections. The advantage of this approach is that it encourages the client to have a voice in what is usually regarded as professional territory. It also provides an opportunity to privilege the issues and concerns of clients in negotiating priorities in physiotherapy practice. Practitioner reflexivity is just as central to the conduct of research as it is to practice. Indeed, Schön (1983) suggests that practice and research are inextricably linked through the process of reflection. 'When someone reflects-in-action he becomes a researcher in the practice context' (Schön 1983: 20). Adopting a reflective approach to physiotherapy allows the therapist to question the power relations of practice and influence the process of therapy at each stage.

14.6 CONCLUSION

Physiotherapy is essentially a process of opening up channels for people to express and explore their feelings, understandings and aspirations through physical therapy. For a reflective practitioner it is also a process of reflecting on questions of the why, what and how of communication. The recognition of touch and physical manipulation as alternative channels of communication is a good starting point for reflecting on the practice of physiotherapy. There are, as indicated above, many other possibilities which can only be mentioned here:

- The use of sign language is the clearest example of a communication mode or channel other than speech. Sign languages, as developed by deaf people, are actual languages with their own syntax. Clients may be fluent in or use British sign language. The onus on physiotherapists is the difficult task, if they are not fluent themselves, to learn what is essentially a foreign language, or at least use the services of a translator. It is important, too, not to make simplistic assumptions. There is a linguistic diversity among deaf people and there are also pros and cons to using translators. The book by Corker (1994) provides an excellent introduction for anyone seeking greater self-awareness and skills in this area.

- Slightly less obvious, but no less important, is the use of translators generally. Though a physiotherapist working, for instance, with a person with learning difficulties may have difficulties understanding him or her, it is often the case that others, including members of a young person's family, other professionals or an advocate, are 'tuned in' to him or her.

- Writing is a mode of communication that is different from speech. Speech is of the moment, but writing can be more deliberate and intentional, and is more permanent, unless speech is recorded.

- Dalton (1994) suggests that other media of communication are essential when working with clients who have what she calls 'impaired communication': she refers to 'drawing and painting, materials which can be handled, and music and movement' (Dalton 1994: 28). All of these can open communication, whether or not the client would be said to have impaired communication. In particular, materials or toys of various kinds can be very useful when working with children using play. Joining children in their play is an effective way of opening channels of communication.

● Finally, in this short list we must include facial expressions and gesture. At their simplest such signals suggest negative or positive feelings towards people, events or experiences. With people who have profound and multiple impairments, for instance, expressions of discrimination and preference can be the basic level of communication within which the physiotherapist needs to be receptive.

Reflective practice is concerned with issues and problems that arise in practice and it aims to bring about change, or influence policy in the practice arena. Below are some pertinent topics for reflecting on practice:

1. Criteria for evaluating physiotherapy, from the viewpoints of both therapists and clients

2. The expectations of clients and therapists

3. The differences between the stories of the therapist and the client

4. The values that therapists bring to their work with clients which predetermine their responses to the client's viewpoint

5. The concepts that therapists bring to bear in the process of physiotherapy (e.g. independence, coping, caring, support, empowerment and partnership) and what they mean in practice

6. The dominant stereotypes of groups of physiotherapy clients (e.g. old, black, disabled people) within our culture.

In this chapter, I have attempted to outline a way of thinking about interpersonal communication within physiotherapy. It is a particular narrative, a particular story of interpersonal communication. It is told to offer grounds and foundation for physiotherapists in critically reflecting on their practice. For further discussion of the ideas presented in this chapter, see Swain et al (2004).

Chapter **15**

Fundamentals of moral decision–making

Julius Sim

15.1 INTRODUCTION

This chapter is to do with the place of health care ethics within physiotherapy. It is, therefore, appropriate to start by trying to outline what is to be understood by 'health care ethics'. For the purposes of this chapter, this term is taken to mean the application of moral reasoning to the context of health care, so as to identify those courses of action that are morally right, and those which are morally wrong. We are dealing, therefore, with a decision-making procedure, but one that is primarily guided by moral criteria, as opposed to clinical, legal, bureaucratic or other considerations. Moral and legal considerations may give rise to different conclusions, and care should be taken not to confuse the relevance of these two types of consideration. A physiotherapist may be under certain legal duties in a particular situation, but simultaneously subject to different, and possibly conflicting, moral duties.

A number of important points follow from this initial statement. First, ethical reasoning is applied to health care, it does not spring from within it. Consequently, there is no such thing as 'physiotherapy ethics', or for that matter 'medical ethics' or 'nursing ethics'. The particular situations with which we are dealing may 'belong' to physiotherapy, but the ethical principles that are applied to them are universal. It follows that health care practitioners can claim no specific moral authority on the basis of their professional expertise (Veatch 1973, Kennedy 1981). To be sure, such expertise will often be relevant when dealing with moral dilemmas, but it does not itself confer any special authority in ethical matters. Second, the ultimate end of the process is to take action. We are not engaged in abstract contemplation or philosophical speculation for its own sake; ethical reasoning in health care is an action-oriented business. Third, we are concerned with what is morally right. The fact that a certain course of action may be correct in terms of clinical judgement does not in itself guarantee that it is the right thing to do morally. What may seem an appropriate decision on clinical grounds may be morally objectionable, and, conversely, what may seem a dubious decision purely in terms of clinical judgement may have much to recommend it as a moral course of action. This further reinforces the point that professional expertise does not carry with it moral expertise. It is also worth noting that, as we will see, the processes of ethical and clinical decision-making may be quite similar, even though they sometimes yield very different conclusions. Finally, it should be stressed that we are dealing with matters of ethics, not etiquette. Professional courtesies are important, but they do not necessarily raise ethical issues. The notion of 'professional ethics' has come to embrace wider concerns.

In the remainder of this chapter, health care ethics, and the specific process of moral decision-making, will be examined within the context of clinical physiotherapy. In the process, the question as to the 'objectivity' of ethics will be considered, and the role of professional codes of ethics will be addressed. In Chapter 16, some specific ethical issues and conflicts will be explored, and the general concepts and principles dealt with in the current chapter will be applied and illustrated.

15.2 ETHICS AND PHYSIOTHERAPY

There has been a growing concern with the ethical issues associated with medicine and health care; numerous texts have been written in this area, and there are a number of academic journals devoted to ethical and other philosophical questions in health care. The literature has traditionally focused on ethics within medicine and nursing, but more recently a number of texts have specifically examined legal and ethical issues associated with physiotherapy and occupational therapy (Bailey & Schwartzberg 1995, Sim 1997a, Swisher & Krueger-Brophy 1998).

Swisher (2002) has recently published a comprehensive review of the ethics literature in physiotherapy. This body of work contains discussion of a number of ethical issues in physiotherapy, and in rehabilitation more widely. In addition to papers discussing the philosophical and practical aspects of these issues, a number of studies have examined the role of ethics in physiotherapy practice from an empirical standpoint. In an early study, Guccione (1990) surveyed physical therapists in New England,

USA, and identified concerns around such issues as establishing priorities for treatment, discontinuation of treatment for non-compliant patients, the moral implications of the patient–therapist relationship, and economic issues to do with third-party payers. More recently Triezenberg (1996, 1997) surveyed members of the Judicial Committee of the American Physical Therapy Association, using a Delphi approach. In addition to some of the issues identified by Guccione, the areas of informed consent, confidentiality, the use of human subjects in research, and the maintenance of clinical competence emerged as prominent issues. In the UK, Barnitt (Barnitt & Partridge 1997, Barnitt 1998) has studied the way in which physiotherapists and occupational therapists perceive and attempt to resolve ethical conflicts, while Cross & Sim (2000) have focused on physiotherapists' understanding of, and attitudes towards, the issue of confidentiality. It is clear, therefore, that matters of ethics are becoming more prominent in professional discourse within physiotherapy.

15.2.1 WHAT ISSUES ARISE IN PHYSIOTHERAPY?

It might seem that many of the dramatic issues that appear in the newspapers, and which are the subject of television documentaries, have little to do with the practice of physiotherapy. Indeed, matters such as embryo research, organ transplantation, abortion and in vitro fertilization are scarcely the everyday concern of the clinical physiotherapist. The sort of ethical questions that arise in physiotherapy tend to be of a more everyday nature:

- Are some patients more deserving of treatment than others, and if so on what grounds?

- How should we set treatment priorities within a caseload?

- Should we obtain informed consent before treating a patient, and if so how 'informed' must this consent be, and what form should it take?

- Can we justify persevering with treatment that is proving ineffective, just because continued treatment has been recommended?

- Under what circumstances is it permissible to cause patients discomfort or pain?

- Should we ever deliberately mislead patients as to their diagnosis, or the nature of the treatment they are being given?

- With whom is it permissible to discuss the details of a patient's case?

- What weight should be given to the wishes of carers or relatives within a patient's rehabilitation programme?

- What action should we take with respect to colleagues whom we perceive as incompetent, or whose conduct we regard as unethical?

However, the fact that these are not generally 'life and death' matters does not mean that they do not require careful examination. Some comments on ethics in nursing are equally applicable to physiotherapy:

'Moral dilemmas of the "do or die" variety help us to focus upon the moral choices we must make, and so debating ethical dilemmas is a useful exercise. We should not, however, allow the big dilemmas to detract from the more routine moral choices involved in nursing' (Melia 1989: 1). The impact of these seemingly more minor issues on the patients whom they affect can easily be underestimated, particularly by health professionals, to whom they may become somewhat 'routine' considerations.

This having been said, it is important to remember that there are in fact some 'high-profile' ethical matters in which physiotherapists may be involved, even if only in an indirect way. It may be the consultant who takes the initial decision to withdraw treatment from a gravely ill patient, but the physiotherapist is very much involved in the subsequent process. As a member of the team, he or she must decide the extent to which physiotherapy treatment should also be limited or withdrawn, and in what way. If antibiotics and other 'active' means of medical care have been abandoned, does this mean that chest physiotherapy should also be curtailed? If no further attempts are to be made to restore functional independence, should mobility still be maintained for reasons of comfort and pain relief? Similarly, physiotherapists are rarely involved in enlisting patients' participation in potentially hazardous drug trials, but while such patients remain under their care the therapists involved may have to face associated ethical problems. For example, it may become clear that the patient was insufficiently informed as to the nature of the drug being tested, or the patient may express a desire to withdraw from the study that he or she is unwilling to voice to the physician conducting the research. In such instances, the physiotherapist, although not directly involved in the affair at the outset, may feel a moral obligation to take an active role, perhaps as an advocate for the patient.

15.3 THEORETICAL ISSUES

Before turning to the specific process of reaching decisions on ethical questions in physiotherapy, it is necessary briefly to address some basic theoretical issues to do with ethics and ethical reasoning.

There are a number of different ways in which philosophers have approached the business of making moral decisions, but they can broadly be grouped into three categories: deontology, consequentialism and virtue ethics.

15.3.1 DEONTOLOGY

Deontology is a system of ethics that has at its core certain fundamental ethical principles. An ethical principle can be regarded as the statement of a fundamental ethical value or belief (see Table 15.1). Thus, broadly speaking, the principle of beneficence states that one should strive to confer benefits on others, while the principle of non-maleficence states that one should seek to avoid inflicting harm on others. The classic expression of non-maleficence is the famous medical maxim *primum non nocere* ('above all, do no harm'), which suggests that there is a paramount

Table 15.1 Basic ethical principles

Principle	Description	Comment
Beneficence	The positive requirement to promote the interests and well-being of others	Includes actions that will protect a person from harm, as well as those that will directly confer benefit
Non-maleficence	The negative requirement not to harm others	Often thought to be more stringent than beneficence
Respect for autonomy	The requirement to respect the self-determination of others	Usually only covers persons who are, or have previously been, autonomous
		May require the enhancement, as well as the preservation, of a person's self-determination
Respect for persons	The requirement to respect the dignity and individuality of others	Closely linked with the principle of respect for autonomy, but covers both autonomous and non-autonomous persons
		Requires that we should not use people solely as a means to an end
Justice	The requirement to treat others fairly	Differential treatment of others must be morally justifiable – based on morally relevant similarities or differences between individuals

prohibition in health care against causing harm. The principle of respect for autonomy requires us to preserve, and where appropriate to promote, the self-determination of others – in relation to both decisions and action – while the principle of justice insists that we should deal with others in a way that is fair and in accordance with their individual merit. According to this principle, we should treat everybody in the same way, unless there are morally relevant differences between individuals; it is legitimate to provide a greater level of care to some patients if their clinical needs are greater than those of others, but not on the basis of one's personal feelings towards them. The principle of respect for persons – which is in some respects similar to that of respect for autonomy – demands that we should deal with others with due regard for their dignity as individuals (Downie & Telfer 1969). Given the potential for 'depersonalization' that exists in busy hospitals and other health care settings, this last principle is of considerable importance. It can be seen as grounded in ideas such as these: 'Respecting the patient as a person calls upon us to regard patients as unique individuals and to see them in the totality of their being, with physical, psychological, social, and spiritual dimensions alike … it is as persons that we are all fellow human beings, fellow members of the human community' (Corr & Corr 1986: 23).

From these general principles, secondary principles or duties can be derived which are somewhat more specific in their application. For example, the duty of confidentiality can be extracted from the wider principle of non-maleficence (Sim 1996a), and the principle of truthfulness, or veracity, can be derived from both the principle of respect for autonomy and the principle of respect for persons (Sim 1986b). The aim of deontology, therefore, is to determine the specific actions that one should perform in order to fulfil certain duties, which are grounded in one or more general moral principles (Table 15.2).

Table 15.2 Approaches to ethical decision-making

Deontology	Consequentialism	Virtue ethics
Focuses predominantly on actions	Focuses predominantly on actions	Focuses predominantly on agents
Concerned primarily with the observance of certain duties, based on basic moral principles	Concerned primarily with the consequences of action	Concerned primarily with the cultivation of moral dispositions or virtues
Moral conflicts are settled by determining which is the 'weightier' duty	Moral conflicts are settled by determining which alternative outcome is better for those concerned	Moral conflicts are settled by determining which course of action exemplifies the more desirable moral character
Attaches special moral weight to relationships between individuals, and the commitments that these imply	Recognizes that relationships between individuals can be morally significant, but does not attach a special moral weight to these	Attaches special moral weight to relationships between individuals
Will countenance an outcome that is less than optimal if this is the only way to honour a fundamental moral duty	Will countenance the breach of a fundamental moral duty if this is the only way to produce the optimal outcome	Not primarily concerned with the honouring of moral duties or the production of good consequences

A person who subscribes to a deontological approach would use these principles as the criteria for ethical decision-making, and as the final test of an ethical conflict. Accordingly, a physiotherapist working within this sort of framework would ensure that all patients were fully consulted as to the form that their rehabilitation is to take, in order to remain true to the principle of respect for autonomy, would decline to inflict unpleasant or painful treatment on a patient, so as not to infringe the principle of non-maleficence, and would allocate treatment according to considerations of justice. Given that a number of different principles are at stake, the situation will sooner or later arise where two or more principles come into some degree of conflict; in such a case, some means of prioritizing among them will be arrived at. Thus, in the second example above, it might be felt that it is justifiable to cause the patient discomfort because this is ultimately to the individual's benefit (i.e. fulfils the principle of beneficence), and that because this benefit is likely to be enduring, while the discomfort is perhaps only transitory, considerations of non-maleficence are outweighed in this instance by those of beneficence.

15.3.2
CONSEQUENTIALISM

An alternative approach is that of consequentialism. In common with deontology, its focus is on the actions that it is appropriate for a person to take in a moral situation. However, in contrast to deontological theories, where there are a number of ethical principles, consequentialism has a single supreme principle which we could term the principle of best outcome. Here, courses of action are chosen not on the basis of the various ethical principles that they either fulfil or contravene, but strictly in terms of the consequences that they will bring about. Moral duties are thus determined not in terms of the *intrinsic* value of actions that fulfil certain principles, but in terms of the *extrinsic* value of those actions, as judged by their consequences. A particular course of action is not right or wrong in itself, but is assessed in terms of its outcome; the same action could be right in one situation and wrong in another, in relation to the different consequences that it may produce. Such consequences are often judged in terms of benefits and harms, and there is thus a consequentalist justification for the principles of beneficence and non-maleficence (Singleton 1996a). None the less, the separate foci of deontology and consequentialism remain – the former privileges beneficent actions, the latter beneficent outcomes (Table 15.2).

Thus the justification for insisting that the truth be told in a certain situation would be that to do so produces better consequences for all concerned, rather than because this is required by a wider ethical principle such as respect for autonomy. Similarly, confidentiality would be observed because to do so leads to a better state of affairs for all concerned, not because of the grounding of confidentiality in principles such as respect for autonomy or non-maleficence. Indeed, when deciding between two actions, the consequentialist will choose the one that produces the best consequences, even if this involves breaching certain ethical principles that the alternative course of action would have left intact. To return to an earlier example, a physiotherapist using a consequentialist framework might deliberately exclude patients from the planning of their rehabilitation, or withhold certain information from them, if he or she felt that more patients would be successfully rehabilitated in this way. The infringement of patients' autonomy involved would not be totally discounted, but in the final analysis it would take second place to the desirable consequences brought about. Indeed, there is a sense in which the infringement of autonomy would just be regarded as one consequence among many of the course of action followed. To the extent that respecting autonomy produces desirable consequences, this may count against a course of action that threatens a person's autonomy. However, the principle of respect for autonomy will have no special status in the calculation, and if other factors that involve infringing autonomy produce better consequences, all things considered, it is legitimate to override notions of autonomy.

To return to deontology, we can note that precisely the opposite situation may obtain. The deontologist can insist that a certain course should be pursued because it best fulfils certain fundamental ethical principles, even if it produces less desirable consequences, on balance, than the alternative. Thus, it would be claimed that the truth should always be told to patients, even when demonstrably better consequences would flow from the telling of a lie, or that confidentiality should be upheld, even if a net balance of harm results from so doing. This is similar to the popular notion that good ends cannot justify a bad means.

In consequentialism, therefore, the ultimate criterion for moral decision-making is the likely consequences of an action, whereas in deontology it is the extent to which certain fundamental ethical principles are observed, through performing or avoiding specific actions that uphold or transgress these principles, respectively. Although the distinction between consequentialism and deontology is often made by reference to situations in which the two ways of thinking generate opposite conclusions in terms of the course of action to be followed, in many situations the recommended course of action will be the same. A consequentialist may favour strict observance of confidentiality on the grounds that this is likely to produce the best consequences, and the deontologist may adopt the same policy because of considerations of autonomy or non-maleficence – it is only the justification for the course of action that differs between them.

15.3.3 VIRTUE ETHICS

The emphasis so far has been on determining the right thing to do in a particular situation. However, many ethicists have also stressed the need to be the right sort of person. In other words, it is important to possess certain virtues or character traits, in addition to performing actions that are morally right (Purtilo 1986, Pellegrino & Thomasma 1993, Johnstone 1994, Nicholson 1994, Oakley 1998). Among these morally desirable character traits are compassion, sensitivity, discretion, integrity, altruism, self-lessness and courage. It is not difficult to see their importance. Unless therapists are compassionate and sensitive to the needs of patients, it is likely that they will be unaware of many situations in which the interests and welfare of their patients are under threat. If they do not possess the virtue of discretion, they may not recognize those situations in which confidentiality is called for. Unless therapists possess a certain measure of courage, they may lack the resolve to carry through morally appropriate courses of action in circumstances where doing so may make them unpopular, or place their own interests at risk. Downie & Telfer encapsulate the importance of character traits in health care, alongside more intellectual aspects of the professional role: 'What is required … is not only intellectual or scientific understanding, but the sort of compassionate help and advice which one human being experienced in life's miseries can give another. This does not come from *having knowledge* (however desirable that may be) but from being *a certain kind of person*' (Downie & Telfer 1980: 160; original emphasis). There is an argument, therefore, that possessing certain moral character traits is a prerequisite for acting morally. Unless a practitioner has the sensitivity and responsiveness that come from virtues such as compassion or altruism, he or she is unlikely to perceive the moral dimension in clinical situations. So, it might be argued, without moral character traits, the more rational processes of moral decision-making – whether consequentialist or deontological – will not be set in motion.

Central to virtue ethics in health care is the concept of caring. Wright-St Clair (2001: 196) argues that 'caring ought to be the moral framework within which clinical and ethical reasoning occurs and from which clinical and ethical competence emerges'. A seminal text on caring is Noddings's (1984) book *Caring: a Feminine Approach to Ethics and Moral Education*. There has been much debate subsequently on the role of caring within health care ethics, especially in the nursing literature – see, for example, Cooper (1991), Hanford (1994), Allmark (1995), Fealy (1995),

Kuhse (1995), Bradshaw (1996), Gormley (1996), and Wright-St Clair (2001).

Thus, moral virtue plays an important part both in the initial recognition of a moral situation, and in the pursuit of action that has been identified as morally appropriate. However, as virtue ethics is not directly concerned with action, it may be less useful in determining the precise actions to take in a specific situation (Rachels 1993). This suggests that moral character traits and action-oriented processes of moral decision-making are interdependent, and that a balance should be struck between the two (Sim 1997a). Pellegrino & Thomasma (1993) provide a comprehensive discussion of the role of virtues in health care. Gauthier (1997) and Loewy (1997) discuss and illustrate some of the issues currently debated on this topic.

15.4 OBJECTIVITY AND ETHICS

It is important to address the common fallacy, identified by Gillon (1985a), that ethics is 'just a matter of opinion', and that, consequently, there is no rational basis for deciding between competing views. There is indeed a subjective element in ethical reasoning, and this explains why there is not necessarily a single correct answer to an ethical conflict or dilemma. However, what we are dealing with here are certain fundamental, subjectively-held moral convictions. These must be distinguished from matters of taste or personal bias: 'Taste involves matters of choice which are, though value-laden, essentially morally neutral. This, indeed, is what we *mean* by a matter of mere taste – that it pertains simply to preference, to matters without moral import' (Callahan 1988: 13; original emphasis).

Reaching a conclusion on an ethical issue is not just a matter of personal preference. Crucially, we are obliged to provide reasons for our decisions on moral matters in a way that we are not when deciding on questions of personal taste. In other words, morality involves us in a process of justification; but, we may ask, if there is a subjective element in ethics, how can we achieve any sort of objective process of justification? Here, it is important to realize that, although we cannot always justify our fundamental moral beliefs or principles according to any objective criteria, when we apply these principles to specific cases in the process of reaching a decision on a course of action, we are subject to certain stringent demands. If we fail to fulfil these demands, we can indeed be criticized. Just because ethical principles have an essential subjectivity about them, this is not to say that the whole process of ethical reasoning is subjective.

The first of these demands is that the way in which we link the particular situation to fundamental moral principles must be logically sound. In other words, when we seek to justify our decision in a certain case in terms of one or more of these principles, the steps we take in this justification must be logically defensible. Beauchamp & Childress (1994) see

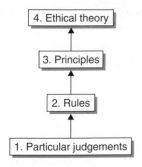

Figure 15.1 Hierarchical levels of ethical justification. Reproduced, by permission of Oxford University Press, from Beauchamp & Childress (1994), p. 15.

this as a hierarchical process (Fig. 15.1). Our particular judgements and actions are logically derived from certain rules, which are themselves derived from the principles that they seek to support (and these principles may be further derived from certain wider ethical theories). The second requirement is that this process of justification should be based on an accurate assessment of the facts of the specific situation. We have to justify our decision-making process in terms of the empirical evidence. Finally, there is a requirement of consistency. If a particular decision is taken in one situation, the same decision should be taken in any other situation that is similar to it in all morally relevant respects. In other words, a failure to adopt the same approach in two apparently similar situations must be justified by pointing to morally relevant differences between this situation and the other situation.

To take an example to illustrate these ideas, you may wish to justify a case of truth-telling in terms of the principle of respect for autonomy. Now, there is no conclusive way in which others can invalidate this principle (or the wider ethical theory on which it is based) as the starting point for your decision. Admittedly, from their own subjective standpoint they can disagree with the moral weight which you attach to it, and relegate it in importance below certain other principles, but it cannot be dismissed out of hand on any objective grounds. The way in which you proceed to base a course of action on this principle, however, must stand up to objective scrutiny on a number of counts, and may well show itself flawed. Each of the steps in the process of justification in Figure 15.1 must be defended. If you choose to formulate a specific rule concerning truth-telling in order to uphold the principle of respect for autonomy (i.e. moving between levels 2 and 3 in Fig. 15.1), you must demonstrate that this rule does indeed bear a strong relationship to the principle it is designed to fulfil; it is always open to somebody else to claim that a somewhat different rule is more appropriate. Similarly, when you enact this rule and take a specific course of action such as conveying certain information to a particular patient (i.e. moving between levels 1 and 2), the onus is once again on you to show that your action is faithful to the rule. Your critics may claim that modifications to your course of action, for example in its timing or the manner you presented the information, would have allowed it to conform better to your rule. Finally, your action must conform to the facts of the situation. It might be argued that you misread these. Perhaps what you took to be an apparent desire for information was in fact an implicit request to be shielded from unpleasant facts. As a result, your decision may have done more to breach the patient's autonomy than to preserve it.

Thus, while your adherence to the fundamental principle of autonomy cannot be refuted, none the less the procedure whereby you derive a moral rule from this principle, the way you translate this rule into concrete actions, and how you justify this process in terms of the external evidence are all areas where you can potentially be accused of being mistaken. Furthermore, you may be taken to task if you have failed to demonstrate consistency in your decision in relation to other, morally equivalent situations involving truth-telling.

Indeed, the demands of ethical decision-making are very similar to those of such processes as clinical diagnosis and treatment planning. In both cases, there is a need for logical thought processes and close attention to the specific facts of the case in question, followed by the formulation of a systematic plan of action.

15.5 CODES OF ETHICS

It is characteristic of occupational groups that have attained, or aspire to, professional status that they formulate a code of ethics (Sim 1985). Both altruism and accountability are central to the concept of professionalism, and codes of professional ethics can often be seen to affirm these notions. An ethical code generally consists of a number of ethical principles or rules, intended to guide the practice of members of the profession. The code is also often the basis for any disciplinary actions taken by the profession against one of its members.

In what sense, it may be asked, can a code of ethics be expected to provide such guidance? What exactly can physiotherapists gain from a code, and, just as important, what can they not gain from it? Above all, an ethical code is a consensus document. It represents the outcome of careful deliberation, by representatives of the profession as a whole, as to the sort of conduct that is required from individual practitioners. As such, it seeks to highlight the fundamental principles upon which one's professional life as a physiotherapist should be conducted, and to alert one to possible dilemmas and areas of conflict. The question remains, however, whether codes of ethics successfully fulfil this function.

In the first instance, it is not immediately clear whether codes of ethics are specifically concerned with ethics, if by 'ethics' we mean an examination of what is morally right or wrong. In many ways, ethical codes tend not so much towards ethics in this sense, as towards a sense of ethics that has 'a specific content which refers to codified procedures, but lacks the prescriptive force of morality' (Downie 1980). Singleton (1996b: 231) argues that: 'There is no explained underlying rationale to these codes. There is an implicit relation to ethical principles but no explicit account of the precise grounding of the codes. Without the philosophical underpinnings of these codes being made explicit, there is no way to assess adequately the resulting codes.'

The American Physical Therapy Association was in many ways ahead of its time when it drew up its first 'Code of Ethics and Discipline' in 1935. However, as Ruth Purtilo (1987) has argued, the code's requirements had more to do with procedural notions of etiquette than with specifically ethical concerns. More recently, the Chartered Society of Physiotherapy's revised *Rules of Professional Conduct* (Chartered Society of Physiotherapy 2002b) have stated that 'Chartered physiotherapists shall respect and uphold the rights, dignity and individual sensibilities of every patient' (Rule II), and that they 'shall ensure the confidentiality and security of information acquired in a professional capacity' (Rule III). These strike at the heart of genuinely moral concerns. However, Rule IV in the same document requires that physiotherapists should avoid inappropriate criticism of other professional staff, while Rule VI insists that advertising should be 'professionally restrained'. Meanwhile, Rule VIII reads: 'Chartered physiotherapists shall adhere at all times to personal and professional standards which reflect credit on the profession'. This is not to say that no ethical justification can be adduced for such requirements, but that they seem to reflect more of a focus on the profession's own public image than a concern for patients' welfare. The therapist who relies on a code of ethics must keep in mind a clear distinction between those aspects of the code that safeguard the interests of patients, and those that are geared towards the protection of professional interests. The former will almost invariably relate to genuinely ethical concerns, whereas the latter may not necessarily do so. Hence, the guidance that can be gained from an ethical code will not be necessarily, or wholly, on strictly ethical matters, such as we have defined them.

Having identified those parts of a code of ethics that deal with areas of genuine ethical import, the physiotherapist should be aware that the help that can be derived from the code can only be of a very general nature, and will inevitably be expressed in fairly clear-cut terms. Those cases that are most ethically perplexing will be far too complex and individual to be adequately catered for by a set of rules or principles. Unfortunately, an attempt to make codes of ethics more specific will not necessarily remedy the situation:

> First, the code will not be able to avoid controversial precepts and hence will be unlikely to win widespread acceptance. Second, it will probably fill many thick volumes, and thus lose the advantages of brevity and simplicity. And third, no matter how detailed it is, such a code will always be incomplete if its aim is to give unambiguous guidance in all possible situations (Benjamin & Curtis 1986: 7–8).

Furthermore, the sensitive and intricate nature of the patient–practitioner relationship is ill-suited to regulation by a standard set of rules: 'No set of rules could encompass all the subtle complexities of even the most ordinary relationship between two persons, much less the special dimensions peculiar to the medical transaction in which one person in special need seeks the assistance of another who professes to help' (Pellegrino 1979: 51).

There may be a tendency for practitioners to shelter behind a code to avoid thinking through the real issues (Johnson 1990). Indeed, Purtilo (1987) suggests that a 'code of ethics' is more appropriately understood as a 'code of morality'. By this she means that the code serves to highlight certain key moral concepts, such as duties and rights, but does not necessarily aid the individual in analysing these concepts, or applying them systematically and critically to concrete cases. In fact, while granting its value in drawing attention to important general ethical norms, one can see a way in which a code of ethics may actually impede an analytical approach to ethics. There is a danger that its codified nature, and the rather definitive terms in which it is expressed, may encourage the practitioner to think that 'the job has been done' in terms of ethical decision-making, and that further reflection on the issues concerned is redundant. As a result, decisions on ethical questions may become unreflective and stereotyped, and individual cases that are subtly but significantly different may be subsumed under a single category. It is vital that ethical 'rules of thumb' are re-examined, and even fundamentally questioned, every time they are invoked to deal with a specific situation.

A further shortcoming of codes of ethics is that they tend to consist of a series of dos and don'ts, and pay little heed to the idea of character traits (Sim 1997a). Such traits were identified earlier as playing an important role in ethical conduct within health care, and codes of ethics play little part in this respect. Finally, professional codes of conduct may reinforce notions of professional demarcation, in a way that goes against interprofessional working (Hewison & Sim 1998).

The above should not be taken as a dismissal of codes of ethics. Rather, it is intended to draw attention to some of their shortcomings, and to suggest that they are at best a partial solution to ethical dilemmas. If we refer back to Figure 15.1, we can see that any sort of rule represents only one level in the process of ethical justification. Moving up the hierarchy, these rules must be justified in terms of overall ethical principles of autonomy, beneficence, the best outcome, etc. Meanwhile, moving in the opposite direction, we see that the general guidance afforded by an ethical code should be augmented by a more critical and individualized examination of the specific ethical demands of the case in question. In the light of these specific demands, broad guidelines must be modified and prioritized, and supplemented by the physiotherapist's own individual ethical deliberation.

15.6 CASE STUDY

Hitherto, the discussion of ethical decision-making has been in somewhat general terms. In an attempt to crystallize some of the issues considered, the following case study will be examined.

Case study

A 54-year-old single woman, otherwise fit and healthy and previously employed as a clerical worker, has undergone an above-knee amputation following a road traffic accident a short distance from her bungalow. She arrives at the rehabilitation unit to take delivery of a temporary prosthesis and to begin walking training. The physiotherapists soon gain the impression that she is poorly motivated, and shows little interest in learning how to use the prosthetic limb. She views the prospect of life in a wheelchair with apparent equanimity. The rehabilitation team feel, however, that she has the prospect of a high level of functional independence with an artificial limb, but seem to be unable to convince her of this. Where should they go from here?

There are two broad approaches that could be taken to this situation:

1. One approach would be essentially to ignore the patient's expressed wishes, and seek to persuade, inveigle or cajole her into taking part in a gait-training programme. This could be justified in two ways. From a deontological standpoint, one could point to the principle of beneficence. In accordance with this, the therapist has a duty to act in the patient's best interests. In this case, these best interests could reasonably be understood as achieving functional independence, and this therefore becomes the goal at which the therapist should aim. If the patient seems a reluctant partner in this enterprise, the therapist must take steps to secure her participation, for her own ultimate good. Alternatively, if we adopt a consequentialist view of things, it could be argued that functional independence is a desirable – indeed the most desirable – possible outcome of the situation. Not only will it improve the patient's future quality of life, but it will also bring benefits to others (she will, for example, be less reliant on formal or informal carers for support). In line with consequentialist thinking, the utility of this outcome more than compensates for any acts of apparent coercion performed on the way. Thus, in both variants of this approach, the focus is on the ultimate goal of rehabilitation, either because this represents the best interests of the patient herself, or because it is overall the best of all the alternative outcomes for all concerned.

2. Others, however, might raise objections to this first approach, and adopt a different strategy. An alternative line of action would be to accept the patient's view, cease gait training, and begin a programme of wheelchair rehabilitation. Such a decision could be justified, in deontological terms, by the principle of autonomy. The sort of beneficent action outlined in the first approach, it might be argued, has been carried to the point at which it violates the individual's self-determination. As such, it would be seen as an example of paternalism:

> Physical therapists who believe that it is their *primary* duty to benefit patients and protect them from harm – including harm from patients' own choices – feel justified in acting paternalistically (Coy 1989: 828; original emphasis).

In other words, paternalism would suggest that the autonomy of the patient may be overridden so as better to serve her own interests, on the basis that the therapist can judge these interests better than she (see Section 16.2.2 for a fuller discussion of paternalism). In contrast to this stance, the present option places autonomy above competing principles such as beneficence, perhaps on the grounds that freedom of self-determination is part of what it is to be a person. An individual who is rendered non-autonomous loses something of his or her personal dignity. This is not to say that no value is attached to the principle of beneficence, simply that it should be regarded as prima facie – that is, it can be made to yield if it is at variance with another principle, such as respect for autonomy or respect for persons, which carries more moral weight in the given situation.

It is important to realize that this second course of action might very well lead to seemingly undesirable consequences for the patient – loss of mobility, greater dependence on others, reduced social contact, and so forth. However, seeking to avoid such consequences would not necessarily justify contravening the principle of respect for autonomy. As was noted earlier, it is maintained within a classic deontological approach that an ethical principle should be upheld, even if doing so seems likely to produce worse consequences overall than an alternative action which would breach this principle. Moreover, it should be remembered that the right to choose for oneself implies the right to make unwise choices, and that full respect for autonomy may involve allowing individuals to come to some degree of harm (Loewy 1989). In any case, therapists should be wary of assuming that the patient's view of a desirable or an undesirable outcome necessarily corresponds to their own.

So far, we have seen how these alternative approaches to the situation might be justified in terms of the various ethical principles and values at stake. However, it will be recalled that ethical decisions must also be justified empirically. It is not enough to produce ethical arguments that are internally coherent, they must also be in accordance with the external evidence of the case. We must ask, then, whether the approaches we have considered are compatible with the facts of the situation (bearing in mind, of course, that we have here only a few of the facts which would be available in the real case). The first approach, in both its deontological and consequentialist versions, relies on the value of achieving functional independence, either because this is in the patient's best interests, or because it is the most favourable set of possible consequences overall. Implicit in these arguments is the idea that, on the available evidence, functional independence is a likely outcome. Given what we know of the patient – that she is comparatively young, and otherwise fit and well – this seems to be a reasonable assumption. Additionally, the fact that she is single – and thus presumably without the constant availability of a partner as a source of help – serves to reinforce the need for independence. The fact that it is a demonstrable benefit lends support to any beneficent action undertaken to secure it.

On the other hand, when we consider the alternative approach that may be taken to this situation, we can find some support for the contention that the patient could attain a reasonable level of independence even if obliged to use a wheelchair. It is perhaps fair to assume that she could meet the demands of her job adequately in a wheelchair, and we know that she lives in a bungalow, thus obviating the need to climb stairs. However, a much more fundamental factual question may arise within this approach. The strategy adopted is founded on the patient's expressed wish not to proceed with gait rehabilitation. It is crucial that this is indeed the correct interpretation. It could be argued that what seemed to be an unwillingness to participate in rehabilitation was in fact only an expression of apprehension as to the hurdles that she will face in the process, and mistrust of her own ability to succeed (particularly if no such reluctance had been expressed by the patient previously). Another alternative is that the patient could be undergoing a reactive depression following the loss of her leg, and is thereby unable to make fully autonomous choices. If either of these were indeed the more plausible interpretation, much of the justification for the autonomy-based approach falls away.

This case illustrates how a situation may present the physiotherapist with fundamentally different ethical alternatives. Each of these has its merits, but in each case there are also possible difficulties. The question as to which is the option to be favoured cannot be settled definitively, but will always remain an open question. What matters is that, whichever course of action is adopted, it can be justified in terms of ethical reasoning and in the light of the particular facts of the case.

Whatever approach is taken, it is clear that a full and open dialogue between therapist and patient will aid the process of ethical decision-making. In this way, a clear picture of the patient's needs and desires, and an understanding of the likely effects of various possible courses of action, will usually emerge. Basically, it is hard to respect the interests and preferences of the patient if one hasn't made the necessary effort to find out what they are.

15.7 CONCLUSION

In this chapter, I have endeavoured to examine the place of health care ethics in physiotherapy, and to explore the means through which ethical decisions can be reached. Although there are often no definitive answers to ethical conflicts and dilemmas, reaching a conclusion on such matters is a rigorous process, and certainly not a mere matter of opinion. Codes of ethics may give help on the way, but ultimately it is for the individual therapist to evaluate each case on its merits, and to justify the course of action decided upon. It is crucial to realize that ethical decision-making is not an optional element in the practice of physiotherapy. Just as one cannot perform competently as a therapist if one is unwilling to assess one's patients, so there is an ethical commitment that is integral to the role of the health care worker (Sim 1983). To undertake a patient's treatment is to enter into a 'moral transaction' (Coates 1990), with all the ethical problems that this may entail. This is inescapable, for failing to confront these problems is itself a decision with far-reaching ethical implications.

In Chapter 16, the ideas introduced in this chapter will be applied to a number of specific issues that are likely to arise in physiotherapy practice.

Chapter 16

Moral decision–making in specific contexts

Julius Sim

16.1 INTRODUCTION

In Chapter 15, the broad concepts and principles of ethical decision-making were explored. In the current chapter, these will be used to examine some specific ethical issues that may arise within physiotherapy practice. Three such issues will be explored: informed consent, truthfulness and confidentiality. Rather than attempting a comprehensive discussion, certain key aspects of each of these topics will be addressed, with suggestions for further reading.

16.2 INFORMED CONSENT

Perhaps because it also has important legal implications, the topic of informed consent is a prominent one in discussions of ethics in physiotherapy (Purtilo 1984, Sim 1986a, 1996b, Coy 1989, Barnitt & Fulton 1994, Vines 1996). Broadly, informed consent may be defined as: 'the voluntary and revocable agreement of a competent individual to participate in a therapeutic or research procedure, based on an adequate understanding of its nature, purpose, and implications' (Sim 1986a: 584). It follows from this that there are a number of elements within the concept of informed consent (Fig. 16.1).

Figure 16.1 Elements of informed consent.

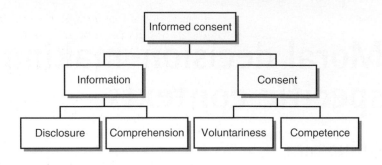

The element of *disclosure* concerns the account of a procedure or other proposed course of action that is provided to the patient by the therapist. The adequacy of disclosure is therefore judged by the content of this information – it should cover those issues that the patient is likely to find relevant in reaching a decision. For consent to be 'informed', disclosure alone is not sufficient. There also has to be *comprehension* on the part of the patient. This has implications for the way in which the information is communicated. Lesser points out that the standard of comprehension must be patient-based: 'the right to be informed must be a right to be informed in a way that one can understand; it is for the professional to adapt to the layperson as far as possible' (Lesser 1991: 156). Hence, the therapist must choose terminology and phraseology carefully, in order to maximize comprehension. Professional jargon or technical terminology may impede this, though it is important not to underestimate some patients' understanding of professional discourse, especially in view of the rapid rise of information available on the internet.

The question of *competence* refers to the individual's capacity to make decisions. Patients may lack competence for a number of reasons. Lack of competence may be temporary (for example, young children, the influence of alcohol or drugs, a confusional state), or intermittent (periodic amnesia, mental illness characterized by alternating periods of confusion and lucidity), or permanent (for example, learning disabilities, severe brain injury, irreversible coma). Individuals deemed incompetent are not necessarily so in a global sense; although they may not be competent in decision-making in some aspects of their lives, they may remain competent in others. Beauchamp & Childress (2001: 70) stress that competence 'depends not only on a person's abilities but also on how that person's abilities match the particular decision-making task he or she confronts'. Similarly, the degree of competence required may depend upon the 'weight' of the decision: 'a patient with some degree of cognitive and emotional disturbance following a head injury may be deemed competent to agree to a session of dressing practice or to the provision of feeding aids, but not sufficiently competent to consent to being rehoused, or to some other intervention which is likely to have irreversible effects' (Sim 1997a: 63).

Finally, *voluntariness* is the extent to which the individual feels genuinely free either to grant or refuse consent. In other words, it refers to the absence of inappropriate pressure or inducement to agree. A lack of voluntariness on the part of the patient may result from particular words or actions on the part of the practitioner, or may arise from the nature of the unequal power relationship between the two. Goodyear-Smith & Buetow (2001) discuss some of the ethical implications of power in patient–practitioner relationships.

Informed consent is based firmly within the principle of respect for autonomy (see Section 15.3.1). Making one's own decisions is core to a person's autonomy, and consent recognizes the importance of such self-determination. Cardol et al (2002: 973) maintain that 'respect for autonomy requires a client-centred rather than a biomedical perspective'; it involves taking the viewpoints and values of patients seriously, and endeavouring to discover what they are for the individual concerned; see also Clapton & Kendall (2002) and Kersten (2002).

16.2.1 PROBLEMATIC ISSUES SURROUNDING COMPETENCE

There are a number of situations in which a decision as to a patient's competence to decide may be problematic. Lack of competence may be temporary or intermittent. It may therefore be hard to decide at precisely what point competence has been lost, or at what point it has been regained. Thus, dementia characteristically leads to a gradual diminution of decision-making capacity. It is important, however, not to assume that the patient can no longer make decisions for him- or herself before this point has actually been reached (Sailors 2001). Equally, following a head injury or other acute trauma leading to loss of consciousness, an individual may no longer have the capacity to make rational decisions. In due course, however, this capacity is likely to return, and a careful judgement must be made as to when this has occurred, so that full decisional authority can be returned to the patient. It is important to judge competence at a particular time and context, and in relation to a particular patient, not in terms of the broad application of a diagnosis (Van Staden & Krüger 2003).

Clearly, newborn infants are not competent to make rational decisions, but when does such competence develop? Although there are legal thresholds for competence to consent to medical treatment, these are necessarily global, and individual children may develop competence at different ages. Research by Alderson (1990, 1993) suggests that children's ability to make rational and autonomous decisions is liable to be underestimated.

Physiotherapists often deal with patients in pain. Where pain is particularly severe – as may occur, for example, in the case of burns – it may be unclear whether an apparent refusal of treatment should be taken at face value. Has the pain in some way distorted the patient's values and priorities, such that the practitioner is justified in overriding the refusal of treatment? It is important not to do so too readily. First, it should be remembered that pain is a normal part of life, and the fact that a patient may be considerably distressed by pain does not mean that his or her judgement is necessarily impaired as a result. Second, there is a danger that the therapist's view that a patient is not competent to decide may actually represent a difference in perspective between practitioner and patient. The issue may have little to do with the rationality of the patient's decision, and much more to do with the therapist's disapproval or incomprehension of the choice being made. A *rational* decision (i.e. one based on consistent and logical reasoning) does not have to be a *reasonable* decision (i.e. one that strikes others as prudent or sensible); autonomy implies the right to make unwise decisions (Haas 1993).

Although it is often clinical aspects of patienthood that impair an individual's competence – symptoms or aspects of treatment that interfere with the usual process of rational decision-making – in some cases it is other aspects of the person's life, concerning his or her career or high-level sports participation (Sim 1993), that may cast doubt on the authenticity of a patient's decision.

Finally, it is unclear how competence should be assessed. There seems at present to be no accepted test of competence that can form part of routine clinical assessment. Furthermore, given that competence is not a global phenomenon, no single test of competence is likely to be applicable to the spectrum of situations in which the patient's capacity to decide may be at stake.

16.2.2 PATERNALISM

Caplan (1988: 315) argues that:

> rehabilitation professionals may be justified in overriding or ignoring the autonomous wishes of patients upon entry to a specialized unit for treatment if there are reasons to believe that the person either has not adapted to the traumatic realities of impairment, or that the patient will require some time to fully appreciate the possibilities available for coping with and adapting to chronic impairment.

Such a view essentially puts the demands of beneficence, at least temporarily, over those of respect for autonomy. This is an example of paternalism, which may be defined as 'interference with a person's liberty of action justified by reasons referring exclusively to the welfare, good, happiness, needs, interests, or values of the person being coerced' (Dworkin 1972: 65).

The notion of paternalism, grounded in notions of beneficence, thus provides a potential justification for ignoring or overriding a patient's wishes. Although something of a 'dirty word' nowadays, paternalism is a natural expression of the virtues of benevolence and altruism, and is generally motivated by a deep concern for patients' welfare. The problem, however, is that paternalistic actions involve some element of substituted judgement. Although in such a situation practitioners should try to view the situation from the patient's perspective, they will almost inevitably use their own beliefs, values and priorities in determining a course of action rather than those of the patient, and there is ample evidence that professionals' values do not necessarily reflect those of patients themselves (Sim 1998). There are, however, different categories of paternalistic action. In general, a distinction is made between acts of paternalism that wholly and expressly disregard a patient's competent wishes and intentions ('strong' paternalism), and those that endeavour to incorporate the patient's intentions, and are limited to those situations in which the patient cannot carry through such intentions him- or herself ('weak' paternalism); see Pellegrino & Thomasma (1988) and Buchanan & Brock

(1989). Beauchamp & Childress note that 'the paradigmatic form of *justified* paternalism starts with incompetent children in need of parental supervision and extends to other incompetents in need of care analogous to beneficent parental guidance' (Beauchamp & Childress 2001: 177; emphasis added). The implication here is that paternalism involving persons who *are* competent is not justified. Thus, weak paternalism is clearly easier to justify than strong paternalism. Highlighting the need to keep sight of patients' own priorities, Ellos (1990: 171–172) argues that:

> We should listen to patient preferences in terms of their own perceived quality of life. We should not be too aggressive in attempting to change or influence the patients' own life plans, goals and aims into which medical intervention fits as only one part or aspect ... the clinical diagnostic and therapeutic indications must be fitted prudently in the frame of the patients' larger scheme of perceived priorities and values.

See Buchanan (1981), Gert & Culver (1981), Childress (1982), and Gert et al (1997) for detailed analyses of paternalism. Shinebourne & Bush (1994) and Veatch & Spicer (1994) provide two sides of the contemporary debate.

16.3 TRUTHFULNESS

The issues relating to truthfulness have much in common with those covering the element of disclosure in informed consent. However, truth-telling is wider in its scope; it is not restricted to instances in which a particular therapeutic intervention is being proposed.

According to Bok, honesty from health professionals 'matters more to patients than almost everything else that they may experience when ill' (Bok 1978: xvi). She also points out that health professionals may not realize the impact upon the patient when they fail to tell the truth: 'many physicians talk about such deception in a cavalier, often condescending and joking way, whereas patients often have an acute sense of injury and loss of trust at learning that they have been duped' (Bok 1978: xvi). Honesty is generally regarded as a key character trait of professionals – especially in health care – and an assumption of the professional client relationship (Veatch 1981, Ellin 1982).

There are a number of ways in which a person can fail to be truthful (Sim 1997a):

- By failing to disclose some or all of the relevant information
- By disclosing all relevant information, but doing so in a way that creates a misleading impression
- By lying.

To the extent that these means stem from the same motive and lead to the same outcome – deception of the patient – there may be little to distinguish them morally. However, if the patient realizes that he or she has been deceived, a lie may be more harmful than withholding the truth (Beauchamp & Childress 2001), perhaps because lying is generally perceived as a more hurtful form of deception for the individual. None the less, professionals should not shelter behind rather dubious moral distinctions between different types of deception. Jackson (2001: 79) argues that: 'if doctors and nurses do have a general duty to inform, doing anything short of that is disreputable: be it lying, deceiving, concealing or simply, not disclosing. Hence, fine distinction drawing between lying and other ways of deceiving will already sound irrelevant and suspect.'

16.3.1 FOR AND AGAINST TELLING THE TRUTH

The principle of respect for autonomy supports the requirement of truthfulness in much the same way as it justifies the requirement for informed consent. In addition, to deceive somebody is to ignore their essential dignity, and may constitute using him or her purely as a means to an end. As such, truth-telling is supported by the principle of respect for persons. A number of more specific arguments can be proposed to support truthfulness, and equally a number of arguments can be advanced to justify deception. Some of these will be briefly considered.

As noted above, honesty is an assumption within the professional relationship. Accordingly, truthfulness can be seen as part of what this relationship means, and it can be argued that without honesty – on both sides – the relationship is likely to fail. There is, therefore, a starting assumption that the truth should be told, and in most instances it is deception, not truthfulness, that requires special justification.

A second reason why truthfulness is important is that it is a precondition for autonomous action and decision-making on the part of the patient. Without certain information, patients cannot make informed decisions, either within the context of health care or in their lives more generally. Thus, the patient with severe back pain who is not told of the full range of alternative treatments cannot make a rational choice between them, and the patient with paresis following a stroke who is not informed of the likely functional recovery cannot make decisions about future education, employment or living arrangements.

Effective management or treatment of the patient depends upon the patient being able to rely on what the therapist says, and vice versa. More specifically, if patients are expected to be involved and to cooperate in their rehabilitation, they must understand the nature of their problems and the purpose of whatever treatment is instituted. Moreover, the patient may well discover an act of deception sooner or later. This will tend to destroy trust in the relationship and the patient will be left wondering what to believe and what not to believe (Sim 1986b). Almost certainly, this will undermine the effectiveness of future care. Much the same effect may arise even before an act of deception is discovered, as the physiotherapist will find it hard to communicate freely with the patient for fear of revealing the information that he or she is trying to conceal.

An essentially fallacious justification for withholding the truth is to claim that the truth need not be told because, ultimately, the truth is not known – we only have a limited proportion of the facts about any situation, and we can never be sure that the information we do possess is correct. Furthermore, the argument may run, even if we have the full picture, the patient cannot be expected to understand it all, so the requirement to tell the truth does not arise. In the first instance, this view almost certainly underestimates patients' ability to understand medical and other technical information about their health, especially in the internet age. It also overlooks the fact that patients may grasp the implications of the facts of their situation, even if they cannot necessarily comprehend every technical detail: 'It is not necessary to comprehend the detailed histopathology of multiple sclerosis to appreciate the effect this condition will have on one's life, the likely prognosis, the probable effectiveness of alternative treatments, etc.' (Sim 1997a: 46). Finally, this argument ignores the fact that what matters is not the *actual* truth, in some omniscient sense, but what the practitioner *believes* to be the truth. Furthermore, the complete truth may not be relevant: 'There is a difference between being fully informed and adequately informed to make a decision, however. A patient is adequately informed if he or she has just enough relevant information to make a decision' (Kyler-Hutchison 1988: 286).

Another of the arguments sometimes advanced to justify deception is that knowing the truth can be harmful to the patient, especially when the truth consists of bad news. Accordingly, either a consequentialist argument, or deontological considerations of non-maleficence, may be adduced to support deception, as a justified form of paternalism. There is, however, strong evidence that what harms patients is not the nature of the truth, however drastic it may be in its implications, but the way in which the truth is told, if this is insensitive or clumsy (Wright 1973, Goldie 1982, Higgs 1994). Patients cope surprisingly well with bad news, providing it is delivered with care. 'Patients and families usually find ways to cope with and adjust to whatever picture reality paints, especially if clinicians deal with them sensibly, sensitively, and supportively. They rarely, if ever, recover from being deceived' (Scofield 1993: 344).

It may be, however, that *temporarily* deceiving a person may prevent harm. Thus, keeping a person in ignorance about their diagnosis or prognosis at a painful or distressing stage in the illness, and postponing disclosure to later may minimize the negative impact of the information while still respecting the patient's right to know.

16.3.2 CASE STUDY

The case below illustrates some of the troublesome issues that may arise in relation to truth-telling, and the situation in which therapists may find themselves. Most notably, the issue of harm is raised. The surgeon may have decided not to convey either the full details of the operation or her prognosis to Mrs Merrick in the belief that such information would adversely affect her recovery. In the event, the opposite seems to have occurred. Believing that she has had a successful operation and yet feeling no better appears to have created a distressing feeling of perplexity that has undermined Mrs Merrick's ability to regain her independence.

Furthermore, Mrs Merrick's attempts to gain additional information from the surgeon have been met by a paternalistic silence. Consequently, questions are now directed to Marielle Coton. This creates a problem for Marielle. Conveying details of the operation and the likely prognosis are ordinarily the prerogative of the surgeon. However, considerations of

Case study

Elizabeth Merrick is 70 years old. She was admitted to a medical ward in a malnourished state, jaundiced, in pain, and too weak to walk independently. After a number of investigations, a malignancy in the abdominal cavity was suspected, and surgery was carried out. Although a primary growth was removed during the operation, secondary growths were found. The message given to Mrs Merrick, however, was simply that the operation was a success. Marielle Coton was the physiotherapist caring for Mrs Merrick after the operation.

Rehabilitation was slow, and the patient constantly asked why she was feeling little better after an apparently successful procedure. Over a period of 10 days, Mrs Merrick became increasingly distressed at her lack of recovery – she was still unable to walk on her own – and began to disengage mentally from her rehabilitation. Having been unable to get further information from the surgeon, Mrs Merrick on several occasions asked Marielle if there was any reason for this; on one occasion she asked: 'The operation was successful, wasn't it?'

respect for autonomy suggest that disclosing such information is also the duty of the surgeon when the patient requests it. If one person fails to do what is morally required, another person may feel impelled to 'fill the gap' by taking up the moral responsibility. Thus, although the duty to inform would normally reside with the surgeon, Marielle may now feel that she has the duty. In the first instance, fulfilling this duty would entail efforts to persuade the surgeon to provide the information requested. As a last resort, however, if such efforts fail, Marielle may feel impelled to disclose the information herself. This raises the issues of the 'ownership' of information. Are the details of the operation Marielle's to give, and is she capable of explaining their implications appropriately? This highlights the problem of deciding at what point moral demands oblige one to step outside the normal functions of a professional role. It may also give rise to strained relationships with colleagues, and in a situation such as the one described in the case study every effort should be made to persuade the surgeon to provide the information before undertaking to do so oneself.

This case also illustrates the issue of requests for information. Mrs Merrick has specifically asked Marielle for additional information about her condition. Does this mean that the moral requirement to tell the truth depends to some degree on whether the details in question have specifically been demanded? Of course, a request for information provides fairly sound evidence that the patient needs to know, and may identify the particular facts that are of concern to him or her. However, if the practitioner feels that the patient needs certain information, a failure to provide it cannot be justified by saying 'but she never asked'. The fact that a person does not seek information does not mean that this information is not needed, or even that it is not wanted. Patients may be fearful specifically to ask for information they inwardly wish to have. On the other hand, enquiring of patients whether they want certain information is difficult without revealing such information in the process (Sim 1986b). Relatives may provide guidance on patients' likely wishes, but it may be hard to justify revealing confidential information to others before doing so to patients themselves. Furthermore, relatives may ask that the patient is not told, and it is important in such a situation to judge whether this for the patient's own sake or because they themselves find it easier to cope if the patient is kept in ignorance. The problem of paternalism may arise here, just as in situations of informed consent. Determining patients' information needs is a difficult and demanding process, requiring tact, sensitivity and a degree of empathy.

When dealing with a situation in which truthfulness is at issue, the physiotherapist may find it helpful to consider the following questions (Sim 1997a: 57–58):

- Is there reason to think that the patient genuinely does not wish to have such information?

- Would it normally be my responsibility as a therapist to deliver such facts, and if not, am I nevertheless justified in doing so?

- Have I discussed the issue with other members of the multidisciplinary team, and if so what light do their thoughts shed on the decision to tell?

- Do I have the appropriate communication and interpersonal skills, and the necessary background knowledge, to inform the patient effectively?

- If the information is likely to have an unsettling or distressing impact, have preparations been made to assist the patient in dealing with this?

16.4 CONFIDENTIALITY AND PRIVACY

Issues of confidentiality and privacy are currently of great concern in health care (Chalmers & Muir 2003, O'Brien & Chantler 2003). A recent study has shown that physiotherapists regard confidentiality as an important legal and ethical issue in their practice (Cross & Sim 2000).

Truth-telling is one side of the notion of trust in the patient–therapist relationship; confidentiality and privacy are the other side. The concepts of confidentiality and privacy are closely allied, but are none the less distinct. Privacy is concerned with access to other people. This may be physical access, but more commonly in health care it is access to information that is crucial. Gert et al (1997: 186) define privacy as follows: 'An individual or group has privacy in a situation with regard to others if and only if in that situation the individual or group is normatively protected from intrusion, interference, and information access by others.' Whereas privacy is to do with persons, confidentiality refers to information. Specifically, confidentiality relates to the use we make of information that we have about a person. Thus, privacy is something that can be *invaded*; confidentiality something that can be *violated* (Gert et al 1997). Privacy and confidentiality impose negative duties – we should not intrude into another's life in a way that the individual would not wish us to and we should not reveal information that we possess about that person. However, privacy and confidentiality may also be seen as imposing positive duties – they may oblige us actively to prevent access to others' lives, and to take specific measures to safeguard and protect information relating to them. Sometimes we have information about a person, but do not know who that person is.

This is a distinct but allied issue of anonymity; the degree to which information is attributable to a specific individual.

Confidentiality does not prevent the sharing of information about a patient; rather, it prevents the *inappropriate* sharing of such information. Communicating the details of a patient's condition to other practitioners involved in the patient's care is clearly legitimate, whereas divulging such information to people with no such direct involvement with the patient is not. The relevant criterion here is the 'need to know'. In almost all cases, members of the public most definitely do not have a need to know the details of a particular patient's medical condition. It is sometimes overlooked, however, that health professionals who are not directly engaged in the care of a patient do not usually have a need to know. Physiotherapists must therefore be very circumspect in the way they handle patient information, even when in the company of fellow practitioners. Above all, they should avoid what Siegler (1999: 492) calls 'the wanton, often inadvertent, but avoidable exchanges of confidential information that occur frequently in hospital rooms, elevators, cafeterias, doctors' offices, and at cocktail parties'. Ubel et al (1995) provide empirical evidence of breaches of confidentiality in elevators.

In terms of the ethical principles outlined in Section 15.3.1, confidentiality and privacy can be grounded chiefly in the principles of respect for autonomy and respect for persons, and confidentiality is also supported by the principle of non-maleficence. Given that autonomy centres on the ability to control one's own life, this idea can be extended to control over information about oneself. Some people, however, are unable to think or act autonomously, and the principle of respect for persons can be used to support privacy and confidentiality in such a case. For example, an individual who is comatose or severely mentally ill may not be capable of autonomous action, but may still possess an essential dignity as a human being that would be undermined by a breach of privacy or confidentiality (Sim 1997a). If information about a person is disclosed inappropriately, this may lead to harmful consequences for the person concerned – for example, information about HIV infection (Sim 1997b) or certain psychiatric diagnoses could lead to a person being stigmatized. Hence, confidentiality also derives support from the principle of non-maleficence.

16.4.1 CASE STUDIES

The following are three cases typical of those that might arise within physiotherapy practice:

Case study 1

Siân Allen is treating a woman, Mary Sorrell, referred by her general practitioner for a frozen shoulder, when she notices swelling in the axilla around the pectoralis major muscle and a puckering of the skin over the lateral aspect of her breast. On questioning the woman about this, she learns that she has found a lump in her breast. Siân asks the woman whether she has seen her doctor about this, but she says that she hasn't, and will not do so as her mother underwent a radical mastectomy at her age and she does not wish to undergo the same experience. Siân cannot persuade her to change her mind on this.

Case study 2

Colin Gray is treating a young woman, Marie Davies, for a haematoma on her arm. During treatment she admits that the injury is the result of her husband hitting her in a fit of temper. Grateful for somebody to talk to, she tells him about problems at home, and comments 'It's not really me I worry about, it's those times when he goes and hits the kids that I get frightened'.

Case study 3

Joan Burrage is treating a 42-year-old man, Graham Murray, for severe back pain. Mr Murray is currently off work from his job as a music shop manager, and is receiving sickness benefit. One evening, Joan goes bowling with some friends and colleagues, and notices Mr Murray taking part enegetically in a game a few aisles from her.

Before analysing specific aspects of these cases, it should be noted that the initial assumption would almost certainly be that confidentiality should be respected; just as with truthfulness, this is a prima facie duty placed on the therapist. Confidentiality is also an implicit assumption of the patient–therapist relationship; patients expect what they tell a health professional to be treated in confidence, by virtue of the professional role, without necessarily seeking or receiving an explicit assurance that this is the case. Acting in the professional role is to make an implicit promise of confidentiality (Cain 1998).

However, there may be specific aspects of a situation that justify a breach of this prima facie duty. Two possibilities exist. First, it may be argued that the information in question is not confidential, and thus falls outside the scope of the duty; for example, certain trivial items of information that have no relationship to personal or private aspects of the individual's life. Cain (1998) gives the example of a nurse being told by one patient that he was a keen golfer and then mentioning this fact to another patient whom she knew also to be a golfer. Hence, Gillon (1985b: 1635) argues that 'there can be no transgression of confidentiality if the information is not regarded as secret by the person giving it' (though this should not be taken to mean that only information revealed directly by the patient comes under the aegis of confidentiality). A person may therefore consent to information concerning him or her being revealed. This removes the requirement of confidentiality – though only in respect of the specific information concerned, and only in the context in which disclosure has been permitted. Second, it may be conceded that the information in question should normally be retained in confidence, but there are factors that override this requirement and thus justify revealing the information. The second argument is the one to be pursued here.

One important question when analysing cases such as these is to ask whose interests are at stake. Broadly, the first case involves the welfare of the patient alone; the second involves the welfare of both the patient herself and her children; and the third involves the interests of society. In addition, one can try to quantify those interests. In the first two cases, issues of personal safety and even life or death are involved; there is no disputing the seriousness of the situation in either case. Moreover, in Case 2, concerning Marie Davies's children, those at risk are especially vulnerable and defenceless. In the third case, the stakes are much lower; many people would argue that a possible fraudulent benefit claim is a relatively minor matter. In contrast, where a patient is deemed to constitute some sort of threat to public safety, much more vital interests of society would be under threat (for example, a patient liable to epileptic fits who continues to drive a minibus).

In terms of the magnitude of the issues at stake, therefore, Cases 1 and 2 might constitute a strong case for a breach of confidentiality. If we assume that all attempts to persuade Mary Sorrell and Marie Davies to seek appropriate help have failed, it might be argued that disclosing information might be the only way to prevent serious harm. This argument might be particularly strong in relation to harm that threatens a third party. So even if it acceptable for Marie Davies to place her own welfare at risk, on the basis that interference would be an inappropriate act of 'strong' paternalism (see Section 16.2.2), there might be a requirement for others to act in order to protect her children.

There are, however, counter-arguments to those supporting disclosure. In some cases, it might be claimed that the reasons for breaching confidentiality are simply not strong enough. Although the argument for disclosure in Case 3 might also be based on the interests of others – fraudulently claiming sickness benefit could be seen as harmful to genuine claimants – the argument is less strong than in Cases 1 and 2 because there is unlikely to be serious harm to any one individual. Another factor that might be adduced here is that the therapist has a direct therapeutic relationship with Mary Sorrell and Marie Davies (and an indirect relationship with the latter's children), but no direct relationship with potential benefit claimants in society at large. In other words, the duty of confidentiality derives some of its strength from the relationship that has been established between patient and practitioner.

The idea of a special relationship would be a deontological argument; consequentialism would not attach any special value to a moral requirement on the basis of its existing within a particular relationship. Rather, the focus would be on outcomes (see Section 15.3.2). It might at first appear that a consequentalist approach would support disclosure. When the welfare of all concerned is considered, breaching confidentiality is likely to produce a better outcome than maintaining it. However, whereas this may be so when a case is examined in isolation, the opposite conclusion may be reached on a long-term perspective. Even if revealing confidential information on a particular occasion might seem to have beneficial consequences, in the long term such a policy would be counterproductive. Thus, if patients do not feel sure that confidentiality will be upheld, they may be unwilling to reveal important pieces of information to health professionals, or may even fail to seek professional help in the first place

(Kottow 1994, Sim 1996a). A dissenting judge in a tragic case involving a psychiatric patient who killed his girlfriend (Tarasoff *v.* Regents of the University of California) commented:

> Given the importance of confidentiality to the practice of psychiatry, it becomes clear the duty to warn imposed by the majority will cripple the use and effectiveness of psychiatry. Many people, potentially violent – yet susceptible to treatment – will be deterred from seeking it; those seeking it will be inhibited from making revelations necessary to effective treatment (California Supreme Court 1994: 178).

Confidentiality can face the physiotherapist with an acute moral conflict, with both disclosure and silence supported by strong moral reasons. In seeking to resolve such a dilemma, it may be helpful to consider the following:

- The 'default' assumption should be that confidentiality is to be maintained; specific arguments are required to override this requirement in a specific case.

- The fact that there may be legal or contractual constraints against breaching confidentiality in a particular case does not necessarily mean that it would be *morally* wrong to do so (see Section 15.1).

- Other strategies for averting harm should be fully explored before resorting to a breach of confidentiality.

- The issues at stake, and the conclusion reached, may differ according to whether it is the interests of others or of the patient him- or herself that are at risk if confidentiality is maintained.

- The likelihood of harm if confidentiality is upheld should be calculated carefully in the case concerned; sometimes there will be certain harm to the patient brought about by breaking trust, but only a probable risk of harm to others if confidentiality is kept (Kottow 1986).

- The consequences of revealing a confidence should be examined in the long term, as well as in the confines of the case concerned.

16.5 CONCLUSION

This chapter has briefly explored three common ethical issues that arise in everyday physiotherapy practice. Fuller analysis of these issues can be found in some of the texts referenced in each section. Other ethical issues – such as those relating to death and dying or resource allocation – also impact on the work of physiotherapists. These are examined in Sim (1997a) in relation to physiotherapy, and from a more general perspective in texts such as Gillon & Lloyd (1994) and Beauchamp & Childress (2001). Some of the theoretical foundations of health care ethics are analysed in detail by Engelhardt (1996).

SECTION 4

Psychosocial aspects of physiotherapy care

Chapter **17**

Defining disability: implications for physiotherapy practice

Sally French

17.1 AIMS AND SCOPE

In the first part of this chapter two central models of disability will be discussed; the individual model and the social model. There are other models of disability, for example those derived from religion where disability may be regarded as a gift or a punishment (Ingstad & Reynolds Whyte 1995, Hughes 1998, Stiker 1999), but these no longer have a strong influence in British society. They do indicate, however, that disability (and indeed impairment) is socially constructed and can change in meaning over time and across cultures. The concept of institutional discrimination will also be examined. Institutional discrimination analyses oppression within institutions, such as hospitals, in terms of attitudinal, environmental, cultural and structural barriers (Swain et al 1998a, Thompson 2001).

17.2 WHAT IS A MODEL?

The terms 'theory' and 'model' are often used interchangeably. Kerlinger (1986: 8) defines a theory as a 'set of interrelated constructs (concepts), definitions, and propositions that present a systematic view of phenomena by specifying relations among variables, with the purpose of explaining and predicting the phenomena.' Models, in contrast, can be defined as a set of assumptions about how an event or process operates. A model usually lies within the framework of a broader theory.

Within every society there are competing models of disability, with some being more dominant than others at different times (Finkelstein 1993, Hughes 1998). These models, although often in conflict, may gradually influence and modify each other. The models put forward by powerful groups within society, such as the medical profession, tend to dominate the models of less powerful groups, such as those of disabled people themselves (Finkelstein 1993, Oliver 1996a, Russell 1998).

It is essential to explore these models of disability, for attitudes and behaviour towards disabled people, policy, professional practice and the running of institutions, including hospitals and rehabilitation centres, are based at least in part upon them. As Oliver states: 'The "lack of fit" between able-bodied and disabled people's definitions is more than just a semantic quibble for it has important implications both for the provision of services and the ability to control one's life' (Oliver 1993a: 61).

17.3 THE INDIVIDUAL MODEL OF DISABILITY

The most widespread view of disability at the present time is based upon the assumption that the difficulties disabled people experience are a direct result of their individual physical, sensory or intellectual impairments (Oliver & Sapey 1999, Priestley 1999). Thus, the blind person who falls down a hole in the pavement does so because he or she cannot see it, and the person with a motor impairment fails to get into the building because of his or her inability to walk. Problems are thus viewed as residing *within* the individual (Swain et al 1993, Hales 1996). The individual model of disability is deeply ingrained and 'taken as given' in the medical, psychological and sociological literature. Even in the literature on the sociology of health and illness, disability, as disabled people define it, is basically ignored (Barnes & Mercer 1996).

The medical model can be regarded as a subcategory of the overarching individual model of disability where disability is conceived as part of the disease process, abnormality and individual tragedy – something that happens to unfortunate individuals on a more or less random basis. Treatment, in turn, is based upon the idea that the problem resides within the individual and must be overcome by the individual's own efforts. Disabled people have, for example, been critical of the countless hours they have spent attempting to learn to walk or talk at the expense of their education and leisure (Sutherland 1981, Oliver 1996a). Caroline, a deaf woman interviewed by Corker states:

> I hated learning speech – hated it – I felt so stupid having to repeat the s, s, s ... Every time I got it wrong, I had to do it all over again and I was asking myself 'Why do I have to keep going over and over it, I don't understand what it all means!' ... It was just so stupid, a waste of time when I could have been learning more important things (Corker 1996: 92).

Priestley (1999) refers to the tendency to individualize disability as the 'culture of embodiment'.

None of these arguments imply that considering the medical or individual needs of disabled individuals is wrong; the argument is that the individual model of disability has tended to view disability *only* in those terms, focusing almost exclusively on attempts to modify people's impairments and return them or approximate them to 'normal'. The effect of the physical, attitudinal and social environment on disabled people has been ignored or regarded as relatively fixed, which has maintained the status quo and kept disabled people in their disadvantaged state within society (Oliver & Sapey 1999). Thus the onus is on disabled people to adapt to a disabling environment (Swain et al 1993, Hales 1996). This is something that disabled people are increasingly challenging. Oliver (1996a: 44) states: 'The disability movement throughout the world is rejecting approaches based upon the restoration of normality and insisting on approaches based upon the celebration of difference.'

Individualistic definitions of disability certainly have the potential to do serious harm. The medicalization of learning disabilities, whereby people were institutionalized and abused, is one example (Ryan & Thomas 1987, Potts & Fido 1991, Atkinson et al 2000). Another is the practice of oralism, where deaf children were prevented from using sign language (Humphries & Gordon 1992, Dimmock 1993, Corker 1996). Disabled children have been categorized into schools according to their impairments, where they have been segregated from society, frequently abused, and usually given an inferior education (Barnes 1991, Humphries & Gordon 1992, French 1996a, French & Swain 2000).

Oliver (1993b), Davis (1993a) and McKnight (1995) are of the opinion that the individual model of disability may serve the needs of professionals more than those of disabled people. Wendell is also suspicious of the involvement of professionals in the lives of disabled people. She states: 'both the charities and most government bureaucracies ... hand out help which would not be needed in a society that was planned and organised to include people with a wide range of physical and mental abilities. The potential resistance created by these vested interests in disability should not be under-estimated' (Wendell 1996: 53).

By individualizing disability, the effect of the environment upon the lives of disabled people is not addressed. Indeed, the environments imposed upon disabled people in the name of treatment – for example, day centres and special schools – can have detrimental effects, leading to greater dependency and an increase in existing problems of function or behaviour (Potts & Fido 1991, French 1996a). Finkelstein & Stuart (1996) are of the opinion that, in the UK, issues relating to disability would be better placed in the Department of the Environment, rather than the Department of Health, and that important new disciplines in engineering and architecture need to be developed in order to make the environment more accessible to disabled people.

As well as experiencing external oppression from disabling environments and other people's attitudes and expectations, disabled people can also become internally oppressed by viewing themselves in the same way as many non-disabled people view them, and behaving as others expect them to behave (Goffman 1968, Mason 1992, Oliver & Barnes 1998). Woolley (1993: 81) explains: 'We are oppressed from without by a society which does not value us and therefore does not give priority to our needs, and we are oppressed from within because we have internalised these same attitudes towards ourselves.' This self-fulfilling prophecy can, in turn, lead to 'proof' that the erroneous attitudes and beliefs about disabled people are correct, which can serve to justify the treatment they receive, thereby creating a vicious circle (Finkelstein & French 1993).

It is not at all surprising that disabled people internalize the views of the wider society as, with the exception of the deaf community (mainly those who are born deaf), there has been very little sense of cultural identity among them until recent times. This makes it difficult for disabled people to reject the expectations and beliefs about how they should think, feel and behave which other people may hold. Disabled children, in particular, are very vulnerable to this conditioning. Their parents are often unwitting oppressors in the process, with their beliefs and expectations being shaped by those of professional 'experts' and society at large (Oliver & Barnes 1998). As Morris states: 'Most of the people we have dealings with, including our most intimate relationships, are not like us. It is therefore very difficult for us to recognise and challenge the values and judgements that are applied to us and our lives. Our ideas about disability and about ourselves are generally formed by those who are not disabled' (Morris 1991b: 37).

These disabling expectations and attitudes are, however, rarely completely internalized and may be quickly dispelled when disabled people are exposed to alternative ideas. It can also be entirely rational to behave in ways that other people expect in order, for example, to gain support, acceptance and approval (French 1993). Such ways of behaving can, nevertheless, give rise to passivity, anxiety and depression and many disabled people spend a great deal of time and energy attempting to reverse such social conditioning (Sutherland 1981, Woolley 1993).

The individual model of disability leads to an expectation that disabled people should play the 'disabled role'. The obligations of this role are to strive for 'independence' and 'normality', to 'accept' disability and to 'adjust' to it (Sutherland 1981, French 1994c). Independence, in the narrow sense of physical self-reliance, is generally considered to be something disabled people desire above all else. Disabled people are admired when they strive for independence, however inefficient, frustrating and stressful it may be. Being able to dress and wash oneself, walk, clean the house and make the bed are frequently considered paramount, however much time and effort are involved, whereas seeking help from others is rarely encouraged and may give rise to disapproval (French 1993). Non-disabled people, in contrast, pay for cleaners, gardeners, mobility aids (in the form of cars and bicycles) and labour-saving devices without any sense of guilt or disapproval from others. Indeed the possession of such assets may serve as powerful status symbols (Shakespeare 2000).

Physiotherapists and other health professionals tend to regard physical independence as a central aim of the rehabilitation programme. But is it always in the best interests of disabled people to strive for independence of this type? Morris (1989) found that many of the women with spinal cord injuries she interviewed chose to rely on personal assistants so that they could concentrate on other things, such as paid work, voluntary work or involvement in political activity. Disabled people are increasingly viewing independence in terms of self-determination and control and are rejecting the narrow, professional definition of independence as oppressive and contrary to their rights. This is reflected in the popularity among disabled people of direct payment, whereby they can buy their own social services following an assessment (Dawson 2000, Holman & Bewley 2000). Ryan & Holman state that '[i]ndependence is not necessarily about what you can do for yourself, but rather what others can do for you, in ways that you want it done' (Ryan & Holman 1998: 19).

Oliver (1993b) contends that the dependency of disabled people is created by a variety of social, economic and political factors. Disabled people are excluded from the workplace in large numbers, which creates economic and social dependency (Burchardt 2000). May (2000) points out that during the 1960s, when jobs were plentiful, far more people with learning difficulties were in open employment than they are today. Similarly, during the Second World War, when many posts were vacant, large numbers of disabled people were given responsible work only to lose it when the war was over (Humphries & Gordon 1992).

Government policy, and failure to enforce policy, can also create dependency. In the 1944 Employment Act, employers who employed 20 or more people were obliged to include 3% who were disabled (the quota system), but this law was never enforced. Health and community policy have created professional services that impose dependency on disabled people through institutionalization and inequality of power. Professionals act as gatekeepers to resources such as aids and equipment and decide, in their role as 'experts', what disabled people can and cannot have. The language of professionals and social policy ('sufferers', 'carers', 'special needs', 'patients') reinforces the notion that disabled people are helpless and tragic (Corbett 1996). Disabled people, after long exposure to these ideas (reinforced by charity advertising and negative imagery in the media) may come to view themselves as dependent, with a subsequent loss of agency and self-esteem (Oliver 1996a, Swain et al 2003a). There has been a failure, at the level of government and within professional education, to analyse disability critically or to learn from disabled people themselves (Finkelstein & Stuart 1996). Davis (1993a), McKnight (1995) and Russell (1998) have pointed out that professionals are dependent on disabled people for their careers, their status and their livelihoods and that many vested interests operate to maintain disabled people in their present situation. They contend that the money spent on professional education and salaries would be better spent directly by disabled people themselves. Similar criticisms have been made against traditional charities. Russell (1998: 90) states:

> charities often do more for nondisabled people. They hire nondisabled employees, appoint nondisabled people to their boards, and contract with nondisabled service organisations who don't employ disabled people. Charities are supposedly set up to do 'for' disabled people; in

reality they are hierarchies of power in which the socio-economic status quo is perpetuated, with disabled people at the bottom.

Although disabled people are usually regarded as the recipients of care, the notion of interdependency applies to them as much as anyone else. As well as providing work for professionals and others in the 'disability industry', disabled people give as much as they receive in their roles as parents, 'carers', employees, volunteers, lovers and friends. There is often an erroneous assumption that disabled people are unable to reciprocate the help they receive whereas, in reality, people who require assistance are often carers themselves (Morris 1991b, Potts & Fido 1991, Walmsley 1993). Institutions for disabled people, for example, could only function because of the work (largely unpaid) of the inmates, not only in cleaning, laundering and tending the garden, but also in assisting those who were younger or more disabled than them. Andrews, who has learning difficulties, explains:

> We worked on other wards too, feeding, washing and dressing. We used to help the nurses …. I used to make the beds, I did night duty too. I was knackered by the time I was finished. There was a tall lady who used to sit in this chair and she couldn't walk, not unless you walked behind her. So I had to put my hands out to stop her from falling backwards and I had to turn her round and put her on the toilet (Andrews & Rolph 2000: 36).

Similarly Gwen, a visually impaired woman, remembered the care she was compelled to give younger children at her special residential school:

> We used to have to help with the bathing of them and putting them to bed. We had no choice but I didn't mind because it was something different. The little children used to like it when we rubbed them dry, they wanted someone to cling to because they were missing their parents. We had to clean their shoes and if your little one went off to church with dirty shoes you were told off (French 1996a: 27–28).

We are, of course, all dependent on each other to a large extent, and we all use aids such as washing machines, scissors, motor cars, aeroplanes, eating utensils and computers, to save time and to overcome physical limitations such as our inability to move fast or to fly. We are also dependent on other people to produce and repair these aids. As Oliver points out, the dependency of disabled people 'is not a feature that marks them out as different in kind from the rest of the population but as different in degree' (Oliver 1993b: 51). Despite the interdependency of us all, the dependency of disabled people tends to be regarded as 'special' and qualitatively different.

The problems disabled people face and the equipment they need, such as wheelchairs, visual aids and hoists, are also regarded as exceptional. This creates beliefs among physiotherapists and others that disabled people should 'manage' in as 'normal' as way as possible and that 'unnecessary' aids may harm them by reducing the amount of exercise they take or making them lazy and dependent. These beliefs, and the control of professionals over resources, exacerbate the considerable practical difficulties disabled people face in acquiring the aids and equipment they need (Davis 1993a).

The physical and psychological stress involved in gaining independence in basic tasks, as well as the wasted time and reduced social opportunities incurred, are rarely given much attention by anyone other than disabled people themselves. Yet we do not insist that people walk 6 miles or even 1 mile rather than use their motor cars, or that they dispose of labour-saving devices in case they become lazy or dependent on the people who produce or repair them. Indeed, to attempt to enforce such a plan would be considered extremely patronizing and a serious breach of human rights, even if it were motivated in terms of the person's 'own good'.

Closely associated with the concept of independence is that of normality. Drake (1996), Russell (1998) and Swain & French (1998) assert that the concept of normality merely reflects dominant values in a particular community at a specific time, and Fawcett believes that 'normality is confirmed by being compared to abnormality, to the "other". Devalued groups by default confirm the validation of other groupings' (Fawcett 2000: 15).

The pressures placed upon disabled people to appear 'normal' can give rise to enormous inefficiency and stress. If people with severe visual impairments attempt to walk around busy towns without a white stick, for example, they are likely to feel more stress and be less efficient than if they use them. Yet despite this, many schools for visually impaired children discouraged their use. Many disabled people are well into adulthood before they realize what is happening or before they find the courage to abandon attempts to be 'normal' (Campling 1981, French 1993). The pressure to be 'normal' is often at the expense of the disabled person's needs and rights. For example, if a person with a motor impairment who can walk short distances is denied a wheelchair, he or she may become isolated or unable to engage in certain types of education or employment. Mason (1992: 27) believes that '[a]lmost every activity of daily living can take on the dimension of trying to make you less like yourself and more like the able-bodied' and Ryan & Thomas (1987) contend that the conventional and conformist lifestyles forced upon disabled people can be an exaggeration of normality. Munro & Elder-Woodward (1992: 29) state: 'Service users should not have to conform to the standards and values of the majority of society, nor to the expectations of service providers, they should have access to the full range of possibilities so that they can make choices using their own values and interests.'

The goal of 'normality' can also be physically dangerous as when the person with a marked visual impairment avoids using a white stick. Similarly the use of crutches over many years (rather than using a wheelchair) can put excessive strain on upper limb joints, and rendering an impairment less visible can produce social problems which are equally or more difficult to manage than when the impairment is exposed (Thomas 1999). As a disabled woman in Sutherland's book explains, 'I'm happier with something that isn't a deception than with something that is' (Sutherland 1981: 75). Sutherland, drawing heavily on the experiences of disabled people in encounters with health professionals, talks at length of this:

> There's a tremendous emphasis on a child who's had polio or whatever to walk, to be as able-bodied as possible. It's like standing up is infinitely

better than sitting down, even if you're standing up in a total frame –
metal straps and God knows what – that weighs a ton, that you can't move
in, which hurts, takes hours to get on and off and looks ugly. It's assumed
that that's what you want and that's what is best for you (Sutherland
1981: 73).

Because of the negative attitudes towards disability that prevail in
society, disabled people, and those who live and work with them, may
come to the conclusion that attempting to be 'normal' is the only way to
succeed; the goal of normality is thus justified in terms of social acceptance. For example, it can be argued that one of the objectives of deaf
people learning to talk, blind people learning to use facial expression,
and people with Down's syndrome having cosmetic surgery, is that they
will be more socially acceptable, less socially isolated and better able to
compete with non-disabled people. Although these ideas contain some
truth, the problem with this approach is that disabled people are left to
deal with disability entirely on their own, while society learns nothing of
its true nature and therefore does not need to change.

The expectation of normality leads many disabled people to attempt to
become 'super-human' so as to avoid the negative stereotypes of helplessness and inadequacy. Morris (1991b) contends, however, that those
who play the role of 'honorary non-disabled person' do little to further
the interests of disabled people as a whole. This type of behaviour is,
however, often rewarded by health professionals, by praise for example,
and encouraged in the professional literature and the media.

Morris (1991b) believes that the assumption that disabled people want
to be 'normal', rather than just as they are, is one of the most oppressive
experiences to which they are subjected. She rejects the view that it is
progressive and liberating to ignore difference, believing that disabled
people have a right to be 'equal but different'. She states, 'I do not want to
have to try and emulate what a non-disabled person looks like in order to
assert positive things about myself, I want to be able to celebrate my difference, not hide from it' (Morris 1991b: 184).

Within the individual model, disability is viewed as an individual
tragedy to which disabled people must 'adjust' (Oliver & Sapey 1999,
Thompson 2001). The period of adjustment is frequently depicted in
terms of the typical stages of grief (denial, anger, depression and acceptance), outlined by Kubler-Ross (1969) in relation to terminal illness.
According to Oliver & Sapey (1999), non-disabled people have imagined
what it must be like to be disabled, have assumed it would be a tragedy,
and have decided that it would require a difficult psychological adjustment. Some disabled people, on the other hand, while recognizing that
disability may be a cause of psychological distress, reject the suggestion
that this is inevitably the case. Many disabled people find that becoming
disabled does not lead to unhappiness and that new and satisfying
opportunities may be opened up by becoming disabled (Swain & French
2000). This is illustrated in the following quotations:

As a result of becoming paralysed life has changed completely. Before my
accident it seemed as if I was set to spend the rest of my life as a religious

sister, but I was not solemnly professed so was not accepted back into the order. Instead I am now very happily married with a home of my own (Morris 1989: 120).

I was horrified by what I imagined to be the experience of disabled people, which I encountered in my practice. Now 15 years after becoming disabled, I find myself completely at home with the concept, of effectively being me! ... Now I know that my assessment of the potential quality of life of severely disabled people was clearly flawed (Basnett 2001: 453).

MS has been something I've used. Having MS has been an added dimension in my training, in my understanding of people, and in the development of my expertise and skills (disabled doctor, quoted in French 2001: 44).

I cannot wish that I had never contracted ME, because it has made me a different person, a person I am glad to be, would not want to miss being and could not relinquish even if I were cured (Wendell 1996: 83).

Even those who do mourn may be mourning the loss of their easy interaction with the social and physical environment rather than the loss of bodily function, a situation that could to a large extent be eliminated by concerted political action.

In many cases physiotherapists and other health professionals have viewed their role as that of helping disabled people accept their situation and adjust to it. Disabled people have been urged to overcome what are viewed as *their* problems, to learn to live with them and never to complain. Any anger or depression concerning lack of access, hostile attitudes, inappropriate rehabilitation, poor housing or non-existent educational or job opportunities has been viewed as evidence of maladjustment, denial and a 'chip on the shoulder'. Individualistic conceptions of disability have been severely criticized by disabled people, who have concluded that they serve the interests not of themselves, but of the non-disabled majority. It is very convenient for society that disabled people should accept what are viewed as *their* problems, and adjust to them, for in that way the status quo is maintained. All aspects of this conception of the disabled role are now regarded by disabled people as oppressive on the grounds that it individualizes and depoliticizes disability and maintains a disabling physical and social environment.

17.4 THE SOCIAL MODEL OF DISABILITY

The social model of disability is often referred to as the 'barriers approach', where disability is viewed not in terms of the individual's impairment, but in terms of environmental, structural and attitudinal barriers which impinge upon the lives of disabled people, and which have the potential to impede their inclusion and progress in many areas of life, including employment, education and leisure, unless they are minimized or removed (Oliver 1996a). The social model of disability has arisen from the thinking and writings of disabled people themselves (Oliver & Sapey 1999). As Priestley asserts, 'the development of the disabled people's movement is inextricably bound up with a social model of disability' (Priestley 1999: 35). Before exploring the social model of disability in more detail, therefore, it is necessary to place it within its historical context within the disabled people's movement and to examine briefly the origins and growth of that movement.

17.4.1 THE DISABLED PEOPLE'S MOVEMENT

Social movements arise as a result of specific or widespread grievances and unrest; their goal is usually to reorganize society in some fundamental way (Fulcher & Scott 1999). Social movements have been defined by Giddens (1989: 624) as: 'a collective attempt to further a common interest, or secure a common goal, through collective action outside the sphere of established institutions'. They are led and controlled primarily by oppressed people themselves when, through sharing their experiences with similar people, they come to attribute the source of their concerns to social conditions and seek to find political solutions. Davis (1993b: 287), talking of the disabled people's movement, states: 'The movement came when disabled individuals first faced up to the fact that they could achieve more for themselves through collective action than they could on their own.'

Oliver (1996a) places the disabled people's movement among the 'new social movements' that have emerged during the second half of the twentieth century: the women's movement, the black civil rights movement, gay pride and mad pride are other examples. The aim of these movements is to gain equality and social justice.

The disabled people's movement comprises organizations *of* disabled people. Organizations of disabled people are those where disabled people are in positions of control. Although such groups have proliferated in recent years, it is a mistake to imagine that the resistance of disabled people to oppression is a recent phenomenon. Two early organizations of this type in the UK were the British Deaf Association (founded in 1890) and the National League of the Blind (founded in 1899). These early groups were militant, focusing on the particular problems deaf and blind people faced within an environment designed for non-disabled living. Other social movements, for example the women's movement, were also active at this time (Summerfield 1996).

Over the next 60 years, many other organizations of disabled people developed. They usually focused on specific impairments or single issues, such as lack of state provision. The National Federation of the Blind, for example, was formed in 1947. During the 1960s and 1970s, organizations of disabled people that crossed impairment boundaries began to develop; the issue that drew them together was poverty. For example, the Disablement Income Group (DIG), formed in 1965 by two disabled women, aimed to secure a disability allowance from the state for all disabled people to compensate them for the extra costs of disability; its appeals and campaigns were notably unsuccessful.

Perhaps the most significant turning point for the disabled people's movement in Britain was the formation in 1974 of the Union of the

Physically Impaired Against Segregation (UPIAS). Davis (1993b) explains how UPIAS fought to change the definition of disability from one of individual tragedy to one of social oppression. This paved the way for the development of the social model of disability that is at the intellectual heart of the disabled people's movement (Priestley 1999) and is referred to by Hasler (1993) as the 'big idea'. The Liberation Network of Disabled People, which was led by disabled women, also developed at this time. It challenged disabling barriers at a more personal level, focusing, for example, on internal oppression. It provided a less overtly political forum for the discussion of ideas and experiences (Campbell & Oliver 1996).

In 1981 a group of disabled activists came together to form the British Council of Disabled People (BCODP), which is an umbrella organization for organizations of disabled people. A large number of BCODP's member organizations comprise coalitions of disabled people and Centres of Integrated Living, which offer a range of services for disabled people, such as advocacy, counselling, information and advice on independent living, and are run and controlled by disabled people themselves. Other member organizations include those that focus on specific impairments or single issues, for example GEMMA (an organization of disabled lesbians) and the Association of Blind Asians.

During the 1980s, BCODP grew and continues to expand; in 2001 it represented 130 organizations and is recognized as the representative voice of disabled people in Britain. It articulates its demands through formal political channels and lobbies and advises both central and local government. It undertakes research and organizes and supports demonstrations and campaigns of direct action.

Disabled People's International (DPI) was also formed in 1981. It is an international umbrella organization of organizations of disabled people. In 2001 it represented 158 national assemblies of disabled people, including BCODP, and is recognized by the United Nations as the representative voice of disabled people internationally.

An important element in the struggle of disabled people for equality and social justice is the disability arts movement. Disability arts is a relatively recent, though well established, branch of the disabled people's movement. A wide variety of activities are encompassed within disability arts including theatre, dance, poetry, photography, comedy, music and visual art. Although disability arts is concerned with gaining access for disabled people to mainstream artistic facilities and opportunities, its main function is to communicate the distinctive history, skills, customs, experiences and concerns of disabled people, which many believe constitute a distinctive lifestyle and culture (Vasey 1992). Disability arts gives disabled individuals the opportunity to express their views and experiences of impairment and disability which often run counter to mainstream ideas and stereotypes. A central feature of disability arts is, however, collective experience. Disabled people are increasingly coming together to help each other express themselves in art and to share information and ideas. Barnes et al (1999: 205–206) define disability arts as: 'the development of shared cultural meanings and the collective expression of the experience of disability and struggle. It entails using art to expose the discrimination and prejudice disabled people face and to generate group consciousness and solidarity. Disability cabarets can empower people in much the same way as going on a direct action demonstration.' Disability arts is a political as well as an artistic endeavour. It involves making the implicit theories of disability explicit by exposing the derogatory nature of disablist images and stereotypes and challenging negative attitudes, discrimination and oppression. Through their art disabled people are promoting very different images of disability. Oliver & Barnes (1998) believe that disability arts produce, at one and the same time, a culture of resistance and celebration.

17.4.2 THE ORIGIN OF THE SOCIAL MODEL OF DISABILITY

The social model of disability has arisen directly from the disabled people's movement and the growing cultural identity of disabled people. This radical interpretation of disability offers disabled people affirmation and support as they redefine their situation. In the past it was thought unnecessary to discover how disabled people viewed the circumstances of their lives. Very little had been written by disabled people themselves until the 1980s, but with the growth of the disabled people's movement and the introduction of disability studies as an academic discipline in universities, this situation has changed. Oliver (1990: 3) states: 'From the 1950s onwards there was a growing realization that if particular social problems were to be resolved, or at least ameliorated, then nothing more or less than a fundamental redefinition of the problem was necessary.'

The following definition of impairment and disability is that of the Union of the Physically Impaired Against Segregation (UPIAS). Its major importance is that it breaks the link between impairment and disability:

Impairment

Lacking part or all of a limb, or having a defective limb, organ or mechanism of the body.

Disability

The disadvantage or restriction of activity caused by a contemporary social organization which takes no or little account of people who have physical impairments and thus excludes them from participation in the mainstream of social activities. Physical disability is therefore a particular form of social oppression (Union of the Physically Impaired Against Segregation 1976: 14).

The word 'physical' is now frequently removed from this definition so as to include people with learning difficulties and users of the mental health system (and 'survivors', as many people who have been through the system like to be called) (Oliver & Barnes 1998). This, and similar definitions, breaks the connection between impairment and disability which are viewed as separate entities with no causal link. This is similar to the distinction made between sex (a biological entity) and gender (a social entity) in the women's movement (Saraga 1998b).

The World Health Organization's *International Classification of Impairment, Disability and Handicap* (ICIDH; 1980) and the revised version (ICIDH-2; 2000) have been rejected by the disabled people's movement because, despite taking social and environmental factors into account, the meaning of disability is still underpinned by the medical model of disability and the causal link between impairment and disability remains intact (Hurst 2000, Pfeiffer 2000).

Disability is viewed within the social model in terms of barriers (Swain et al 1993). There are three types of barriers, which all interact:

Structural barriers which refer to the underlying norms, mores and ideologies of organizations and institutions which are based on judgements of 'normality' and which are sustained by hierarchies of power.

Environmental barriers which refer to physical barriers within the environment, for example steps, holes in the pavement, and lack of resources for disabled people, for example lack of Braille and lack of sign language interpreters. It also refers to the ways things are done which may exclude disabled people, for example the way meetings are conducted and the time allowed for tasks.

Attitudinal barriers which refer to the adverse attitudes and behaviour of people towards disabled people.

The social model of disability locates disability not within the individual disabled person, but within society. Thus the person who uses a wheelchair is not disabled by paralysis but by building design, lack of lifts, rigid work practices, and the attitudes and behaviour of others. Similarly the visually impaired person is not disabled by lack of sight, but by lack of Braille, by cluttered pavements, and by stereotypical ideas about blindness. Finkelstein (1981, 1998) has argued that non-disabled people would be equally disabled if the environment were not designed with their needs in mind, for example if the height of doorways only accommodated wheelchair users. Human beings fashion the world to suit their own capabilities and limitations and disabled people want nothing more than that.

Attitudinal barriers are regarded within the social model of disability as very significant, but only in the context of environmental and structural barriers (Swain et al 1998a). It is believed that an exclusive focus on attitudes will never be successful, yet this is where most focus lies (Swain & Lawrence 1994), for example in the government's campaigns to change the attitudes of employers, which have been notoriously unsuccessful, and its great reluctance over the years to introduce comprehensive disability discrimination legislation. Oliver contends that '[d]iscrimination does not exist in the prejudiced attitudes of individuals but in the institutionalised practices of society' (Oliver 1996a: 76). If the focus is solely on individuals' attitudes, then the structural and environmental barriers, and the systems of power that maintain them, are ignored.

The social model of disability arises from the collective experiences of disabled people themselves. It has engendered personal and political empowerment, self-confidence and pride (Morris 1991b). Crow, for example, states:

> For years now the social model of disability has enabled me to confront, survive and even surmount countless situations of exclusion and discrimination. It has been my mainstay as it has been for the wider Disabled People's Movement. It has enabled a view of ourselves free from the constraints of disability (oppression) and has provided a direction for our commitment to social change. It has played a central role in promoting disabled people's individual self-worth, collective identity and political organisation (Crow 1996: 207).

Disabled people are thus engaged in a struggle to replace the individual model of disability with a model couched in terms of human rights. Oliver talks of its considerable success:

> For the past fifteen years the social model of disability has been the foundation upon which disabled people have chosen to organise themselves collectively. This has resulted in unparalleled success in changing the discourse around disability, in promoting disability as a civil rights issue and in developing schemes to give disabled people autonomy and control in their own lives (Oliver 1996a: 40).

One of its achievements was the passing in the UK, in 1995, of the Disability Discrimination Act after many years of campaigning. This act is, however, far from comprehensive and cannot be regarded as full civil rights legislation, although it has been strengthened by the present Labour government and will possibly be supplemented and enhanced by the Human Rights Act (1998).

In recent years, a number of disabled people, particularly women, have pointed out some limitations of the social model of disability and have sought to extend it. Their major concern has been the neglect of impairment (Morris 1991b, Abberley 1996, Crow 1996, Wendell 1996, Garland Thomson 1997, Hughes & Paterson 1997, Thomas 1999, Thomas 2001). Crow (1996) believes that it has been necessary for disabled people to provide a clear, unambiguous model of disability to bring about political change. Admitting that there may be a negative side to having an impairment or being disabled, or highlighting problems which cannot be readily solved by social and environmental manipulation, may undermine the campaign. This, it is argued, has led to disabled activists ignoring impairment, which has become something of a taboo subject. Shakespeare (1992: 40) states:

> The achievement of the disability movement has been to break the link between our bodies and our social situation and to focus on the real cause of disability i.e. discrimination and prejudice. To mention biology, to admit pain, to confront our impairments has been to risk the oppressive seizing of evidence that disability is 'really' about physical limitations after all.

Hughes & Paterson (1997: 326) also see the danger of focusing on impairment:

> the social model has succeeded in shifting debates about disability from biomedically dominated agendas to discourses about politics and citizenship. However, debates about the body and impairment are beginning to

re-emerge within the disability movement ... This is a highly contentious debate since it tugs – somewhat disconcertedly – at the key conceptual distinction which lies at the heart of the transformation of disability discourse from medical problems to emancipatory politics.

Garland Thomson (1997: 283) believes that rather than neglecting impairment, 'the embodied difference that using a wheelchair or being deaf makes should be claimed, but without casting that difference as lack'.

Hughes & Paterson (1997) have been critical of the neglect of the body in the social model of disability on the grounds that the body can be viewed in psychological, social, historical and cultural terms and is not, therefore, merely a biological entity. They argue, for example, that physical pain is a biological, psychological, social, cultural and historical phenomenon; that it is 'clearly far more than a carnal sensation' (Hughes & Paterson 1997: 335; see Section 9.2). Hughes & Paterson point out that there has been little or no debate between theorists of disability studies and theorists of the sociology of the body and that the social model of disability understands impairment only in terms of medical discourse. They argue that 'there is a powerful convergence between biomedicine and the social model of disability with respect to the body. Both treat it as a presocial, inert, physical object' (Hughes & Paterson 1997: 329).

Hughes & Paterson (1997: 335) believe that impairment structures the experience of disabled people and that they encounter impairment and disability 'as part of a complex interpenetration of oppression and affliction'. Crow agrees, and states that '[e]xternal disabling barriers may create social and economic disadvantage but our subjective experience of our bodies is also an integral part of our everyday reality' (Crow 1996: 210).

Wendell (1997) draws parallels between the oppression of women and the oppression of disabled people, which is built around attitudes towards the body in patriarchal society – attitudes that Hughes & Paterson (1997) refer to as 'tyrannies of perfection'. Wendell (1997) believes that in a society that idealizes the body, physically disabled people are marginalized and that disabled women are the most likely to be affected, as women are judged by their bodies more than men. The fitness and health of the body are also greatly valued in our society today and this may serve to oppress disabled people, for example in their employment, if their bodies do not meet these ideals. Wendell explains:

> When you listen to this culture in a disabled body you hear how often physical health and vigour are talked about as if they were moral virtues. People constantly praise others for their 'energy', their stamina and their ability to work long hours ... when health is spoken of as a virtue, people who lack it are made to feel inadequate (Wendell 1997: 260).

Wendell believes that, if given a voice, the unique experiences disabled people have about their bodies could help to dismantle cultural mythologies about the body that oppress almost everyone.

One reason for the neglect of impairment by the disabled people's movement, and its concentration on disabling barriers, is that the latter affects all disabled people and has the potential, therefore, to draw them together into a powerful political force. This is particularly important as the diversity of impairment is often used as a reason for leaving disabling barriers intact (Barnes 1991). Oliver (1996b) believes that collectivizing the experience of impairment would be far more difficult than collectivizing the experience of disability and that the social model is a model, not a full theory of disability:

> If we expect models to explain, rather than to aid understanding, then they are bound to be found wanting. Many of those arguing for the incorporation of impairment have confused models and theories. I suggest that the continuing use and refinement of the social model of disability can contribute to rather than be a substitute for the development of an adequate social theory of disability … an adequate social theory of disability must contain a theory of impairment (Oliver 1996b: 50).

The representativeness of the disabled people's movement, and hence the consensus among disabled people concerning the meaning of disability, has also come under scrutiny. The disabled people's movement has been fashioned by men, particularly men with motor impairments (Morris 1991b). This may be one reason why the more personal aspects of disability and impairment have been neglected. It has largely been feminists who have emphasized personal experience and its important role in political analyses:

> Like other political movements, the disability movement both in Britain and throughout the world, has tended to be dominated by men as both theoreticians and holders of important organisational posts. Both the movement and the development of a theory of disability has been the poorer for this as there has been an accompanying tendency to avoid confronting the personal experience of disability (Morris 1991b: 9).

Not all disabled people are equally well represented in the disabled people's movement, for example old people and people with learning and communication disabilities. In addition, some people in the deaf community do not regard themselves as disabled but as a linguistic minority (Ladd 1990). The disabled people's movement has been accused of élitism and of failing to represent the views of all disabled people (Oliver 1996a). Most disabled people are not actively involved in disability politics and some may view disability in a similar way to non-disabled people – that is, as an individual problem. This has led to questions concerning the right of the disabled people's movement to represent the views and interests of disabled people. Bury states, for example, that 'disability theorists are themselves arguing a case which reflects the experiences of a small and unrepresentative minority of the disabled' (Bury 1997: 139). Oliver is, however, irritated by such arguments. He states:

> In representative democracies, representation is always less than perfect. The Conservative Party does not represent all conservative voters nor does the British Medical Association represent all doctors … and yet the right of the Disability Movement to represent disabled people is continually questioned by politicians, policy makers and professionals alike … if

the legitimate claims of the movement to represent the interests of disabled people are denied, who else will represent our interests – doctors? politicians? the Royal Institutes and Associations? (Oliver 1996b: 150)

Oliver (1996b) points out that these concerns are rarely raised in relation to other democratic organizations, and objects to the way in which the right of the disabled people's movement to represent disabled people is constantly queried. Oliver argues that: 'The "emerging" politics of disability is still emerging, and has still to move from concepts and minority activism to the hearts and minds of disabled people more generally' (Oliver 1996b: 106).

Proponents of the social model of disability have also been accused of failing to take account of multiple and simultaneous oppression, for example that of black disabled people, disabled women and lesbian and gay disabled people (Stuart 1993, Keith 1994, Morris 1996, Vernon 1996). These issues are, however, slowly being addressed and can be explained, at least in part, in terms of the disabled people's movement being a young social movement.

Shakespeare & Watson (1997) believe that the social model of disability will continually undergo refinement and development and that thousands of disabled people are constructively debating the best ways to theorize disability through their writings, conferences and organizations. They believe that the differing views among disabled people are minor compared with those between disabled and non-disabled people: 'As with any other area of political debate, or sociological theory, there is a constant process of criticism, self-criticism and development ... No theory emerges into the world fully formed, and getting the balance between the experience of impairment, and the experience of disability is a continuing endeavour' (Shakespeare & Watson 1997: 298).

17.5 INSTITUTIONAL DISCRIMINATION

Swain et al (1998a: 5) define institutional discrimination as: 'Unfair or unequal treatment of individuals or groups which is built into institutional organisations, policies and practices at personal, environmental and structural levels.' Disabled people face institutional discrimination in a social and physical world that is geared by, for and towards non-disabled people. The concept of institutional discrimination in relation to disabled people (institutional disablism) has been articulated by disabled people themselves and has been influenced by the social model of disability. As Priestley (1999: 9) states: 'The disabled people's movement has struggled hard to gain acceptance for the idea that disability can be considered as a form of institutional discrimination or collective social oppression.'

The notion of institutional discrimination has played an important role in the development of disability theory. The commonalties in issues of racism, sexism, homophobia and disablism can be explored through themes such as attitudes, power relationships, the denial of rights and discriminatory language, while also highlighting differences in the forms of discrimination faced by different groups (Thompson 2001). To see discrimination as institutional is to recognize that inequalities are woven into the very structure and fabric of British society including its organizations such as universities, hospitals and professional bodies.

People with impairments are disabled by institutional barriers that prevent their full participative citizenship within society and their access to and participation within organizations. Figure 17.1, the SEAwall of institutional discrimination, depicts these barriers as the bricks in a wall. In this model of institutional discrimination, attitudinal barriers are constructed on environmental barriers that are themselves built on structural barriers. Ideology (beliefs and dogma) plays a key role in the inter-reliance between each layer (Swain et al 1998a).

At the structural level, institutional discrimination is built into what might be called the macro-systems of British society, for example economics, education and welfare. Oliver (1991) and Finkelstein (1993) argue, for example, that disabled people are largely excluded from labour market participation because of changes in the work processes that came with the coming of our industrialized, capitalist society, which relies on speed and competition. Many disabled people have also been excluded from mainstream educational provision, which has had the effect of reducing their subsequent life chances in terms of employment and wealth (Barnes 1991, Armstrong & Barton 1999, Moore 2000, Rieser 2001). In recent years, the concept of citizenship has been drawn upon in understanding structural barriers (Oliver 1996a). Disabled people, as a group, are denied political, social and human rights that many non-disabled people take for granted (Barton 2001).

Disablism is built into the environment of institutions and organizations through arrangements such as fire regulations, timetables and assessment and examination procedures, which restrict certain groups of people including disabled people. Discrimination is also encountered by disabled people in their daily interactions with the physical world of transport, housing and equipment, and physical barriers, such as cars parked on the pavement and the position of furniture in a classroom. Equipment is geared to the needs and norms of non-disabled people

Figure 17.1 The SEAwall of institutional discrimination (cemented by ideologies of 'normality' and 'independence').

Attitudinal	Cognitive prejudice: assumptions about the (in)abilities, emotional responses, needs of disabled people	Emotional prejudice: fear	Behavioural prejudice: individual practice and praxis	
Environmental	Disablist language	Institutional policies, organization, rules and regulations	Professional practices: assessment, care management	Inaccessible physical environments
Structural	Hierarchical power relations and structures: disempowerment of disabled people	The denial of human, social and welfare rights	Structural inequalities: poverty	

(steps, taps, cars, buses, etc.), with the needs of disabled people being marginalized as 'special'. The picture is complex, in that the needs of disabled people are diverse (for instance, a lack of curbs is advantageous to people who use wheelchairs but is problematic for blind people who use them to distinguish between the pavement and the road). Very little attention is given to such human diversity.

Attitudinal discrimination refers to negative feelings, beliefs and behaviours towards disabled people. Attitudes are complex. They are generally viewed as having three components: a cognitive component, an emotional component and a behavioural component. Attitudes are complicated further because there is a loose connection among these three components (Reber 1985); people's understandings, feelings and behaviour do not necessarily relate closely to each other. Nevertheless, each of the three components plays a part. A negative attitude towards deaf people might include a lack of understanding about deafness, fear of deaf people and negative labelling which may in turn lead to discrimination in, for example, employment. The concept of institutional discrimination is related to the social model of disability in that both emphasize the ways in which external barriers create disability.

17.6 DEFINITIONS OF DISABILITY IN RELATION TO PHYSIOTHERAPY

While physiotherapists may feel constrained by their working role or the administrative procedures required in carrying out assessments, there usually remains some degree of flexibility in which they can work in partnership with disabled people. For example, they can share power by sharing 'expert' knowledge and information, and they can encourage clients to participate actively in the writing of reports and case files, so that their voices are heard and their viewpoints represented in 'official' documents.

Awareness of disability by all those who work in physiotherapy departments can be encouraged and developed through disability equality training, run by skilled disabled people. Disability equality training 'is primarily about changing the meaning of disability from individual tragedy to social oppression; it emphasises the politics of disability, the social and physical barriers that disabled people face, and the links with other oppressed groups' (French 1996b: 121). Another way in which physiotherapists can work in partnership is by recognizing and acknowledging the disabled person's expertise in relation to the meaning and experience of being disabled. This means encouraging disabled people to exercise choice of services appropriate to their desired lifestyles. Physiotherapists can work in partnership with disabled people by regarding themselves as a resource (expertise, information, advocacy) so that disabled people can work towards achieving their own goals. This would include clarifying the goals to which the disabled person aspires, identifying the barriers that may prevent the realization of those goals, and working towards removing the barriers.

Counselling skills may also be employed in the service of enabling disabled people to overcome disabling barriers or to counteract painful and oppressive experiences at the hands of a disabling society. However, counselling disabled people to 'come to terms' with the 'limitations' of their impairments or with the lack of resources to achieve a desired lifestyle is inappropriate if physiotherapists wish to practise within the social model of disability.

Physiotherapists and managers can actively encourage disabled people to become involved in fora where they can influence the development of relevant services. This includes ensuring that meetings are held in accessible venues and that disabled people are not excluded by lack of transport or inappropriate methods of communication.

From the perspective of the social model of disability, professional power can be used to highlight the shortfall in resources for disabled people, to ensure that the subjugated voices of disabled people are heard and responded to, and to encourage and support disabled people to assert themselves so that their expertise about disability is at the centre of the development of services and support. It is important that physiotherapists, and all other staff in physiotherapy departments, make a conscious decision to heighten their awareness of disability as an area of enquiry. It is also essential that more disabled people become physiotherapists, if the profession is to reflect the community it serves.

17.7 CONCLUSION

The relationship between disabled people and health professionals has never been an easy one, for it is an unequal relationship with the professional holding most of the power. Traditionally, the professional worker has defined, planned and delivered the services while the disabled person has been a passive recipient with little if any opportunity to exercise control (French & Swain 2001). Disabled people's definitions of the problems they face, and the appropriate solutions to such problems, are generally given insufficient weight, thereby seriously hampering the rehabilitation process; for if there is no consensus little real progress can be made.

Over the last 20 years disabled people have become increasingly organized and politically active, and Centres of Integrated Living, coalitions of disabled people and international organizations, run and controlled by disabled people themselves, now flourish. There are radio and television programmes promoting the views of disabled people and an increasing number of conferences, courses, journals and books on disability issues organized and produced by disabled activists and academics.

Professionals may, understandably, find these developments threatening as their status, power, role and even their jobs no longer seem secure. There are some disabled people who, disillusioned with the help they have received in the past, reject any professional involvement in their lives or in the new services they are developing. Others, however, believe that partnership and collaboration with professional workers are important.

Disability studies (the social, political and cultural analysis of disability) have barely touched the curriculum of health professionals, including physiotherapists. This has given rise to countless problems between disabled people and professionals and to inappropriate, oppressive and damaging services (Linton 1998). With the growing impact of the social model of disability, and changes such as the implementation of the Disability Discrimination Act, physiotherapists will need to extend their viewpoint beyond the individual model of disability and to work with disabled people as equal partners. This may mean moving away from the traditional approach of 'helping' and working with a much broader brief. Physiotherapists need to join forces with disabled people and to use their professional power, in collaboration and partnership with disabled people, to dismantle every aspect of disablism and to further the fight for full citizenship for all disabled people.

Chapter **18**

Psychological interventions in chronic illness

Nicola Adams

CHAPTER CONTENTS

18.1 INTRODUCTION

The aim of this chapter is to provide an overview of psychological interventions used in the management of chronic illness. The way in which psychological approaches may be integrated into physiotherapy management will also be discussed.

A biopsychosocial model of chronic illness will be introduced and psychosocial factors mediating pain and disability reviewed. As one of the primary symptoms of chronic illness is often pain, the psychological management of pain will be detailed. Additionally, approaches to address other symptoms such as fatigue will be addressed. Management approaches to chronic illness, particularly with regard to chronic pain, will be presented and discussed. The chapter will also include current examples of rehabilitation and self-management programmes.

18.2 BIOPSYCHOSOCIAL MODEL OF PAIN AND ILLNESS

Illness, like health, is the result of a complex interaction of biological, psychological and social variables. From this perspective, diversity in illness expression is accounted for by the interrelationships among biological changes, psychological status and the social and cultural contexts that shape patients' perception of, and response to, illness (Gatchel & Turk 1996).

Biological factors alone cannot explain reports of pain, pain-related disability or depression associated with chronic illness. For example, not all patients suffering with chronic illness and pain are depressed or disabled to the same degree. The association between pain, depression and disability appears to be mediated by psychosocial variables and a multidimensional biopsychosocial model of pain emphasizes the influence of these variables (see Chs 8 and 9). Psychological and social factors can all play a role in the aetiology, severity, exacerbation and maintenance of pain, suffering, disability and response to treatment in chronic illness conditions (Waddell et al 1993, Fordyce 1995, Romano et al 1995, Gatchel & Turk 1996, Lackner et al 1996). These have been found to include factors such as the meaning of the situation, perceived life control, attentional focus, prior learning history, cultural background, appraisals, beliefs and expectations, environmental contingencies, social support and financial resources (Skevington 1995, Adams 1997, Gatchel & Turk 1999). Detailed discussions of psychological and social factors have been presented in other chapters and thus the following is intended only to illustrate the rationale of using psychological interventions in the management of chronic illness. Psychological interventions focus upon emotional, cognitive and behavioural aspects of illness, such as addressing patients' beliefs by educating them about the condition, reducing anxiety and stress by teaching stress management techniques, and increasing personal control by teaching coping skills. Thus, biopsychosocial approaches address the range of physical, psychological and social components of chronic conditions (Nielson & Weir 2001).

18.3 EMOTIONAL AND COGNITIVE ASPECTS OF ILLNESS

18.3.1 EMOTIONAL ASPECTS OF ILLNESS

Most patients experience emotional distress to a varying degree, the most commonly reported being feelings of anxiety and depression. The latter has been reviewed in detail in Chapter 8, and has been implicated as a psychosocial risk factor for developing long-term disability in low back pain (Pincus et al 2002). Anger, frustration and resentment are also reported to a lesser degree, and have received less attention in the research literature. Various factors contribute to the extent of emotional distress, such as the nature and prognosis of the condition, coping abilities, social support, attitudes and behaviours of health professionals and patients' beliefs (Skevington 1995). For example, Crisson & Keefe (1988) found that patients with strong beliefs that their health was controlled by chance or misfortune were more likely to be depressed, anxious and obsessive-compulsive compared with patients who believed they could exert a measure of control over their own health outcomes. Physiologically, anxiety and distress may maintain autonomic arousal with consequent physical symptoms, which may thus confirm beliefs that some underlying condition exists. Anxiety and depression may also increase the likelihood of patients making cognitive errors or negative appraisals, which may result in avoidance of activity. Thus negative emotional responses affect biological and behavioural responses and these feed back to negatively affect the emotional response to pain, and vice versa (Truchon 2001). High levels of anxiety and distress not only affect the experience of pain, but also affect processing and recall of information. The above factors should be borne in mind when providing patients with information regarding the management of their condition.

Addressing emotional factors is therefore an important part of the management of any chronic condition. In the case of chronic musculoskeletal pain, psychological approaches address maladaptive cognitions and behaviours associated with pain. An active self-management approach is often adopted, with emotional distress addressed by education, improving coping abilities and group support.

In the case of pain due to cancer, a more empathic individualistic approach is required. Anxiety and distress can be at least partially relieved by reassuring patients that they will receive adequate analgesia as required and that sufficient emotional support will be provided to them and their family (McDonald et al 1999).

A high incidence of depression among individuals with chronic pain has been well documented (Geisser et al 1994) and has been reported to be associated with higher levels of self-reported pain and pain behaviour, lower levels of physical and psychosocial functioning and poor response to treatment (Haythornthwaite et al 1991). Depression has been associated with feelings of helplessness and loss of control (McDonald et al 1999) and thus restoring a sense of control to the patient often assists in alleviating symptoms of depression which confound chronic pain conditions, resulting in poor motivation and inactivity which further exacerbate the condition.

Geisser et al (1994) have suggested that catastrophizing – i.e. a tendency to think the worst possible outcome will occur in any given situation – may be more important than depression in terms of how patients with chronic pain ultimately evaluate their pain experience and may impact upon how they cope with chronic pain. Those who report high negative affect have been found to be more hypervigilant to bodily sensations and report more health complaints (Bacon et al 1994). Further, Pincus & Williams (1999) have reported that chronic pain is associated with biases in the processing of information. In a controlled study investigating the interpretation of ambiguous homophones, patients with pain were found to exhibit a recall bias towards pain stimuli but not towards depression-related stimuli. The authors suggested that depression in chronic pain is qualitatively different from that of other depressed groups in that the focus and self-image of patients with chronic pain appear to be related to suffering, dependency and invalidity (Pincus et al 1996). This has implications for the management of depressive symptoms in this group of patients in that a cognitive-behavioural approach to reduce dependency and increase activity and coping ability may be more appropriate than a psychodynamically orientated approach.

18.3.2 COGNITIVE ASPECTS OF ILLNESS: COPING

Many of the variables that influence pain intensity and physical and psychosocial disability fall under the construct of coping, and many models of pain and illness give coping responses an integral role in understanding and predicting adjusting to pain and illness (Turner et al 2001). Identification of the pain coping strategies that have greatest influence on adjustment provides the clinician with an empirical rationale for deciding which coping strategies to teach and encourage and which to discourage.

According to Endler et al (2001), individuals use four main types of coping with health problems: distraction; palliative; instrumental; and emotional preoccupation. *Distraction coping* involves thinking or engaging in activities unrelated to the health problem. *Palliative coping* includes soothing strategies aimed at alleviating the unpleasantness of the health problem. *Instrumental coping* is analogous to task-orientated or problem-focused coping in the general coping literature and involves strategies such as finding out more information about the illness or seeking medical advice. *Emotional preoccupation* is similar to emotion-focused coping and involves focusing on the emotional consequences of the illness. Endler et al (1998) have shown that patients with chronic illnesses often use more emotional preoccupation coping strategies and instrumental coping strategies than those with acute illnesses. Perceived control and higher self-efficacy have been shown to be positively related to lower levels of state anxiety and greater use of more adaptive coping strategies (i.e. task-orientated rather than emotion-focused coping), which in turn have been positively related to psychological and functional outcome measures (Scharloo & Kaptein 1997). Perceived self-efficacy (i.e. an individual's belief that they can succeed at something he or she wants to do) has been shown to be positively related to quality of life in patients with cancer (Cunningham et al 1981).

Coping is influenced by a number of factors including mood, disability, beliefs, other symptomatology, level of support in the marital relationship and locus of control, i.e. the extent to which individuals believe that they are in control of outcomes and the extent to which they believe in chance or misfortune (Skevington 1995). Patients who are most adaptive are those who have strong internal beliefs, strong beliefs in the powers of others such as health professionals, and weak beliefs in chance. Pain beliefs may affect treatment outcomes and patients' beliefs about their illness affect their attitudes to coping skills, adherence and compliance with treatment, for example if patients believe they are not in control of their condition they are less likely to adhere to a self-management programme (Williams & Keefe 1991). In addition, they may believe that a certain course of treatment is effective and another ineffective. Waddell et al (1993) suggest that coping strategies may be an important mediator between pain and depression and thus disability in low back pain.

Coping skills can be developed by teaching cognitive techniques such as problem-solving, correction of distorted cognitions by education and encouraging physical activity. The provision of information is important in that it enhances perceived control about pain and thus anxiety and distress are reduced (Arntz & Schmidt 1989). Affleck et al (1992) found that the two most frequently used coping strategies by patients with rheumatoid arthritis were direct action to reduce pain and the use of relaxation.

Positive coping strategies – i.e. related to 'good' adjustment (active coping) – that have been identified for coping with chronic illness include positive coping self-statements, pacing, positive social comparisons, regular exercise, distraction, seeking social support and task persistence (Gatchel & Turk 1996).

Fernandez (1986) has suggested that coping strategies can be classified into physical, behavioural and cognitive coping strategies. Physical strategies include surgery, medication, physical therapy and the use of electrotherapeutic modalities. Cognitive strategies such as problem-solving and cognitive restructuring all involve attempting to modify pain by cognitive processes, and behavioural strategies attempt to modify behaviours through, for example, operant conditioning, pacing and goal setting. These are reviewed in a later section.

Maladaptive coping responses, which have been related to 'poor' adjustment, have been found to include pain-contingent rest (i.e. rest taken in response to the level of pain experienced), guarding, wishful thinking, avoidance of activity, catastrophizing, and the use of sedative hypnotic medication.

Catastrophizing has been found to be significantly related to pain severity and depression among people with chronic pain (Swimmer et al 1992) and has also been found to be related to lower pain thresholds and pain tolerance levels in those without pain (Geisser et al 1994). Although there is debate as to whether catastrophizing is best characterized as an appraisal rather than a coping response (Jensen et al 1991b), it has been found that reducing catastrophic thoughts is useful in terms of increasing adjustment to osteoarthritis pain (Keefe et al 1990a).

Lethem et al (1983) developed a fear-avoidance model of chronic pain where catastrophizing leads to fear of pain, leading in turn to avoidance of activity, hypervigilance, depression and disuse, resulting in disability. Fear-avoidance beliefs and fear of movement/(re)injury in particular have been shown to be strong predictors of physical performance and pain disability (Waddell et al 1993, Crombez et al 1998b, Vlaeyen et al 2002). Therefore, reducing catastrophizing through education and coping skills training and increasing activity according to this model will reduce depression and disability. The reader is referred to Chapter 8 for a fuller discussion of cognitive aspects of pain.

18.4 BIOPSYCHOSOCIAL APPROACH TO MANAGEMENT OF CHRONIC ILLNESS AND PAIN

Psychosocial factors can be integrated with physical factors within a biopsychosocial framework in a way that can address these factors within a treatment programme (Jensen et al 1994b, Nielson & Weir 2001). Psychological and social factors may act indirectly on pain and disability by reducing physical activity, flexibility, strength and endurance. Cognitive factors may have a direct effect on physiological variables associated more directly with the production or exacerbation of nociception. Cognitive interpretations and affective arousal may directly affect physiology by increasing sympathetic nervous system arousal, production of endogenous opioids and elevated levels of motor activity.

According to this model, treatment approaches should therefore not only address the biological basis of symptoms but should also incorporate psychological and social factors that have been found to affect pain distress and disability. Thus, treatment approaches should be designed not only to address the physical contributing factors but also to address patients' behaviours, regardless of the specific pathophysiology. In chronic conditions, treatment should focus on providing the patient with techniques to gain a sense of control over the effects of pain as well as modifying the affective, behavioural, cognitive and sensory aspects of the pain experience. Behavioural techniques can help patients to show that they are more capable than they may have thought, and cognitive strategies help to place affective, behavioural, cognitive and sensory responses under a patient's control. The assumption here is that long-term maintenance of behavioural changes will only occur if the patient has learned to attribute success to his or her own efforts. It has been suggested that these approaches can result in changes in beliefs about pain, coping style and reported pain severity as well as direct changes in behaviour. Treatment approaches that result in increases in perceived control over pain and decreases in catastrophizing have also been associated with reductions in pain severity ratings and functional disability (Severeijens et al 2001).

It is important first to identify the relevant physical, psychological and social characteristics of patients and then develop treatments matched to these characteristics. One should also evaluate their efficacy, as different treatment components have been shown to maximize outcome for different subsets of patients. For example, Turk et al (1996) found that fibromyalgia patients ($n = 105$) could be classified into three subgroups based on psychosocial and behavioural characteristics using standardized inventories. The authors refer to these groups as 'dysfunctional', 'interpersonally distressed' and 'adaptive copers'. The dysfunctional group were characterized by high levels of pain, life interference, emotional distress and functional limitation; the interpersonally distressed group were characterized by low levels of social and personal support; and the adaptive copers group were characterized by low levels of pain, functional limitation and emotional distress. The authors concluded that treating fibromyalgia patients as a homogeneous group may deter development of effective management. It is suggested that treatment approaches may be adapted for different groups of patients. In particular, patients who exhibit high levels of distress and have low levels of support may require greater training in coping skills than patients who are already coping adequately with their pain.

In terms of evidence, a systematic review by Guzman et al (2001) of 10 trials involving 1964 patients with chronic pain found that intensive multidisciplinary biopsychosocial rehabilitation with a functional restoration approach improved pain and function when compared with out-patient non-multidisciplinary rehabilitation or usual care.

18.5 PSYCHOSOCIAL ASPECTS OF PHYSIOTHERAPY MANAGEMENT

Although physiotherapy is ostensibly viewed as a primarily physical treatment, therapists often address psychosocial factors as part of their management of patients' conditions (Sim 2002). Physiotherapists routinely educate and teach self-management and relaxation skills as part of their repertoire of skills, particularly in chronic conditions such as arthritis, chronic obstructive airways disease or cancer, where there is no cure. The aim of physiotherapeutic management is therefore to teach patients to cope more effectively with their pain, disability and quality of life. To this end, the importance of the therapist–patient interaction is paramount in teaching self-management skills and providing support, empathy, reassurance and encouragement.

Physiotherapy thus has a cognitive component and a counselling component. Also, many physiotherapy treatments, such as exercise, are behavioural in nature. The importance of these aspects of treatment will be highlighted in what follows.

18.5.1 PATIENT–PRACTITIONER INTERACTION

There are a number of psychological factors in patient–practitioner interactions that may influence the process and outcomes of treatment. The attachment and collaboration between patient and practitioner is an important element in any therapeutic process. Communication is an integral part of the patient–practitioner relationship and is a significant factor in influencing patient satisfaction or dissatisfaction with treatment (Audit Commission 1993; see also Chs 4 and 14). Communication involves both verbal and non-verbal behaviours, such as provision of information, listening, empathy and use of touch. Physical contact, in addition to its physiological benefits, also has a psychological component in that patients often feel they are being individually cared for. In addition to their physical treatment, it is important that patients feel they have been listened to and experience a feeling of caring. Provision of information is important to ensure patient adherence and prepare patients for treatment; adequate preparation and explanation will reduce anxiety, which can otherwise limit recovery. It is argued that communication is as important as the treatment itself, and the practitioner in this way is a powerful mediator of improvement (Klaber-Moffett & Richardson 1995). Good communication skills and empathy are described as being the two main aspects affecting satisfaction and have been associated with health outcome and compliance (Fitzpatrick 1991). A questionnaire study of patients with cancer ($n = 36$) found that patients felt that good communication involved the ability to give good advice, answer questions, problem-solve, inspire confidence, actively contribute to discussion and pass on relevant information to other parties involved in their care (Bailey & Wilkinson 1998). It has been suggested by Skevington (1995) that the social interaction between the patient and practitioner influences who stays in treatment and who leaves. Addressing patients' anxiety and uncertainty has been found to affect ratings of satisfaction more than technical ability, though future research is required to investigate the relationships between treatment efficacy and patients' and practitioners' expectations and beliefs.

While different approaches are required depending upon the nature and stage of the presenting condition, Raue & Goldfried (1997) suggest that a working alliance should consist of agreement between the patient and practitioner regarding the type of therapy employed, the goals of therapy and the development of a therapeutic bond.

18.6 PSYCHOLOGICAL APPROACHES

There are a number of psychological approaches that can be used in the management of chronic pain conditions. The most popular and readily adapted for physiotherapeutic management is the cognitive-behavioural approach. Recently this model has been reformulated with regard to chronic pain (Sharp 2001) and will be discussed in a later section.

There is general agreement that psychological approaches adopted in the management of chronic pain and disability can make a contribution to the management of chronic illness (for example, Astin et al 2002). As stated previously, a cognitive-behavioural model, which combines two major psychological approaches, can be readily applied to physiotherapeutic management within rehabilitation programmes for chronic pain such as low back pain and fibromyalgia. It is important to realize the contribution of factors that may be addressed by other approaches for other conditions, such as the application of counselling skills in cancer.

18.6.1 PSYCHO– PHYSIOLOGICAL APPROACHES

These models consider the interaction of physiological and psychological factors in the development of chronic pain. Psychophysiological studies examine the influence of psychological events (thoughts, memories and emotions) on physical changes that produce pain (Gamsa 1994). The possible role of physical responses such as muscle activity, vascular changes or autonomic arousal has been studied extensively in relation to pain disorders such as headaches (Andrasik & Holroyd 1980), myofascial pain and low back pain (Flor et al 1991), with inconsistent findings.

In explaining the mechanisms that link abnormal psychophysiological patterns with pain, two general models are proposed. First, general arousal models propose that frequent or prolonged arousal of the autonomic nervous system, including sustained muscle activity, generates and perpetuates pain. In contrast, specificity models explain the development of specific types or sites of pain in relation to inter-individual differences in psychophysiological responses to environmental stressors due to genetic predisposition, previous experiences and personality type. The mechanisms involved, however, are not well understood.

Treatments such as static electromyography (EMG) biofeedback and relaxation techniques are designed to reduce levels of muscle activity and autonomic arousal, thereby reducing pain. Psychophysiological therapies (PPT) attempt to change cognitions through the manipulation of physiological responses. Such treatments have been found to be effective in reducing pain in muscle contraction headache (Andrasik & Holroyd 1980), migraine and back pain, although not necessarily more so than other psychophysiological interventions (Gamsa 1994). Developments in dynamic paraspinal EMG monitoring have extended these concepts to include correction of dynamic muscular activity with subsequent reduction in subjective pain report and increased function.

These studies demonstrate that it may be possible to control autonomic and physiological responses to pain. However, physiological response has not been shown to correlate closely with subjective pain report (Taylor & Lee 1991). In terms of perception of pain, this lack of correlation may be due to an individual's psychological state, beliefs and expectations and may not reflect the ineffectiveness of a strategy in controlling the physiological component of the pain.

Relaxation

Relaxation enables the individual to cope with the symptoms of the stress response in particular situations. Relaxation techniques have been found to reduce anxiety and thus pain (Linton 1982, Philips 1988) and are often used in rehabilitation programmes, in obstetric care, in palliative care, and in the management of asthma (Ritz 2001). Furthermore, such techniques have become popular with complementary practitioners in treating symptoms of anxiety and depression, with anecdotal reports of success.

Physiological relaxation

Progressive relaxation (Jacobson 1938) and modifications of progressive muscular relaxation (Bernstein & Borkovec 1973) involve systematically contracting and then relaxing various muscle groups throughout the body, one group at a time, while paying close attention to the feelings associated with both tension and relaxation. This exercise reduces skeletal motor activity while sensitizing the individual to subtle differences in muscle tone which denote a tense or relaxed state as they appear in everyday situations, enabling release of tension where it is noted (Bernstein & Given 1984). Progressive relaxation has been reported to be effective in inducing relaxation (Danton et al 1984), but there have been methodological problems in assessing its therapeutic effectiveness. Reviews of literature have shown an almost universal reliance on subjective self-assessments of relaxation as the principal outcome measure, despite evidence demonstrating a lack of correlation between self-report measures and objective outcomes (Taylor & Lee 1991). Further, in studies where objective measures have been used as outcome variables (Carey &

Burish 1987), progressive relaxation was used in conjunction with other techniques, making it hard to examine its differential effects.

Rationale for the use of relaxation

There are three main models postulated to explain the mechanism by which relaxation can assist in pain alleviation. The reflex-spasm model and the stress-causality model (Collins et al 1982) both conceptualize the pain relief mechanism in physiological terms, while the cognitive factors model (Flor et al 1983) views pain relief in psychological terms. Relaxation is an important coping skill and is often used as part of a cognitive-behavioural programme.

The reflex-spasm model suggests that, in response to tissue injury, inflammation and subsequent pain, increased muscle tension occurs to protect and immobilize the injured area, preventing further tissue damage. When increased muscle tension is prolonged, muscle fatigue can occur, with associated physiological changes, and contributes to the pain experience. Using such a model, the aim of treatment is to reduce muscle tension in the affected area, thereby breaking a cycle of pain and spasm. The model received some support from early EMG biofeedback studies; however, the lack of findings of increased motor activity in areas of pain has not always supported this model. Findings of abnormal (asymmetrical) EMG patterns in chronic back pain have been supported by more recent literature (for example, Larivière et al 2000).

The stress-causality model postulates that a person responds to perceived pain or external stress by undergoing a generalized physiological response, as seen in arousal states (Collins et al 1982). Local and general muscle tension levels are elevated, along with other physiological parameters. The aim of treatment using this model would be to assist the person to reduce the arousal state and to attain a relaxation response.

Finally, the cognitive factors model postulates that relaxation methods alleviate pain through cognitive factors. Relaxation methods are seen as a technique to reduce feelings of general anxiety and increase feelings of control. Treatment using the cognitive factors model emphasizes the importance of teaching stress reduction and coping skills.

Autogenic training

Autogenic training (Schultz & Luthe 1969) is a system of psychosomatic self-regulation designed to support the central mechanisms responsible for homeostatic processes and involves the entire neurohumoral axis. This system is based on regular practice of short periods of passive concentration on self-generated psychophysiological stimuli and is designed to facilitate relaxation in different somatic systems such as the neuromuscular and vascular systems It involves steps to concentrate on heaviness and warmth in the legs and arms, the regulation of breathing and cardiac activity, abdominal warmth and forehead cooling. While thorough research has not been completed on its mechanism, a listing of the disorders that are reported to benefit from autogenic training can be found in the second volume of Luthe (1969). A recent meta-analysis of clinical outcome studies found positive effects of autogenic training for tension headache/migraine, mild-to-moderate essential hypertension, coronary heart disease, somatoform pain disorder (unspecified type) as well as anxiety, depression and functional sleep disorders (Stetter & Kupper 2002).

Efficacy of relaxation

A number of studies have examined the efficacy of relaxation techniques (Engel & Rapoff 1990, Engel 1992, Engel et al 1994). These authors examined the use of relaxation for the treatment of children with headaches. In addition to finding short-term benefits, they also found beneficial effects at long-term follow-up. However, small subject numbers limit the external validity of the research. Other studies have shown mixed results. Linton & Gotestam (1984), in comparing applied relaxation and applied relaxation plus operant conditioning for chronic pain, found that the applied relaxation group had a significantly lower pain intensity over time, while the applied relaxation plus operant conditioning group had a significantly better result on analgesic reductions. In comparing relaxation training, relaxation training plus cognitive-behavioural therapy and a control, Turner (1982) found that patients with chronic low back pain in both active conditions showed significant improvement. A randomized controlled trial of four groups of cancer patients receiving bone marrow transplants ($n = 94$) found that relaxation and imagery training reduced treatment-related pain as compared with usual treatment or therapist support (Syrjala et al 1995). A review of nine studies of relaxation training for adult asthma did not find any significant contribution of relaxation to the standard treatment of asthma (Ritz 2001). The author commented on the methodological deficiencies of studies available. Huntley et al (2002) similarly concluded that, while there is some evidence that muscular relaxation improves lung function of patients with asthma, there is no evidence to date for the efficacy of any other relaxation technique in the management of asthma.

Other issues associated with this type of intervention principally involve client motivation and individual patient characteristics, which can affect treatment outcome. Since these interventions rely on regular home practice, compliance can become an issue in unmotivated clients.

In summary, results suggest that relaxation may be of value in pain management, though longer-term benefits have not yet been studied. Further research is needed in this area to provide definitive scientific evidence of therapeutic efficacy.

18.7 BEHAVIOURAL APPROACHES

Behaviour theory defines pain by the presence of 'pain behaviours' (Fordyce 1976, 1986). Pain behaviours are verbal and non-verbal signs of distress that are independent of subjective report. Using an operant learning theory framework, Fordyce postulated that a pain problem becomes chronic because the pain behaviour is positively reinforced while what might be termed 'well' behaviour is not reinforced (Adams et al 1996). However, the question of what the patient is actually experiencing is avoided in this model (Gamsa 1994). Behavioural treatment specialists recognize that pain behaviour patterns are learned. The appropriate treatment of a patient with chronic pain based on behavioural principles requires that pain behaviours are unrewarded and well, normal or healthy behaviours are positively reinforced. Pain behaviours are believed to be instrumental in the development of avoidance of activity, which then also becomes a pain behaviour (Waddell & Turk 2001). Main et al (1992) found that scores on the non-organic signs test evaluating some specific 'inappropriate' pain behaviours in the clinic increased with the amount of failed treatment. If behavioural treatment is to be effective, a careful analysis of historical influences on pain behaviour is essential (Keefe & Lefebvre 1994). Thus, more recent approaches to this model have acknowledged the effects of biological and psychological variables on behaviour. It should also be remembered that, although it may be possible to reduce pain behaviours by controlling their reinforcers in pain management programmes, this is more difficult in the patient's own environment where there may be difficult family dynamics and interpersonal and social problems (Adams et al 1996).

A systematic review of 24 randomized controlled trials of behavioural treatment for chronic low back pain found strong evidence that behavioural treatment had a moderate effect on pain intensity and a small positive effect on generic functional status and behavioural outcomes of patients with chronic low back pain when compared with a waiting list control or no treatment (van Tulder et al 2000b). However only 25% of studies in the review were rated as high-quality. The authors concluded that behavioural treatment was effective for patients with chronic low back pain but it is unknown what type of patient benefits most from what particular behavioural treatment.

18.8 COGNITIVE APPROACHES

Cognitive theory examines constructs such as expectations and beliefs about pain, personal control, problem-solving abilities and coping skills (Gamsa 1994). Cognitive models make a clear statement about the relationship between cognition, affect and behaviour. Cognitive models are usually subsumed under the cognitive-behavioural model because cognitive processes and behaviour are intricately linked.

The assumption of cognitive models of pain is that cognitive activity and an individual's emotional distress or behavioural difficulty is not a direct reaction to an untoward life event but rather a consequence of how that event is perceived.

Cognitive treatment and assessment involve identifying those dysfunctional thought processes and irrational beliefs that lead to emotional distress and increase pain perception and experience. Cognitive interventions to control pain attempt to increase patients' self-efficacy, i.e. ability to cope with the problem. Ciccone & Grzesiak (1984) found that cognitive events that amplify pain syndromes included catastrophizing, over-generalization, low frustration tolerance, external locus of control and mislabelling of somatic sensations. Thus the focus of the cognitive approach to treatment is to change the way individuals think about their pain. As cognitive therapy is generally used in combination with other techniques, empirical assessment of its differential effects is difficult.

18.9 COGNITIVE–BEHAVIOURAL APPROACHES

In this approach, the behavioural model is expanded to incorporate cognition and affect within behavioural therapy. It draws upon such areas as behaviourism, social learning theory and cognitive psychology (Grzesiak & Perrine 1987). A variety of psychological interventions are combined within this framework and it emphasizes education, control by patients and coping strategies. Cognitive-behavioural therapies consider the cognitive effects on behaviour and attempt to change physiological responses through the manipulation of cognitions. Cognitive-behavioural therapy helps patients to identify and modify maladaptive beliefs and behaviours and use adaptive coping strategies to manage their condition (Turner et al 2001). Treatment is usually a combination of cognitive and behavioural interventions such as education, acquisition of coping skills and operant conditioning. Although not offering a model of the cause of the pain, it views the way in which individuals react to pain as a complex, multidimensional response. However, Sharp (2001) claims that cognitive-behavioural theory has continued to be founded on behavioural principles, and that interventions have continued to be dominated by behavioural components. He has offered a reformulated cognitive-behavioural therapy model which focuses more directly on patients' thoughts about, and appraisals of, their pain based upon suggestions that the relationship between pain and arousal is mediated by appraisal.

Cognitive-behavioural approaches are used extensively in pain management programmes with some evidence of effectiveness in restoring function and mood and reducing pain and disability-related behaviour (Harding & Williams 1995, Morley et al 1999). In a systematic review and meta-analysis of 25 randomized controlled trials of cognitive-behaviour therapy and behaviour therapy for chronic pain in adults, Morley et al (1999) concluded that active psychological treatments based on the principle of cognitive-behavioural therapy were effective. Several theories have been suggested as mediating the efficacy of cognitive-behavioural therapy. These include a reduction of the stress response by increasing control and reduction of fear, closure of the proposed gating mechanism to painful stimuli, disruption of reverberatory neural activity, activation of the endogenous pain control system and a reduction of pain associated with immobility.

18.9.1 PRIMARY ASSUMPTIONS OF COGNITIVE–BEHAVIOURAL THERAPY

Based on Gatchel & Turk (1996), the following are the main assumptions underlying cognitive-behavioural therapy:

1. Individuals actively process information regarding internal stimuli and environmental events. Thus, their behaviours are influenced by their expectations and by the perceptions and consequences of their behaviours.

2. Individuals' thoughts may alter behaviour by their influence on emotional and physiological responses. These thoughts may also be influenced by emotional, physiological and behavioural responses.

3. Individuals' behaviours may be influenced by the environment and may also shape environmental events.

4. Treatment interventions must address the emotional, cognitive and behavioural dimensions of individuals' problems if they are to be effective.

5. Individuals must become active participants in treatment if they are to learn adaptive methods of responding to their problems.

18.9.2 AIMS OF COGNITIVE–BEHAVIOURAL THERAPY

The primary aims of cognitive-behavioural therapy are:

1. To help patients to alter counterproductive beliefs that their problems are unmanageable, i.e. help them to become resourceful problem solvers and enable them to cope effectively with their pain, emotional distress and psychosocial difficulties.

2. To assist patients in learning to monitor their thoughts, emotions and behaviours and to identify relationships between these factors and environmental events, pain, emotional distress and psychosocial difficulties.

3. To teach patients to develop and maintain effective and adaptive ways of thinking, feeling and responding, which can be used to cope with problems that may be experienced after treatment has ended and to maintain any gains resulting from treatment.

4. To teach patients to perform behaviours at appropriate times in order to cope effectively with pain, emotional distress and psychosocial difficulties and reduce dependency on medication. This is particularly applicable to physiotherapy as physiotherapists can help to improve levels of physical fitness, mobility and posture and thus increase ability to perform functional abilities through, for example, graded exercise and postural correction. They may also teach relaxation skills to improve the ability to manage stress.

There are generally four phases within psychological treatment based on cognitive-behavioural principles. These are: education; skills acquisition; cognitive and behavioural rehearsal; and generalization and maintenance

The following section reviews treatment components of cognitive-behavioural therapy. It should be noted that coping skills comprise several treatment components.

18.9.3 COMPONENTS OF COGNITIVE–BEHAVIOURAL THERAPY

Education

Provision of information

Patients' needs for information include information about the nature and course of their illness, treatment plans, and the process and after-effects of diagnostic and therapeutic procedures. The provision of information is important in reducing anxiety and distress and increasing coping abilities (Field & Adams 2001; see also Section 4.4.1). Adherence with treatment has been found to be related to the level of appropriate information provided. Adequate knowledge of the condition can enhance the patient's self-efficacy and develop coping skills, and this has been found to be successful in the management of fibromyalgia syndrome (Scudds & Li 1997). A survey by Sim & Adams (2003) found that these patients were perceived by therapists to be generally ill-informed about their condition.

Providing information to patients about their condition can help them cope more effectively with their symptoms, for example if patients with back pain understand the basic anatomy, physiology and biomechanics of the spine, they will understand the role of posture and movement in the management of their condition. Information concerning basic anatomical and physiological bases of pain and physical activity should be provided and instruction on the use of proper body mechanics. Patients should be informed about the effects of inappropriate posture and distorted gait on pain and the value of active exercise regimes versus passive modalities should be emphasized. The use of self-management strategies should also be discussed. Patients' ability to self-manage their condition when at home may also enhance coping skills and feeling of control over pain. This applies to many chronic conditions where a cure is not possible and the patient has to learn how best to manage symptoms. Information may be provided in oral, written or media form, though there is a lack of studies from which to draw conclusions of their relative effectiveness. A combined approach using written material and oral information appears to be the most successful (Shuldham 1999). Support and self-help groups may also provide a valuable source of information, support and advice.

Reassurance and reduction of anxiety

Patients have a tendency to seek reassurance and many fear that their condition is due to an underlying pathology. Also many patients with pain express fears about experiencing more damage and believe that more investigations are needed. It is important that doctors and therapists do not reinforce these beliefs and unwittingly encourage excessive disability and a passive approach (Pither & Nicholas 1991, Kouyanou et al 1998).

The prospect of undergoing a medical procedure may be anxiety-provoking as patients may be concerned about the pain and discomfort they expect to experience, may be unfamiliar with the procedure, and may have concerns about the diagnosis and prognosis (Edelmann 1992). Various studies have suggested that reducing anxiety results in reduced pain and distress, reduced analgesia consumption and quicker recovery time. Anxiety may be reduced by explaining procedures to patients and by providing reassurance as to what is routine and normal, and also what to expect after the procedure. In the case of patients with chronic pain, cognitive-behavioural techniques such as problem-solving, goal-setting and developing positive coping strategies have been found to be helpful in reducing anxiety (Harding & Williams 1995, Scudds & Li 1997).

Behavioural components

Changing behaviour

It is important to reinforce well behaviours and not to respond over-solicitously to exaggerated staggering and grimacing. Patients often avoid activity for fear of the consequences of the activity. Waddell et al (1993) encouraged the use of exercise and education as part of functional rehabilitation of patients with chronic low back pain to reduce fear of pain, which has been found to be a better predictor of avoidance of activity than pain severity or physical pathology (Crombez et al 1998b). Patients should therefore be encouraged to participate in controlled activity and thus increase their functional abilities.

Reinforcing well behaviours may be viewed from a behavioural perspective and the therapist may also use cognitive strategies to allow patients to reinterpret their pain. Pain may be interpreted as a temporary discomfort from carrying out prescribed exercises, due to stretching little-used muscles and ligaments, rather than as a serious symptom. Patients are encouraged to participate in well behaviours such as increased functional activity, and not reinforced for behaviours such as exaggerated facial expression of pain. It is important that patients also receive encouragement for their efforts and gains. This may be achieved by setting goals for the patient to achieve and maintain.

Exercise

Exercise is an important part of many management programmes for chronic illness. Exercise has been shown to be effective in the management of chronic conditions such as arthritis, chronic fatigue syndrome and fibromyalgia, where it may assist in functional rehabilitation of patients by improving aerobic conditioning and increasing strength and flexibility (Sim & Adams 1999). Exercise is often used in functional rehabilitation programmes for chronic low back pain, as these patients often avoid activity due to fear of pain, with consequent physical deconditioning and loss of strength and flexibility. Aerobic exercise has been found to produce systematic increases in both exercise levels and expectancies of exercise capabilities while reducing worry and concern about exercising (Waddell et al 1993). However, a systematic review carried out by van Tulder et al (2000a) found conflicting evidence on the effectiveness of exercise therapy compared with inactive treatments for chronic low back pain with regard to pain intensity and return to normal activities and work. Exercise therapy was found to be more effective than usual care by the general practitioner.

Exercise therapy is also important as part of the management of heart disease and other chronic illnesses such as asthma (Emtner et al 1998). Further, a randomized controlled trial of early exercise therapy for stomach cancer patients following curative surgery found that early moderate exercise had a beneficial effect on the function of in vitro natural killer (NK) cells (Na et al 2000). Though the study is limited by a small sample ($n = 35$) and lack of follow-up, this is an interesting area for future research.

A number of randomized controlled trials have been carried out into the use of exercise therapy in fibromyalgia. McCain et al (1988) found those patients who received cardiovascular fitness training not only improved in cardiovascular fitness but also showed improvement in pain threshold scores as compared with a control group receiving flexibility exercises. Martin et al (1996) found an exercise programme ($n = 18$) including aerobic strengthening and flexibility components to be superior to a relaxation programme ($n = 20$) in terms of tender point score, total myalgic score and indices of aerobic fitness. However, this study had no follow-up and therefore longer-term differences between these interventions are unclear. In addition to aerobic effects, other reported benefits of exercise are an increased sense of control, an antidepressant effect and relaxation (Bennett et al 1991). White & Naish (2001) found graded exercise therapy to be a clinically useful treatment in about 50% of patients referred to physiotherapy with the diagnosis of chronic fatigue syndrome in terms of exercise capacity, cardiovascular fitness and clinical global impression scores.

Goal setting

For many patients with chronic conditions, pain is the guiding factor and patients tend to carry out an activity until the pain stops them. This is often followed by a period of rest and medication. Patients often report feelings of frustration and lowered mood as a result of being unable to complete their activity. This is a repetitive cycle and each time it occurs, an avoidance method of coping is reinforced, leading to reduced activity levels and consequent physical deconditioning and loss of flexibility and strength. A consequence of this activity cycling is that periods of activity become shorter and periods of rest longer. Goal setting and pacing are techniques that can be used to break this cycle of overactivity/underactivity.

A goal is an activity or aim that the patient would like to carry out or achieve, such as swimming three lengths of a pool or visiting a cinema. To achieve the goal, the individual needs to work towards the goal in a planned and systematic way on a regular basis. Goal setting in the context of pain management is not dependent on level of pain. The target or goal should be set at a low level initially, i.e. at a level that is achievable on a good or bad day. This should gradually be increased as tolerance and practice improve the level of function required for the activity. Having set the overall goal, the goal is split into mini-goals or stages, for example if the individual is able to swim half a length without a break, an intermediate goal of one length could be set, then one and a half, and so on until the long-term goal is achieved. The next stage is only embarked upon when the previous stage becomes easy to achieve regardless of the level of the pain. In this way, fitness, stamina and confidence will improve over a period of time. The aim is to work in small achievable steps towards the long-term goal.

O'Hara (1996) summarizes the process of goal setting as follows:

- Set goals, long-term and short-term, working towards the ultimate goal
- Establish activity baselines, i.e. how much the person is able to do without aggravating the pain
- Adjust the goal-setting process to the person's rate of progress
- If a person's pain is increased through the activity, then the goal or level of activity may need to be reassessed and worked out on a lower level
- Pain can be minimized by setting a low baseline and not increasing too quickly.

To help the process of achieving the goals it may be helpful to encourage reinforcers or rewards to help increase the frequency of the task. For many people the feeling of achievement is a reward in itself.

Social reinforcement when it is planned with another person (for example, friends or family) is helpful, and the presence of another individual doing a similar activity successfully can act as an effective model. This is one of the benefits of participation group in pain management programmes rather than individual therapy.

Pacing

As the term suggests, pacing refers to how patients may learn to pace activities so that they are able to function without becoming overly tired. Prioritizing and planning are also important in pacing the activity to ensure that a cycle of overactivity and underactivity does not occur. For example, a subset of patients with fibromyalgia have a history of excessive work performance and perfectionism and thus a realistic level of priority will need to established without compromising their feelings of achievement and thereby adversely affect their self-esteem.

Planning the activity involves breaking the job down into stages and looking at what is required to carry out the job, for example housework or preparing and cooking a meal. To pace an activity, a baseline first needs to be found for each activity that causes difficulty. A baseline is the level at which an activity can be performed regularly on good and bad days. This level can then be increased gradually (through the goal-setting process) as stamina and exercise tolerance improve. Tolerance levels for activity should be built up gradually and systematically, with regular rests taken between activities. Positions should be changed regularly and activities planned so that rests and changes of position are included. In order to find the baseline for an activity such as sitting, first the individual should time how long he or she is able to sit comfortably at different times during the day, take the average of these times and halve it. This is the individual's baseline for sitting. The same method can be used for walking, standing or carrying out a task.

The patient should select an activity or task that they carry out frequently and work out a baseline for the activity. The baseline is the level at which he or she should be able to carry out the chosen activity each day regardless of any other circumstances. The individual then increases the baseline at his or her own pace. To increase the baseline and maintain it, the baseline must be realistic. It should be set at an achievable level and fit in with the individual's lifestyle.

Cognitive components

Cognitive restructuring

Cognitive restructuring teaches the identification and elimination of maladaptive cognitions such as catastrophizing and encourages a more realistic appraisal of events, so as to decrease depression and to increase functioning among patients with chronic pain. Cognitive restructuring aims to identify patterns of maladaptive coping behaviour, including negative thoughts, pain-engendering thoughts, images, feelings and behaviours, and to use positive coping resources in both pain- and non-pain-related experiences. Significant others may be engaged in the intervention process. Cognitive restructuring is an essential component of chronic pain management, especially for those individuals who demonstrate higher than average levels of catastrophizing.

Distraction

Distraction is when attention is focused on a stimulus other than pain. Often, techniques using mental imagery or slow rhythmic breathing are used as a means of distraction. Distraction may increase pain tolerance and decrease perceived intensity, as pain ceases to be the focus of attention. However, when the distraction stops, pain becomes the central focus of the individual's awareness and is often accompanied by fatigue and irritability (O'Hara 1996). Melzack et al (1980) found that distraction techniques were only effective if pain intensity was constant or increased slowly. Eccleston et al (1997) suggested that where there is high pain intensity and a high somatic awareness, cognitive coping strategies based on distraction might be difficult to apply. Where pain is less intense, however, distraction may be an effective strategy.

Problem-solving

Learning problem-solving skills is an essential part of chronic pain management. Often patients with chronic pain have poor problem-solving abilities with regard to everyday difficulties, becoming easily stressed and overwhelmed. This may result from negative attitudes and low self-esteem. Patients may need help in selecting and prioritizing a realistic set of goals for rehabilitation. Problem-solving may follow the procedure below:

1. Defining the problem or stressor
2. Setting realistic goals
3. Examining alternatives
4. Considering other perspectives and motives
5. Selecting an appropriate strategy
6. Delineating necessary steps to reach a goal
7. Rewarding behaviour for having tried.

Effectiveness of coping skills training

The use of coping skills training for patients with pain is widespread in clinical practice. Such training is usually given as part of an overall treatment package. Hence, while some studies have evaluated the effectiveness of overall treatment programmes, few have focused solely on the coping skills training component. Most of the studies that have focused on the effectiveness of various coping skills have been drawn from an experimental pain paradigm (Tan 1982, Fernandez & Turk 1989) and using healthy subjects; they may not therefore be directly comparable with a clinical situation.

18.9.4 STRESS MANAGEMENT AND RELAXATION

Stress management and relaxation are often included as part of cognitive-behavioural therapy; however, depending on the model used, it can be argued that these are psychophysiological approaches.

Stress management is a frequently used psychosocial intervention in chronic illness and is also a component of many pain reduction programmes (Levenson 1992). Many theories and mechanisms linking psychological factors to physical disorders have been proposed and are beyond the scope of this discussion, for example Cohen & Rodriguez

(1995), McCubbin et al (1991). Prolonged stress can also have psychological sequelae, such as chronic anxiety and depression, which can negatively influence the experience of pain. Further, patients with high pain intensity and high somatic awareness have been found to report greatest affective distress (Crombez et al 1998c).

Stress management techniques include patient education, training in psychophysiological self-control, for example by relaxation and lifestyle modifications in terms of nutrition and physical activity. There are few studies that document the efficacy of comprehensive stress management programmes. Studies of components such as relaxation are more plentiful and are outlined in Section 18.6.1.

18.9.5 CRITICISMS OF COGNITIVE–BEHAVIOURAL THERAPY

A major criticism of using cognitive-behavioural interventions is that the potential exists to provide mixed messages about the nature of the pain problem. Ciccone & Grzesiak (1984) indicated that if patients are receiving a comprehensive programme that includes operant conditioning, relaxation and coping skills training, then they are being told by the operant philosophy that the environment is maintaining their pain behaviour. An assumption inherent in coping skills training, however, is that individuals can modify and self-regulate aspects of the pain problem. Therefore, according to Ciccone & Grzesiak (1984), patients are potentially receiving two opposing messages about the nature of pain and its control. In practice, this does not appear to happen, given the success of such programmes as evidenced by a recent systematic review and meta-analysis by Morley et al (1999). It can be surmised that many aspects are being addressed in this combined approach and this produces a favourable outcome, though it should be borne in mind that some programmes may be eclectic and multimodal in nature.

18.10 GROUPWORK

Groupwork for patients with chronic pain may take the form of therapy groups, structured groups and self-help groups (Corey & Corey 1987). Often, a combined structured group using group therapy processes is used. Such a group would focus upon the specific topic of pain management, utilizing the qualities of caring, support, modelling, role-playing and confrontation. Herman & Baptiste (1990) state that a pain group should incorporate positive expectations, opportunities for mastery and autonomy and a willingness to change attitudes and thoughts. Pain groups provide a safe and supportive environment in which patients can learn more about their pain, gain more realistic beliefs and attitudes regarding their pain and learn more adaptive coping strategies (Strong 1996). Self-help groups are also beneficial for skill maintenance and support with an ongoing problem.

One of the difficulties in determining the efficacy of groups is the frequent use of concurrent modalities – patients may also receive pharmacological and neurosurgical interventions in addition to a range of psychological interventions.

18.11 PAIN MANAGEMENT PROGRAMMES

Multidisciplinary pain management programmes are generally based upon cognitive-behavioural approaches, and their use has been supported by systematic review and meta-analysis (Morley et al 1999). These programmes have become increasingly popular in the UK where around 70 pain management programmes have been identified (Peat et al 2001). They are usually staffed by a medical specialist in pain management, a clinical psychologist and physiotherapists experienced in pain management. The minimum desirable criteria for programme content, according to the Pain Society (1997), are that the programme should include provision of physical reconditioning, posture and body mechanics training, applied relaxation techniques, information and education about pain and pain management, medication review and advice, psychological assessment and intervention and graded return to activities of daily living.

Williams et al (1996) confirmed that initial treatment gains were largely maintained at 1-year follow-up, though a survey conducted by Peat et al (2001) found that there was substantial variability among UK programmes in length of follow-up, attendance rates and outcome measurement. The authors concluded that further research into factors underlying variations in follow-ups and their impact upon patient outcomes was required. They suggested that service providers should consider incorporating follow-ups into existing desirable criteria and agreeing core outcome measures.

However, there are difficulties in overall evaluation of pain management programmes due to factors such as the heterogeneity of the programmes themselves, differences in patient characteristics and assessment instruments, differing outcome appraisal and socioeconomic influences on outcome.

18.12 PSYCHODYNAMIC PSYCHOTHERAPY AND COUNSELLING

There is a subset of people suffering from chronic pain who do not benefit from either behavioural or cognitive-behavioural approaches. They are intractable and prove to be unresponsive to either medical or psychological interventions. These patients may benefit from more traditional psychodynamic psychotherapy, which should be performed by a qualified clinical psychologist or psychotherapist. The theory underlying psychodynamic models of chronic pain is that emotional factors may generate and perpetuate chronic pain (Engel 1959). Psychodynamic themes such as physical and sexual abuse, emotional neglect, loss and abandonment may be explored in relation to this subset of people with chronic pain. The major contribution of these models is that they recognize the individuality of each patient and that past experiences, family dynamics, affect and personality all play a role in each patient's perception and response to pain (Adams et al 1996).

Psychodynamic approaches to psychotherapy that are relational in orientation can be helpful to clinicians working with those with pain because they allow for the application of cognitive-behavioural techniques without interfering with or minimizing the importance of exploring the meaning of a patient's pain and suffering. An increased awareness of these aspects of the patient's life deepens the therapist's capacity to understand the patient's interpersonal needs and conflicts, and in so doing creates a context that can facilitate the implementation of cognitive-behavioural interventions. Such approaches may be helpful in illnesses such as cancer, where it has been found that patients' concerns relate to their desire to be with their loved ones, fear of dependency and of losing their faculties, and fear of uncontrollable pain and of surgical mutilation (Ventafridda 1989). Gaston-Johansson et al (1999), in a correlational study of 883 breast cancer patients undergoing autotransplantation, found a positive correlation between state anxiety and depression and physical role functioning. The authors concluded that health professionals needed to address issues of psychological distress and coping as part of routine patient assessment and management.

18.13 CONCLUSION

Illness is the result of a complex interaction of biological, psychological and social variables. Psychosocial contexts shape patients' perceptions and response to illness. Psychosocial factors can be integrated with physical factors in a way that can address these factors within a treatment programme. According to a biopsychosocial model, treatment approaches should not only address the biological basis of symptoms but should also incorporate psychological and social factors that have been found to affect pain, distress and disability (see Chs 8 and 9). Psychological approaches and interventions focus upon emotional, cognitive and behavioural aspects of illness, such as addressing patients' beliefs by educating them about their condition, reducing anxiety and stress by teaching stress management, and increasing personal control by teaching coping skills. There are a number of psychological approaches that can be used in the management of chronic conditions and each has been reviewed in this chapter. There is general agreement that psychological interventions may be important adjuvant therapies in the medical management of many chronic illnesses. Most scientific evidence exists for cognitive-behavioural approaches, which combine two major psychological models and incorporate education, coping strategies, physical rehabilitation and self-management. These approaches are often used in pain management programmes, though factors such as heterogeneity of the programmes, differences in patient characteristics, assessment instruments and outcome appraisal make evaluation difficult. There is considerable scope for future research in this area.

The main points that emerge from the discussion in this chapter are:

1. Illness is the result of a complex interaction of biological, psychological and social variables. Diversity in illness expression is due to the interrelationships between biological changes, psychological status and th

social and cultural contexts that shape patients' perception and response to illness.

2. Psychological approaches focus upon addressing emotional, cognitive and behavioural aspects associated with pain and disability. Physiotherapists routinely address psychological factors as part of their management of chronic conditions.

3. The importance of the therapist–patient interaction is paramount in teaching self-management skills and providing support, empathy, reassurance and encouragement.

4. Communication is an integral part of the patient–practitioner relationship and is the most significant factor influencing patient satisfaction or dissatisfaction with treatment.

5. There are a number of psychological approaches that can be used in the management of chronic conditions. The most commonly used are cognitive-behavioural approaches, which involve addressing maladaptive thoughts and teaching appropriate coping strategies.

6. Cognitive-behavioural approaches are used extensively in pain management programmes and have been found to be effective in restoring function and mood, reducing pain and disability-related behaviour. Treatment components of cognitive-behavioural therapy include education, exercise, goal-setting and pacing, problem-solving, coping skills, stress management and relaxation.

7. There is little scientific evidence for the use of single treatment modalities. The effectiveness of multimodal strategies may emphasize the multidimensional nature of many chronic conditions.

8. There is a subset of patients suffering from chronic pain who do not benefit from either behavioural or cognitive-behavioural approaches and prove unresponsive to either medical or psychological interventions. These patients may benefit from referral to a suitably qualified clinical psychologist or psychotherapist.

Chapter 19

Counselling and enabling relationships

John Swain

19.1 INTRODUCTION

This chapter looks, in general terms, at how the field of the theory and practice of counselling can inform physiotherapists in enhancing the performance of their role and developing their practice. I shall consider this topic from the dominant 'use of counselling skills' approach but also build on this by taking a broader social approach (as explored in Ch. 14) to develop a specific focus on enabling relationships. The first question to address, then, is why physiotherapists should consider their practice in terms of the relevance of the theory and practice of counselling.

Physiotherapists will inevitably, by the nature of their work, work with clients who are experiencing personal difficulties, coming to terms with serious illness or impairment, and coming to terms with physiotherapy treatment itself. Physiotherapists encounter clients experiencing different kinds of trauma and complex and fraught problems in their lives. This includes clients who regularly experience physical illness and pain; those who are terminally ill; those who have recently become disabled; and those who have experienced physical and mental abuse. These are contexts in which emotions can run high: fear, anger and hostility, shock and guilt, grief and anxiety. How each individual acts and reacts depends on numerous factors including cultural differences, differences in background and previous experiences. Two further general points can be added to this picture. First, the physiotherapist also will have emotional responses to encounters with clients, including the general stresses and satisfactions of the job as well as specific emotional responses towards clients, their experiences and feelings. Second, for both clients and physiotherapists, the communication of emotions and interpersonal attitudes is sometimes fraught with difficulties including threats to self-esteem, misunderstandings and denials. Physiotherapists can be in situations, then, in which clients need and/or request counselling either through referral or within the provision of physiotherapy.

It can be argued, however, that a physiotherapist should no more provide counselling than a counsellor should provide physiotherapy. Furthermore, there are possibilities of role conflicts, as pointed out by Horton & Bayne:

> Doctors, nurses, physiotherapists, occupational therapists and other medical and health practitioners may be effective counsellors with their patients, but it is important to recognise that there are inherent risks. It can be difficult for the health professional in the role of expert, with in-depth knowledge of a particular mode of treatment, efficient and skilled in performing tasks for others, and responsible for the treatment, then to switch roles, and provide a counselling relationship in which the responsibility is on the *patient* to work through and come to terms with painful and emotional aspects of his or her life (Horton & Bayne 1998: 9).

Perhaps even more questionable is the possibility of 'dabbling in counselling' when this involves delving into clients' personal lives without their consent and against their wishes (Swain 1995).

Questions have also been increasingly directed at the provision of counselling itself that can inform implications for physiotherapy practice. One concern is that the provision and practice of counselling can itself be discriminatory. Summarizing some of the evidence, McLeod (1998a: 246) writes: 'An examination of theory and practice in relation to three client groups – working-class, gay and lesbian, and religiously committed – suggests that concerns about inequality and discrimination in counselling are far from empty'. Overall, counselling theory and practice can generally enhance communication and relationships in physiotherapy practice. There is evidence that training in counselling skills can enhance the practice of health care professionals (Ryden et al 1991). The concerns raised above, however, underline the importance of a self-reflective stance on the part of physiotherapists and the importance, too, of training and professional development that addresses such concerns.

A second fundamental question at the outset of this chapter is, why the focus on 'enabling relationships'? In this context, the phrase has two related meanings. First, it refers to the processes of enabling relationships between participants: physiotherapists and clients. How might the arena of counselling inform the development of effective professional–clien relationships? Professional support is an essentially human activity that needs to be understood in terms of the relationships and the dynamics of communication between the people involved. Second, the phrase 'enabling relationships' invokes the power of relationships to empower and construct change. Empowerment involves seeking to maximize the power of clients and to give them as much control as possible over their circumstances. It has meaning within the broader historical and social context and hierarchical power structures within our society. Some people have more power than others, including the resources at their disposal, the opportunities available to them and the choices on offer to them in their daily lives. This, then, invokes the wider social environment in considering the practice of physiotherapy, including discrimination and inequality on grounds of gender, age, disability, sexual orientation, economic background, race, religion, culture and language.

In this chapter I shall first explore the notion of the 'use of counselling skills', its foundation in humanistic psychology and the possibilities it holds to inform enabling relationships. The focus then moves to 'changing power relations', moving towards considering physiotherapy in terms of wider social relations. I then turn to more specific approaches underpinned by a social constructionist perspective, that is narrative approaches. The chapter concludes by summarizing the principles of a social model to physiotherapy as derived from counselling theory and practice.

19.2 THE USE OF COUNSELLING SKILLS

There are numerous texts such as Burnard (1999) that are specifically aimed at encouraging health care professionals to use counselling skills in their work and helping them do so. In relation to physiotherapy Burnard suggests three specific examples of the application of counselling skills:

- Helping clients to adapt to long-term disability
- Helping people to cope with their treatment
- Helping people to regain their motivation in the rehabilitation process (Burnard 1999: 8).

Horton and Bayne reflect the widespread acceptance of the use of counselling and counselling skills by physiotherapists: 'Physiotherapists and other health care professionals can also make use of counselling and communication skills and sometimes work with patients in a counselling mode over a fairly lengthy period, yet it remains part of a wider (medical) treatment plan' (Horton & Bayne 1998: 8). A widely accepted distinction is made between: a) counselling in the formal sense of what counsellors do in their professional capacity; and b) what is sometimes called 'use of counselling skills' in the more *ad hoc* sense of being part of the work of all carers and helpers, professional and informal, and including, of course, physiotherapists.

The notion of the use of counselling skills has drawn on a number of perspectives in counselling theory. It can be argued, however, that the main foundation is found within humanistic psychology and in particular the work of Carl Rogers. Humanistic psychology is a product of many individual efforts and an assimilation of many ideas. It is a multifaceted perspective on human experience that focuses on each person's uniqueness. The following are probably the main characteristics of the work of most of those who maintain a humanist perspective:

1. Attention is centred on the experiencing person and the emphasis is on meaningfulness and significance of experiences to the person.

2. The focus is on such distinctive human qualities as choice-making creativity, valuation and self-actualization. The last of these is not easy to define but involves: 'the attempt to "fulfil one's potential" by freeing oneself and trusting in one's intuitive wisdom to develop towards a sense of "fuller being"' (Stevens 1996: 206).

3. The ultimate concern is the dignity and worth of people and an interest in the development of the potential inherent in every person. Central to this perspective is the person, as he or she discovers his or her own being and relates to other people.

4. The person has one basic tendency and striving: to actualize, maintain and enhance the 'self'.

Rogers believed, first and foremost, that as human beings we are free, and our freedom can transcend all those forces, from within and without, which would determine ourselves and our lives. As in Sartre's existentialism, 'existence comes before essence' and each person is 'responsible for the self one chooses to be' (Rogers 1983: 276). This rejection of the deterministic assumptions and the declaration that 'people are free' is right at the heart of this perspective. Furthermore, freedom as self-actualization is not an underlying or implicit assumption, it is a fundamental, dynamic orientation essential to human survival and fulfilment. Rogers's person-centred approach seeks to facilitate and empower the person 'in the direction of increasing self-government, self-regulation and autonomy, and away from … control by external forces' (Rogers 1961: 488). There is also a strong moral dimension in Rogers's beliefs about human nature in that the person is seen as basically trustworthy. Behaviour has meaning for the person in that it is intentional and the person is: 'capable of evaluating the outer and inner situation, understanding herself in its context, making constructive choices as to the next steps in life, and acting on those choices' (Rogers 1978: 15).

This perspective is directed towards the meaning of experience for the person, the immediacy of experience, and the feelings and values that pervade all experience. The person creates tentative personal truths through action and interaction with the social world. Help, then, is primarily a process of facilitating the other person to define their own problems and identify their own solutions.

To focus on the use of counselling skills in physiotherapy practice, from a humanistic perspective, is to focus on the relationship between the therapist and the client as people and their understanding of themselves and each other as people, rather than as 'therapist' and 'client'. There are four major elements to this.

1. The therapist is first and foremost a person. This may seem so self-evident as to be not worth saying. Nevertheless, the dominant ideology in the literature, training and working context is addressed towards therapists as therapists, with all the expertise, responsibilities and expectations that define the role.

2. The same is true of the client. The physiotherapist, when thinking of the use of counselling skills, is not working with an illness, injury or impairment, or even with a patient or client, but rather with a person with all his or her values, feelings, aspirations, lifestyle and human rights.

3. Physiotherapy is seen as a process of opening two-way communication and establishing empowering relationships between people. It is working *with* rather than *on* people through negotiation and cooperation.

4. The focus of therapy is the person rather than 'the problem': it is person-centred rather than problem-centred.

The central importance of relationships in the use of counselling skills, and counselling *per se*, is emphasized time and again in the literature. The necessary qualities of relationships are often referred to as 'core conditions' of counselling, particularly in person-centred approaches developed from the work of Carl Rogers. Three such qualities have received considerable attention in the literature relating to practice and research. Apart from the first, they are referred to by a variety of possible terms:

- Empathy
- Genuineness/realness/congruence
- Acceptance/respect/unconditional positive regard/trust/warmth.

It is also important that, though it is possible to consider each separately, they are inextricably interlinked. Mearns & Thorne (1999: 63) suggest: 'Just as empathy perfectly integrates with congruence, unconditional positive regard also takes its place as inseparable from the other two – inseparable, that is, except by writers who divide books into chapters!'

19.2.1 EMPATHY

Empathy is a shared understanding and sensitivity between two people. 'Putting yourself in the shoes of another' and 'seeing through the eyes of another' are ways of describing empathy. It involves both feeling and understanding how the other person feels in particular situations. Rogers defines the process as involving:

> entering the private world of the other and becoming thoroughly at home in it … It includes communicating your sensings of his world as you look with fresh and unfrightened eyes at elements of which the individual is fearful. It means frequently checking with him as to the accuracy of your sensings, and being guided by the responses you receive (Rogers 1975: 4).

It is useful to distinguish 'empathy' from the related term 'sympathy', particularly when this is based on one person thinking he or she had the same or similar experience as another. Empathy involves understanding the experience through the other person's eyes, rather than understanding an ostensibly similar experience through your own eyes. There is what has been called an 'as if' quality to empathy, that is feeling and understanding with the other person without ever losing the recognition that the feelings and understandings are uniquely his or hers and that you are a separate person in your own right with your own feelings and understandings. It is a growing together of minds while recognizing that you remain separate.

Bowen, in her interview with Stillwell, emphasizes the 'relational self' (see Section 14.3) as a foundation of empathy: 'Empathy is something someone is – their presence – not what they do. Being in deep empathy requires a therapist to be committed to her own inner journey and experiential self-awareness' (Stillwell 1998: 30).

19.2.2 GENUINENESS/ REALNESS/ CONGRUENCE

Genuineness involves the possibility of 'being yourself' in a relationship and in communication. McLeod (1998a) suggests that the realness, authenticity and willingness of the counsellor set the humanistic, person-centred approach apart from others. Genuineness in communication involves the sharing of true feelings and attitudes, or mutual self-disclosure. In this sense, genuineness implies flexibility of expectations so that neither person is 'playing a role'. When the expectations of both participants are rigidly defined, communication is not genuine. The dictum 'just be yourself' can be reassuring but also frustrating and confusing. I have had it said to me, for instance, before going into an interview for a job. It is not so simple, particularly when my preference in 'being myself' would be to avoid formal interviews entirely. Egan (1990: 69–72) provides a list of suggestions for being genuine in helping clients, including the following:

- *Do not overemphasize the helping role*. This means not hiding behind the role or facade of being a physiotherapist and avoiding stereotyped behaviours of the role.

- *Be spontaneous*. This is being free to communicate 'here and now' feelings, but it does not mean expressing in an uncontrolled way negative thoughts and feelings which may be tactless, disrespectful and even hurtful to the client.

Egan's other suggestions are: be consistent; be open; and work at being comfortable with behaviour that helps clients.

19.2.3 ACCEPTANCE/ RESPECT/ UNCONDITIONAL POSITIVE REGARD/ TRUST/WARMTH

The third of these core conditions involves acceptance and trust in a relationship. It involves communicating that the other person is a worthwhile, unique and capable person. Acceptance in communication also involves accepting that the other person has a point of view which, whether you agree with it or not, is valid to that person and worth listening to. Rogers himself states: 'What I am describing is a feeling which is not paternalistic, nor sentimental, nor superficially social and agreeable. It respects the other person as a separate individual and does not possess him. It is a kind of liking which has strength, and which is not demanding. We have termed it positive regard' (Rogers & Stevens 1967: 64). Judgement is suspended and the therapist is in every way for and with the client and communicates this to the client. Trust is a widely used concept in applying this quality of relationships to the work of health care professionals. Northouse & Northouse (1998) suggest that there are two positive outcomes to trust in a professional–client relationship. First, trust engenders a sense of security and helps individuals feel that they are not alone in coping with their problems. It also creates a supportive climate in which individuals can be more open and genuine about their attitudes, feelings and values. Bennett (1993: 36) provides a typical list of strategies for encouraging trust:

- Being sensitive to the person's needs and feelings
- Demonstrating genuineness and sincerity
- Being realistic, but optimistic, about people's abilities to get to grips with the problems they face
- Maintaining confidentiality
- Making a contract and keeping any agreements made.

19.2.4 ASSUMPTIONS UNDERLYING DESIRABLE COUNSELLING QUALITIES

Though these qualities of relationships are thought to be necessary for effective counselling (Merry 2002), they have been brought into question. It can be argued that they are founded on values and assumptions that are white, Western and middle-class. Corey & Corey (1993) provide examples of assumptions that may interfere with helping in multicultural situations, including the following:

1. Assumptions about trusting relationships

As a physiotherapist you may form relationships quickly and expect yourself and your clients to talk easily about issues that touch on personal lives. This may be difficult for some clients from cultural backgrounds in which meaningful relationships are expected to be slow to form and trust is to be earned rather than assumed.

2. Self-actualization

The belief in the importance of the individual is not shared equally across all cultures. Value systems can differ quite fundamentally in terms of whether self-worth is an individual or collective matter.

3. Assumptions about directness

Corey & Corey (1993: 117) state: 'Although the Western orientation prizes directness, some cultures see it as a sign of rudeness and as something to be avoided. If you are not aware of this cultural difference, you could make the mistake of interpreting a lack of directness as a sign of being unassertive, rather than as a sign of respect.'

4. Assumptions about assertiveness

The ideal of determining your own life and telling others what you think and feel is not shared across all cultures.

Furthermore, counselling and the use of counselling skills from a humanistic perspective concentrate on personal power and empowerment. Rogers has been questioned in terms of recognizing the social bases of authority and power. Smail, for instance, writes of the focus on the microenvironment which is 'completely dwarfed by the events and relations of the world in which the patient actually lives' (Smail 1993: 163). More recently, advocates of this perspective have attempted to address such criticisms. Mearns & Thorne (2000: 217) write:

> We wish to empower and not to disempower through the imposition of our own perceptions and prejudices. For us it is the very cornerstone of our practice that we cherish and respect the uniqueness and the resourcefulness of our clients and seek to facilitate a process whereby they come to recognize and to own their personal power and not to be forever the slaves of the expectations, needs and demands of others.

19.3 CHANGING POWER RELATIONS

Notwithstanding the possibilities offered to physiotherapists through the notion of counselling skills underpinned by humanistic psychology, counselling theory and practice is a broad and varied field. It is also a developing field. Humanistic psychology can be seen as part of a first wave of counselling theories and practice. McLeod (1998a) argues that counselling has emerged within a social, historical and cultural context dominated by an ideology of self-contained individualism and he refers to the 'profoundly individualistic nature' of counselling. The over-individualized response to what are seen as 'personal problems' has ignored the social origins and conditions that ultimately produce these problems. Smail has developed a similar critique over a number of years. He states: 'I have become less and less able to see the people who consult me as having anything "wrong" with them, and more and more aware of the constraints which are placed on their ability to escape the distress they experience' (Smail 1993: 3).

In McLeod's (1998a) view there is now a second wave of counselling approaches, including feminist, multicultural and narrative, which address questions of power in counselling, and the notion that counselling is a social and political act. We turn now to these questions of power and look first at a number of general strategies that have been developed, across a wide range of contexts, in changing power relations. I shall summarize three very general approaches: questioning dominant ideologies; empowerment; and anti-oppressive practice.

19.3.1 QUESTIONING DOMINANT IDEOLOGIES

A starting point for changing power relations can be the questioning of dominant ideologies. This involves the detailed critical scrutiny of taken-for-granted assumptions and beliefs about people, society and social issues. As McLeod (1998a: 256) states: 'Often the first steps in initiating change involve not direct action but creating a framework for understanding what is happening, and how things might be different.'

Section 14.5 outlined social constructionism as a framework for reflecting on physiotherapy practice. Here I shall focus specifically on ideologies that can underpin power relations with clients. Social constructionism has, in some approaches to counselling, provided a theoretical foundation to address power relations. A powerful quotation from Martin Luther King Jr is as relevant today as it was in the 1960s, and sets the scene well for 'questioning dominant ideologies'. He questions notions of maladjustment and, by implication, adjustment:

> Today, psychologists have a favorite word, and that word is maladjusted. I tell you there are some things in our social system to which I am proud to be maladjusted. I shall never be adjusted to lynch mobs, segregation, economic inequalities, 'the madness of militarism', and self-defeating physical violence. The salvation of the world lies in the maladjusted (in Freedman & Combs 1996: 95).

The power relations that characterize all of our social interactions are played out (among other ways) in the language we use to describe our lives. The notion of ideology is important here, that is 'sets of ideas, beliefs and assumptions in general and, more specifically … those that reflect existing power relations' (Thompson 1998: 20). Ideologies are sets of ideas that legitimate inequalities. Dominant ideologies represent and strengthen the position of powerful groups and are shaped and maintained according to distributions of power (Dallos 1997).

The critique of what is sometimes called essentialism is common to all the second-wave approaches to counselling. Essentialism is any way of thinking about human beings and social issues which suggests that behaviour can be attributed to 'essences' or fixed qualities. It can be argued that essentialist discourses legitimate inequality (Thompson 1998). Differences between people are seen as natural and therefore grounds for inequality. Fuss (1989), for example, argues that supposedly natural sexual difference (the division into 'male' and 'female') is used to explain social differences. Inequalities between men and women are justified on the basis that 'men are stronger and more logical', 'women are better at caring' and so on. Saraga (1998c) argues that essentialism implies both the permanence of a condition or identity and the homogeneity of people defined by this characteristic. She analyses a number of examples, including sexual preference, ethnic minorities and disability. Of the last of these she writes: 'Disability is commonly seen as an essential, and hence permanent, characteristic of people, derived from physical/biological/psychological/cognitive traits' (Saraga 1998c: 196).

It is possible to suggest, then, some grounds for anti-essentialism, to depathologize homosexuality, respond to the values, needs and experiences of people from different religious and cultural backgrounds, and recognize disability as a condition of a society dominated by the needs and interests of non-disabled people (Section 17.4). The following are some critical questions in challenging essentialist thinking in physiotherapy practice:

1. What does the concept of 'normal' mean? There is no single meaning of normality that applies across all cultures. Furthermore the concept of

normal can be oppressive when applied to some people, including disabled people, gays and lesbians.

2. In what ways might racism, homophobia and disablism affect the therapy process? Power imbalances between therapists and clients may reflect the imbalances of power between the cultural communities or groups to which they belong, for example, between white therapist and black client, or between non-disabled therapist and disabled client.

3. What does the concept of 'independence' mean? Dependency is not devalued in all ethnic minority communities. The concept of independence can be oppressive to disabled people, particularly when it is conceived in terms of non-disabled norms.

19.3.2 EMPOWERMENT

The concept of empowerment is also central to many approaches to counselling, including, as we saw above, humanistic counselling. It is a term, however, which raises a number of questions and can be defined in different ways. Thompson (1998: 211) recognizes that it is a contested concept but suggests that we 'can identify its core element as a process of helping people gain greater control over their lives and the sociopolitical and existential challenges they face'.

Davey points to a notion of empowerment that is social as well as personal:

> Empowerment must address all their problems together if it is to be meaningful. Poverty, poor housing and the nature of the social security system put a strain on relationships and lead to widespread demoralisation. Depending on the circumstances of individuals they can lead to physical and mental ill health, criminality, addiction and the persecution of individual or collective scapegoats: racism, sexism, picking on individuals (Davey 1999: 37).

He goes on to argue that this is not a question of helping people to adjust to their circumstances. One counselling approach that has addressed empowerment is feminist counselling. It has to be said that there is no single school of feminist counselling and it is questionable whether there is a unified approach. Nevertheless, there are some basic principles that can be identified and the overall direction is towards social empowerment. Present-day feminist perspectives have emerged from collective struggles against oppressive values, expectations and 'man-made' sufferings that disempower and discriminate against women and feminist values: the struggle for equality, civil rights and 'people power'. Problems are seen as having social origins: poverty, bad housing, unremitting child-care and care of old people without adequate support. Growth and change are seen as being fostered in non-hierarchical and cooperative relationships in which differences are accepted and, indeed, celebrated. Such relationships provide a safe and supportive space for people to explore and express their feelings and thoughts and to come to their own understandings of the oppression faced through the inequalities and hierarchies in society. This is empowering women to contribute to the transforming of hierarchical relationships and thus the changing of society. Chaplin writes:

> It is difficult to be 'healthy' in an 'unhealthy' society. And many so-called neurotic patterns that people bring to counselling are vital survival mechanisms in an 'unhealthy' society … Far too often women blame themselves for problems that are not of their own making. By helping them to see the processes actually at work, during counselling, we contribute to their ability to deal with them more effectively and thus contribute to changes in society (Chaplin 1999: 17–18).

Similar notions of empowerment have emerged from disabled people and people who work with disabled people. Standing (1999), a physiotherapist working with people with learning difficulties, writes of the possibilities for empowerment through working in partnership with clients. She states: 'Empowerment is likely to be achieved in situations and within programmes where professionals are not the key actors. The cognitive, motivational and personality changes experienced by those who gain a sense of control are the essence of empowerment' (Standing 1999: 256). She looks towards the role of therapist as enabler, allowing clients to take the lead, as in many approaches to counselling.

Barnes & Bowl (2001: 25) also define empowerment in terms of broad-ranging transformations in people's lives. Their list includes:

● Personal growth and development
● Gaining greater control over life choices
● Resistance to and subversion of dominant discourses and practices
● A means of achieving structural change: reducing inequalities
● A process of developing and valuing different knowledges – linking knowledge and action – praxis.

Dalrymple & Burke (1995) provide a list of principles and assumptions of empowerment which have relevance across all professions. These include:

● Empowerment is a collaborative process
● The empowering process views the client as competent and capable
● Clients must first perceive themselves as able to effect change
● Competence is acquired or refined through life experiences
● Solutions are necessarily diverse
● Informal social networks are a significant source of support.

19.3.3 ANTI-DISCRIMINATORY AND ANTI-OPPRESSIVE PRACTICE

This is again a diverse set of notions that are defined in various ways. Indeed, anti-discriminatory and anti-oppressive practice are often used as umbrella notions that incorporate challenging dominant ideologies and strategies for empowerment. Braye & Preston-Shoot (1995) differentiate between anti-discriminatory and anti-oppressive practice, highlighting some of the issues. In their model, anti-discriminatory practice is reformist, and challenges inequality within officially sanctioned rules, procedures and structures. Specific strategies include: equal access to services; ethnically sensitive services; consultation about services. Anti-oppressive practice, in this model, seeks more fundamental changes in power structures and specific strategies include: rebalancing power relationships between professionals and clients, with client control of services and resources; and identification and challenging of abuses of power experienced by clients. In most of the literature, however, the two terms are used interchangeably, and similar ideas are drawn on.

Reimers & Treacher (1995) have put forward a set of principles for a 'user-friendly' style of counselling, in particular family therapy, which offer a basis for anti-discriminatory practice in physiotherapy. Their proposals, directed towards physiotherapy practice, would include the following:

1. Physiotherapy is essentially a human encounter between people who are human beings first and therapist and client second. Failure to address power differentials, whatever their grounds, opens the door to abusive practice.

2. Physiotherapists must accept that ethical issues are of primary importance in therapy practice. Ethical issues include the daily dilemmas of physiotherapy with decisions about 'how best to give information, how much time to spend with people, how best to offer support, how to find some support for yourself or how to give your attention to someone you do not particularly like or respect' (Murray 1998: 189; see also Section 15.2.1).

3. An effective professional–client relationship is an alliance in which the interests, viewpoints and experiences from both standpoints are the grist of negotiation.

4. Anti-discriminatory practice recognizes difference of class, sexual orientation and other social divisions as part of the warp and weft of individual differences.

5. Clients' experiences of therapy and their satisfaction with therapy must form a crucial part of the evaluation of physiotherapy practice.

6. Notions of anti-discriminatory practice necessitate recognition of the wider social environment in consideration of physiotherapy practice and recognition too of the limitations of physiotherapy. The provision of physiotherapy for disabled children in school, for instance, can play a role in accessing the educational environment.

Addressing the issue of inclusive schools for children with learning difficulties, Whittaker & Potter (1999: 142) argue that: 'Therapists need to examine their own belief systems and how these impinge on their practice; and to enter into constructive dialogue concerning their important role in supporting young people with learning difficulties in their right to inclusive schooling.' As Thompson (2001: 162) points out, 'establishing a basis of equality and social justice in service provision is no easy matter'. In the face of different forms of discrimination and multiple discrimination, and also the vested power interests that obstruct change, there can be no simple formula solutions to developing physiotherapy practice. Successful change will depend on collective commitment and action.

19.4 CHANGING NARRATIVES

We turn now to a particular approach to counselling and its implications in informing physiotherapy practice: narrative or working with stories. The terms 'narratives', 'accounts' and 'stories' are used interchangeably in this approach to denote selected sequences of life that, for some narrative therapists, come into existence through the very act of being told (Payne 2000). In this brief summary I shall characterize the approach, its relevance to physiotherapy practice and general strategies employed.

First, it has to be said that 'narrative' is not a single approach and also it shares common principles and practices with other approaches, including humanistic and feminist counselling. Indeed, it could be argued that all counselling has elements of 'working with stories'. However as McLeod (1998a) points out, the social constructionist approach has most fully exploited narrative ideas. White & Epston (1990) put forward a view of therapy as a process of people 'storying' and 're-storying' their lives and experiences. Therapy, they argue, provides opportunities for people to re-author and create new and possibly liberating narratives.

The constructionist account suggests that the social rather than individual realm is the primary ground from which the human being may be understood. Payne states: 'Narrative therapy embodies an assumption that cultural, social and political factors affect lives, and in particular that power-based relations in Western society are endemic both "locally" (interpersonally) and more widely' (Payne 2000: 12). Often, it seems, problems are such because people feel unable to move them – they have lost agency in their life. What is happening is that the stories people are telling themselves about what is happening are disabling (Drewery & Winslade 1997). Problems, in this sense, are the products of ways of speaking that have placed the person in problematic positions in the story he or she is telling about his or her life. As Riikonen & Smith (1997: 15) suggest: 'A particular feature of the narrative approach is that it allows the naming of the interpersonal politics which support or enforce certain meanings or existing stories'.

How, then, might clients' narratives be incorporated into physiotherapy practice? Atkinson has argued that physiotherapy practice, by its nature, can provide a favourable milieu for narrative:

> Therapists are well placed, through their work and in their relationships with clients, to play an active part in the telling of stories. This starts with recognizing that everyone has a personal past, and acknowledging and respecting that past. It goes further: it means listening to the life story when it is told; helping where possible, with the telling and the researching of that story; and recording the present sensitively, so that today's stories are recorded for the future in ways that people themselves approve (Atkinson 1999: 21).

A narrative approach focuses on the stories that participants tell about their experiences. These stories can give physiotherapists insight into motives, expectations, aims and convictions of the clients involved.

Widdershoven & Smits (1996: 285–286) point out that a narrative 'can make us understand how people give meaning to a concrete situation and why they respond to it through a specific action. Narratives are not just descriptions of feelings and actions; they present these feelings and actions as part of a practice.'

Narratives have the power to illuminate experiences of illness and healing. Narratives give meaning to illness or accident or impairment, the place of physiotherapy within the unfolding story of responses to treatment, and re-telling of life history in the face of illness or impairment. McLeod suggests that:

> With non-professional, lay people, the form of understanding of accounting for illness that is most often employed is the *story*. People tell stories about their health and illness. The sense of 'what made me unwell', 'how I feel today' or 'how I got better' is communicated to others through stories ... People who are ill are often in a period of transition, struggling to make the link between their pre-illness life-narrative and the story of who they are now. Achieving a coherent narrative can help give the person a sense of control and mastery over his or her condition, and can facilitate the process of establishing a viable role within their social group. Telling the story is a way of being known ... Allowing space for telling the story, and creating opportunities for the experience of being heard and understood, are part of effective health care (McLeod 1998b: 51, 62–63).

Mattingly (1998: 13) developed similar ideas in her work: 'Life histories tend to emphasize the need for persons to find coherence and continuity in their lives ... and telling a life story becomes one device by which persons try to interpret disruptive illnesses in life context'. Through narrative, physiotherapists come in contact with participants as people engaged in the process of interpreting themselves. Writing of her experiences using a life story approach in health care research, Smith states:

> Participants were seen to develop new insights into their personal experiences, family relationships, and social world understandings. They declared stronger feelings of self-value and personal rights; expressed increased confidence in the validity of their own perceptions; experienced greater integration of past events into their present sense of self; and presented an overall more centered, grounded, and self-cohering demeanor (Smith 2000: 19).

A particular example is provided by the work of Blanche (1996), an occupational therapist. She explored the effect of cultural differences on the delivery of health care services through a life story approach with the mother of a disabled child. She used a 'cooperative story-making' approach which rejects the ideology of 'observed versus observer' and sees both the interviewer and the informer as building the story together. She concludes that:

> clinicians need to acknowledge the client's and their own culture as well as the perceptions, expectations, values, and beliefs that are inherent in

each … Stereotyping persons and treating them as homogeneous ethnic or racial groups saves time but is not effective. Listening to a client's life story may give us the information we need to place our services within the complexity of his or her life (Blanche 1996: 274–275).

Two key ideas in this type of narrative therapy are *deconstructing* the dominant narrative and *externalizing the problem*. The notion of deconstruction, as discussed above, stems from the idea that people live their lives within the dominant narratives or knowledges of their culture and family, such as the individual medical and tragedy models of disability (see Section 17.3). This dominant narrative can conflict with personal experience (for instance, of the barriers facing people with impairments in a disabling society) and be in itself oppressive. Listening to narratives can involve actively deconstructing the dominant narrative: 'Unlike the Rogerian therapist, whose active listening is intended to reflect back the client's story like a mirror without distortion, the narrative therapist looks for hidden meanings, spaces or gaps, and evidence of conflicting stories. We call this process of listening for what is not said *deconstruction*' (Drewery & Winslade 1997: 43). As McLeod (1998a) explains, the process of externalizing the problem involves the client separating himself or herself and personal relationships from the problem. Furthermore, 'the device of externalization helps to reverse the trend in psychology toward seeking more and more deficits in human character and encouraging clients to relate to themselves as deficient human beings' (Drewery & Winslade 1997: 45). Thus the process of 'changing narratives' can be seen as part of the process of 'changing power relations'.

The notions of both deconstruction and externalizing the problem require physiotherapists to access non-dominant, or what Thompson (1998) calls countervailing, ideologies, such as the social model of disability (see Section 17.4). This has been recognized, for instance, by Donati & Ward, who take a critical stance to both the medical model and educational approaches in their work as therapists and state: 'As a result of disability rights and independent living movements, the traditional view of disability has been redefined as one that locates the barriers within the social and built environment rather than within the individual' (Donati & Ward 1999: 245). Standing, in advocating working in partnership with people with learning difficulties, also looks beyond the medical model and states: 'Working in partnership with people with learning difficulties demands for therapists far more than learning new techniques of treatment; it involves a willingness and capacity to respond imaginatively to every person as a unique individual and to help and support each person in the achievement of his or her own aspirations and desired lifestyle' (Standing 1999: 259).

19.5 CONCLUSION

The development of a social approach to counselling, by McLeod (1999), offers a framework for considering the implications of counselling theory and practice for physiotherapy practice, and a structure for the concluding section of this chapter. As an alternative or complementary approach to the use of counselling skills it is tentative and reflective rather than prescriptive. A social approach aims to draw attention to important social processes that occur in any physiotherapy encounters. It does not prescribe any specific techniques or interventions from the practice of counselling, but offers a set of principles which may be of value to both clients and practitioners.

The following, then, is McLeod's general framework in summarizing the main implications of a social perspective (see also Swain et al 2003b):

The image of the person. McLeod (1999: 221) states: 'People are seen as being human through their membership and participation in a culture and social world'. For instance, as noted earlier, Burnard (1999) suggests that 'helping clients to adapt to long-term disability' is a goal of physiotherapy. The question arises as to whether this is an essentialist view of disability with clients adapting to a pathological, individualized conception of disability, or whether what is being adapted to is a social model view of disability, which argues that people are seen as inhuman (abnormal) through the discrimination and segregation that deny their participation in mainstream culture and social world. The construction of the 'image of the person' is engaged in within and through therapy practice, recognizing the social, historical, cultural and political bases of this construction.

The goals of physiotherapy. In terms of the goals of counselling, McLeod (1999: 221) states: 'The aim is to strengthen the culture within which we live, by enabling persons to participate, contribute, give and receive care, and to belong'. In developing a social approach, the goals of physiotherapy address social change through challenging taken-for-granted ideologies, engaging with the empowerment of clients, and pursing anti-oppressive practices.

The physiotherapy process. Drawing on this model of counselling casts physiotherapy practice in a broader social domain. McLeod (1999: 221) states: 'It is possible to characterize this new approach as *post-psychological* in so far as it recognizes that, in a counselling relationship, a reliance only on psychological concepts and language restricts what can be said and the kinds of stories that can be told.' There are stories to be told, by both clients and therapists, about deconstructing the experiences and understanding of themselves and their lives that bring them to physiotherapy practice.

Physiotherapy theory. In terms of counselling, McLeod (1998a: 25–26) states that: 'within contemporary practice, the alliance between therapy and social action has been made most effectively by feminist and gay counsellors, and practitioners from ethnic and minority groups'. The theory of physiotherapy is again placed in the wider context of people's lives. Physiotherapy can offer the client opportunities to enter into dialogue over problematic aspects of experience and to construct alternative ways of telling the story of events and experiences.

The training and preparation of physiotherapists.   As McLeod (1999: 221) states: 'It is necessary for counsellors to be able to locate their approach within its social and historical context.' One implication is the inclusion of training such as disability equality training (DET) and anti-racism courses within physiotherapy training, as core rather than optional elements. Training and education drawing on counselling theory and practice can prepare physiotherapists to go beyond the medical and locate therapy within its social and historic context.

Chapter **20**

Researching together: a participatory approach

John Swain and Sally French

20.1 INTRODUCTION

Research is a vast and multifarious topic to fit into in a single chapter. None the less, it is of fundamental importance to physiotherapy students and practising therapists for numerous reasons – from the requirements on physiotherapy students to conduct small-scale projects to the general pursuit of research-based practice. In this chapter, we focus on a shift of thinking in research that is centrally concerned with the relations between those who conduct research and those who are research subjects. The crucial shift is from doing research *on* people to doing research *with* people. This is not to suggest that participatory research is the only approach that is of value within physiotherapy. It is rather a shift within social science research generally that challenges thinking within physiotherapy research and offers possible alternatives to more traditional approaches. We shall concentrate specifically on research in the field of disability as a significant context for the development of a participatory approach, though recognizing that the general principles have a wider application.

The chapter begins with an overview of the development of participatory research, what this shift in thinking is, and why researchers have moved towards this approach. We then turn to disability research and discuss why disabled people are dissatisfied with research done 'on' them. In this context we look at what has come to be known as 'emancipatory research' and contrast this with participatory research to pinpoint key issues for researchers and disabled people. In the next section, we highlight examples of research with disabled people that involves them and gives their perspective. Against this background we turn to the implications for physiotherapists. We provide an overview of published physiotherapy research in terms of the principles of a participatory approach and conclude by drawing out the implications for development. Emancipatory and participatory research approaches are relevant to other minority and oppressed groups; disability is being used in this chapter to illustrate the arguments from a health perspective.

20.2 RESEARCH WITH PEOPLE

Brechin (1993: 73) states that research 'tends to be owned and controlled by researchers, or by those who, in turn, own and control the researchers'. Researchers who adopt a participatory approach are attempting to change these power relations and to ensure that research is owned and controlled by research participants as well as researchers. In characterizing participatory research, Cornwell & Jewkes (1995: 1667) argue that 'the key difference between participatory and conventional methodologies lies in the location of power in the research process'.

Participatory methodologies have arisen from qualitative research approaches, which aim to reflect, explore and disseminate the views, concerns, feelings and experiences of research participants from their own perspectives. The realization of participatory research goes beyond this, however, to engage participants in the design, conduct and evaluation of research, with the construction of non-hierarchical research relations (Zarb 1992). Participatory research, then, attempts to change the social relations of research processes.

A crucial tenet of participatory research is that it is research *with* rather than *on* people (Reason & Heron 1986). The research process is viewed as a potential source of change and empowerment for the research participants as well as a process for influencing professional policy and practice by reflecting the views and opinions of service users. Reason & Heron (1986) believe that participatory research invites people to participate in the co-creation of knowledge about themselves. Using the term 'partnership research', Lloyd et al (1996) recognize similar principles: non-hierarchical research relationships in setting the research agenda, data analysis and dissemination.

Participatory research is an approach that has been evolving in recent years, particularly in the developing countries. Chambers (1986: 1) refers to it as a 'new paradigm', 'a coherent and mutually supportive pattern of concepts, values, methods and action amenable to wide application'. Furthermore, there are a number of relevant approaches that claim to be essentially 'participatory', such as 'democratic research' and 'emancipatory action research'. The general change in terminology from 'research subjects' to 'research participants' is indicative of the influence of participatory approaches. Participatory research aims to involve, at every stage of the research process (choice of topics, methods, evaluation and dissemination), those towards whom research is normally directed, people whom Chambers describes as 'the last', for example rural village dwellers in developing countries, patients and disabled people.

There is no place for 'subjects' or passive cooperation in this approach; instead everyone involved is an active participant. Ideally, the expertise and talents of everyone are utilized to the full and training is given if necessary; the approach does not, however, reject expert knowledge or help from outside; rather, it aims to make traditional research more effective and more meaningful.

The development of participatory approaches in research can also be seen as part of wider developments in social and health care. Braye (2000) includes: the involvement of individual service users or prospective service users in their own use of service; involvement in strategic planning for service provision and development; and the development of user-led services (such as centres for integrated living established by disabled people). The trend towards the participation of disabled people in research can be linked with the development of user involvement, citizenship and consumer participation (Zarb 1995). The NHS and Community Care Act 1990, for instance, requires that local authorities should consult with service users in the review and planning of services (Lloyd et al 1996).

The broad notion of 'participatory' in relation to research is associated with other principles in service planning and delivery, such as 'empowerment': 'Practice can be improved, too, by being imbued with clarity of thought, critical analysis and informed choice of approach. Both empowering practice and empowering research depend on being participatory, encouraging participants to "own" the outcome by setting the goals and sharing in decisions about the most desirable process to be followed' (Everitt et al 1992: 50).

Partnership practice is also a model that appears consistently in professional literature. Key objectives include (Braye & Preston-Shoot 1995):

• Open dialogue with service users such that their views and concerns are represented in the definition of problems, prioritization of needs and in decision-making

• Honesty about differences of opinion and how they are affected by the power held by the different parties in the partnership.

Other relevant and much used terms in the general literature would include 'consultation', 'choice' and 'user involvement'.

There is also, however, a widely held belief that terms such as 'empowerment' and 'partnership' have developed into fashionable buzz words and are often used loosely and uncritically (Gomm 1993). Baistow has argued, for instance, that while empowerment may have the potential to liberate, it can also open up regulatory possibilities. She states: 'Far from user empowerment limiting the intervention of professionals into the lives of citizens, in current empowerment discourses we see space being created for new sorts of professional expertise to emerge and for new or transformed "client groups" to be identified as the objects of this new type of professional attention' (Baistow 1994: 41).

It appears, then, that empowerment can be central to the continued legitimacy of professionals and their interventions. Who is being empowered? Braye & Preston-Shoot (1995) discuss the whole notion of user involvement, particularly in terms of users being in a negotiating position from which power can be exercised and where the exercise of that power has the potential to achieve its purposes. There are necessary key qualities and characteristics if 'participatory' is to be more than a mere buzz word and empty rhetoric. In the following list (Braye & Preston-Shoot 1995: 118), we have used the term 'participation' rather than involvement:

- Clarity about what participation is being offered, and what its limits are
- Participation from the beginning in ways which are central to agency structures and processes, but which are also flexible
- Tangible goals for participation
- Participation from black and minority perspectives
- Individual and collective perspectives
- Provision of time, information, resources and training
- Openness to advocacy
- Clear channels of representation and complaint
- Participation of the key participants
- Open agendas
- Facilitation of attendance.

Recognizing the need for critical reflection, Thompson (1998) argues that, as a practice principle, participation occurs not only at the micro level of specific practice situations, but also at the wider levels of service planning, policy development, evaluation, training and so on. He states: 'Developing approaches based on partnership and participation is a challenging task, and one that demands considerable skill and commitment' (Thompson 1998: 213–214).

Having begun by defining what is meant by 'participatory approaches' in research, the next obvious question is, why?

De Koning & Martin (1996: 1) offer two reasons why participatory approaches have grown in popularity. First, 'there is an increasing recognition of the gap between the concepts and models professionals use to understand and interpret reality and the concepts and perspectives of different groups in the community'. Second, 'many factors, cultural, historical, socio-economic and political, which are difficult to measure, have a crucial influence on the outcomes of interventions and efforts to improve the health of people'. Chambers (1997) identifies the following as some of the key features of participatory research: it breaks down the mystique surrounding research; it ensures that the problems researched are perceived as problems by the community to which the research is directed; it helps to develop self-confidence, self-reliance and skills within people to whom the research is directed; and it encourages democratic interaction and transfer of power to the research participants. Participatory research is essentially about establishing equality in research relationships; that is, giving more say in research to people who are more usually subjected to research.

From an ethical standpoint, the justification of participatory research can be founded on the recognition that research is not necessarily a social good. Research is not justifiable simply on the traditional, modernist grounds of furthering knowledge, on the basis that knowledge is intrinsically good. The research process can be detrimental to both research participants and, on a broader basis, people who are not directly involved in the research. Domholdt (2000) lists types of risks for participants in therapy research. There can be physical risks, such as the development of delayed muscle soreness from the use of isokinetic equipment. Psychological risks include adverse emotional reactions to data collection in investigations of sensitive topics. Social risks can emanate, for instance, from a breach of confidentiality. The fourth category of risk is economic, for example lost working hours (including for therapists involved in the research). Prentice & Purtilo (1993) also list legal risks (for example, criminal prosecution).

Research has also been linked to wider issues of social inequality and social injustice, including: sexuality; sexual abuse; race and ethnicity; age; gender; and disability (Truman et al 2000). The research process is bound up with social and political forces of which researchers should be aware. Research findings can affect political decisions, which may be detrimental to various people in society. Research on sensitive issues such as race may increase prejudice and discrimination or create social unrest; research aimed at producing greater efficiency in a particular industry or profession may reduce job satisfaction or give rise to widespread unemployment; and expenditure on medical research may limit expenditure on social research or social action. Furthermore, knowledge is often put to use in ways that are not beneficial to the people to whom the research is directed. Research into the treatment of a particular disease, for example, may serve to maintain the status quo by failing to address the social, economic and political factors involved in its aetiology.

It is likely that therapists beginning to get involved in research will regard research as a good thing: to inform and develop practice; to contribute to knowledge and understanding, and so on. A starting point for thinking about the ethics of research is, however, the possible harm to participants that might result from their involvement in the research.

In the next section of this chapter, we take up the general issues we have raised in the specific context of disability research.

20.3 DISABILITY RESEARCH: TOWARDS PARTICIPATORY AND EMANCIPATORY APPROACHES

In 1992 Oliver laid down the gauntlet to researchers in the field of disability studies. He stated:

> As disabled people have increasingly analysed their segregation, inequality and poverty in terms of discrimination and oppression, research has

been seen as part of the problem rather than part of the solution ... Disabled people have come to see research as a violation of their experiences, as irrelevant to their needs and as failing to improve their material circumstances and quality of life (Oliver 1992: 106).

Since then, it seems, disability research has been in 'a state of transformation and transition' (Moore et al 1998a: 11). Seemingly solid, traditional, modernist grounds have turned to shifting, sinking sands. Research is not justifiable simply on the traditional grounds of furthering knowledge with the presumption that knowledge is intrinsically good. All research is political, and research production and processes can further the oppression of those who are the subjects of research.

Critiques of disability research have analysed the processes through which research maintains and strengthens the status quo within a disablist society, such as Abberley's (1992) evaluation of the Office of Population Census and Surveys (OPCS). As French (1994b) argues, research has traditionally reflected an individualistic stance to disability and served to oppress disabled people by depoliticizing the political. A project with which one of the authors was involved as a research subject serves as an example of research that clearly demonstrated an individualistic, tragedy model (see Section 17.3). In a trial of a newly developed form of insulin, research subjects with diabetes were required to complete a questionnaire about 'you and your diabetes ... the way you feel and how diabetes affects your day to day life'. With each question was a choice of four answers ranging, basically, from 'very much' to 'not at all'. The first question set the scene: 'Do you look forward to the future?', with the implication that the supposed tragedy of diabetes may negate any hope for the future. The 32 questions were peppered with words of tragedy, such as 'fear', 'edgy', 'worry' and 'difficult'. Some questions addressed psychological responses to the tragedy, such as: 'Do you throw things around if you get upset or lose your temper?', 'Do you get touchy or moody about diabetes?' and 'Do you hurt yourself or feel like hurting yourself when you get upset?' Two questions invoked the essence of the tragedy model: 'Do you even for a moment wish that you were dead?' and 'Do you wish that you had never been born?' Thus, the ultimate version of the tragedy model, as conveyed within this research, is that physical death is better than the social death of disability. The agenda within the research is that of the researchers, not the concerns of disabled people. For instance, the causes of any anger are clearly conceived in terms of the person's response to impairment, not to the barriers faced within a disabling society (or, indeed, to completing a questionnaire of this kind).

Many disabled people are of the opinion that medically orientated research has not fundamentally altered their position within society (Abberley 1992, Oliver 1992). The way in which disability has been researched has become a major issue for disabled people and their organizations in recent times. In 1991, a series of seminars on the subject of researching disability were organized by disabled academics (Disability Research Seminars), culminating in a conference (Researching Disability: Setting the Agenda for Change) in 1992.

Disability has generally been defined in an individualistic, medicalized way as an internal condition of the individual, and most research on disability, including the large OPCS government surveys, reflect this orientation. Many disabled people, on the other hand, view disability in terms of social, physical and attitudinal barriers, which could be removed if only the political will to do so were present (see Section 17.4).

If an individualistic stance is taken by researchers, then the questions posed will be based on impairment and not on discriminatory practices and lack of access. Oliver (1990) has reworded some of the questions used in an OPCS survey to illustrate this point. For example, in place of the question 'What complaint causes you difficulty in holding, gripping and turning things?', he substitutes the question 'What defects in the design of everyday equipment, like jars, bottles and tins, causes you difficulty in holding, gripping and turning them?' and in place of the question 'Did you move here because of your health problems/disability?', he writes 'What inadequacies in your housing caused you to move here?' (Oliver 1990: 7). Abberley (1992: 158) believes that 'It is a political decision, conscious or otherwise, to employ questions of the first type rather than the second'. The way in which disability is defined is a serious issue, as findings may be translated into practice (French 1994b).

20.3.1 DISTINGUISHING EMANCIPATORY AND PARTICIPATORY RESEARCH

The more recent developments in disability research have taken two quite distinct directions, though they are often related and, more often, simply confused. They are associated with a number of terms but we shall use the most common: 'participatory research' and 'emancipatory research'. In a previous paper (French & Swain 1997), we argued that these two methodological bases can be traced to distinct historical roots. Participatory approaches have developed from general qualitative methodology. They have been developed, generally, by non-disabled researchers who wish to break down the traditional hierarchical researcher–researched relationship. It is important to understand that the roots of participatory research lie in the development of research methodology itself, rather than the development of a different understanding of disability. Qualitative research is primarily concerned with meaning, interpretation and giving research participants 'a right of voice'. There is a commitment to seeing 'through the eyes' of research participants, and a belief that social behaviour cannot be grasped until the researcher has understood the symbolic world of the research participants. Researchers in the qualitative tradition accept that the research in which they are engaged cannot be independent of their own values and perspectives.

This is not to imply that qualitative approaches are free of conflict, difficulties and ethical dilemmas when it comes to disability research. It can, for example, be difficult to find justifications for undertaking research into intimate, personal matters such as sexual behaviour or feelings of vulnerability following impairment or illness (Swain et al 1998b). It would seem that participatory research reflects the concerns and views of disabled research participants and thus tends to reflect a social model of disability. However, participatory methodology is not inherently associated with a social model of disability. As Oliver (1997: 26) states: 'participatory and action research is about improving the existing social and material relations of research production; not challenging and ultimately eradicating them'. It seems, then, that the participatory research paradigm has arisen from qualitative research approaches and philosophical arguments about social reality. Participatory research has been applied within disability research, but it does not have its roots in a different understanding of disability.

Emancipatory research, in the area of disability at least, has its roots in the growth of the disabled people's movement and the development of a social model of disability. The emancipatory paradigm takes the adoption of a social model of disability as the basis for research production (Priestley 1999, Barnes 2003). It can be argued that emancipatory research, unlike participatory research, is not a research methodology as such, but rather part of the struggle of disabled people to control the decision-making processes that shape their lives and to achieve full citizenship. As Barton (1998: 38) states: 'The task of changing the social relations and conditions of research production is to be viewed as part of the wider struggle to remove all forms of oppression and discrimination in the pursuit of an inclusive society.'

Emancipatory research goes further than participatory research by aiming to change the social relations of research production, with disabled people taking complete control of the research process. In emancipatory research, the social relations of production are conceived as part of the processes of changing society to ensure the full participation of disabled people. Barnes explains:

> Emancipatory research is about the systematic demystification of the structures and processes which create disability and the establishment of a workable 'dialogue' between the research community and disabled people in order to facilitate the latter's empowerment. To do this researchers must learn how to put their knowledge and skills at the disposal of disabled people (Barnes 1992: 122).

Barnes (2001) has pinpointed and discussed what he sees as the core principles of an emancipatory research model. He argues that accountability to the disabled community is a key component of this model, and that the emancipatory model is founded on the social model of disability (Barnes 2003). He further claims that researchers must make their position clear at the outset, 'ensuring that our choice of research methodology and data collection strategies are logical, rigorous and open to scrutiny' (Barnes 2001: 20). In terms of the choice of data collection methods, Barnes argues that from the point of view of the emancipatory model, all data collection strategies have their strengths and weaknesses. In terms of 'the role of experience', Barnes argues that 'what is important is that the discussions of disabled people's experiences, narratives and stories are couched firmly within an environmental and cultural context in order to highlight the disabling consequences of a society that is increasingly organised around the needs of a mythical, affluent non-disabled majority' (Barnes 2001: 23).

In relation to practical outcomes, Barnes (2001) asks whether emancipatory disability research can offer anything different and argues that it can and has. He also suggests that doing emancipatory research cannot be conceived in terms of a single project or even a collection of projects, but is a continuous process, and the organization and content can only be determined by disabled people and their organizations. Furthermore, the evaluation of the effectiveness of the research can also, ultimately, only be determined by disabled people and their organizations.

In emancipatory research, the production of research is part of the liberation of disabled people; that is, part of the process of changing society to ensure full participative citizenship. This is research conceived as political action in which the processes and products are the tools of disabled people in the achievement of their liberation.

Although certain features of participatory and emancipatory research may overlap, one common confusion, it seems to us, is the equating of emancipatory research with the qualitative paradigm. There is no reason inherent within the nature of emancipatory research why it should adopt a qualitative methodology, as long as the research agenda is generated by disabled people themselves. Indeed, it could be argued that a quantitative approach is more likely. For instance, emancipatory research into the housing stock and, in particular, accessibility of housing for disabled people is likely to take the form of a quantitative survey to produce statistics to influence housing policies. Thus, research undertaken at the Policy Studies Institute, *Measuring Barriers within Society*, aimed to make a systematic analysis of physical, social, economic and political barriers using both qualitative and quantitative measures (Zarb 1995). Oliver states:

> If the category disability is to be produced in ways different from the individualised, pathological way it is currently produced, then what should be researched is not the disabled people of the positivist and interpretive research paradigms but the disablement ingrained in the individualistic consciousness and institutionalised practices of what is, ultimately, a disablist society (Oliver 1996a: 143).

Zarb sums up the fundamental difference between participatory and emancipatory research as follows:

> Participatory research which involves disabled people in a meaningful way is perhaps a prerequisite to emancipatory research in the sense that researchers can learn from disabled people and *vice versa*, and that it paves the way for researchers to make themselves 'available' to disabled people – but it is no more than that. Simply increasing participation and involvement will never by itself constitute emancipatory research unless and until it is disabled people themselves who are controlling the research and deciding who should be involved and how (Zarb 1992: 128).

Complicating the matter even further, Walmsley (2001) uses the term 'inclusive research'. Her discussion justifiably addresses the issues of participatory and emancipatory approaches in research with people with learning difficulties. She argues that inclusive research raises questions that have been barely acknowledged in the literature, such as: 'the consequences for non-disabled researchers of acting as allies; which disabled people can and should undertake research; how theory can be shared with or generated by people with mental impairments; and the possible dangers of research as political action' (Walmsley 2001: 203).

We conclude this section by arguing that participatory research and emancipatory research are two distinct, though by no means incompatible, research paradigms. As Stalker (1998) suggests, there are shared 'beliefs' within the two paradigms, but we believe that the differences also need to be recognized. 'Ideal types' are conceived here as a basis for critical reflection in terms of intention and, in particular, the pursuit of social change.

20.4 REFLECTING ON RESEARCH

'Participation' can be seen as an ideal to which researchers can aspire. In this light, there are not two types of research, participatory and nonparticipatory, but an imperative for researchers to reflect critically on projects in terms of the realization of participatory principles. In developing processes of critical reflection, we would suggest that two key questions need to be addressed. The first question is: does the research address the concerns of disabled people themselves? Second: does the research promote disabled people's control over the decision-making processes that shape their lives? The question can be directed at the decision-making processes within the research, and the empowerment of the participants through their involvement in research. Clearly, such critical reflection should itself be participatory and these questions can only be answered with disabled people themselves. In this section we shall look at some projects with disabled people that involve them and give their perspectives. We have selected research that is of direct relevance to physiotherapists.

In relation to the first question, there are now numerous examples of studies that reflect the concerns of disabled people, adopting an openended agenda, flexible to control by the disabled participants. The following projects have been selected to reflect a wide range of topics and participant groups relevant to physiotherapists. Closs (1998) explored the views of children and young people with life-threatening or life-shortening medical conditions. Six young people participated in the study by reflecting on their childhoods, 'responding to questions on key issues identified in the literature and supplemented by them, and criticising drafts' (Closs 1998: 112). From the data she collected a number of themes were considered critical to the quality of children's and young people's lives, including: the individual's understanding of his or her condition; feelings of sameness/difference; educational experiences and attainments; friendships; family; and experience of the medical/paramedical services and hospital life. In relation to the last of these, comments from young people illustrated some distressing experiences, such as: 'If they didn't call it treatment you could call it torture'; 'I could write a book about doctors, good, bad and unspeakable'; and 'I realised I had nothing on under the sheet. Maybe it was easier for them to put in tubes...but I felt really embarrassed' (Closs 1998: 121). There were also some enjoyable experiences: 'I don't think you can live for too long in the dumps. I've had lots of laughs, lots of highs' (Closs 1998: 116).

Fifty people with aphasia were involved in a study by Parr et al (1997). In-depth interviews were adopted to allow important topics and issues to be raised by the participants, in addition to those on the researchers' agenda. One topic was people's experiences of services. From participants' detailed accounts, for instance, attributes of successful services included: availability and accessibility; appropriateness and adequacy; flexibility and responsiveness; integration; reliability and consistency; respectfulness; ability to support communication; and ability to provide relevant and accessible information (Parr et al 1997: 66). The experiences of individual participants varied greatly. Madge felt that she had been supported and that the care she had received had been satisfactory. Rebecca's views were very different:

> Rebecca tried to convey the fact that her field of vision was impaired to one doctor: 'He said: "Explain what you mean" and of course I couldn't and he sat there sort of tapping his fingers. He said: "Well does that mean you can't see countryside?" I said ... I just thought ... I just didn't bother.' Although she had intensive treatment from physiotherapists who were 'like Rottweilers', Rebecca had no contact with a speech and language therapist, despite her impaired communication (Parr et al 1997: 74).

Ahmad (2000) reports two qualitative studies focusing on parents of pre-school deaf Asian children with thalassaemia major or sickle cell disorder and their interactions with professionals, from the points of view of both parents and professionals. Atkin et al (2000) report on parents' perspectives. There were 62 parental interviews, 21 of which were in languages other than English. Semi-structured interviews were adopted, as 'this approach is particularly recommended for the study of the ways that individuals express their understanding of themselves, in the context of their social, cultural and personal circumstances' (Atkin et al 2000: 108). They found, for example, that parents face many problems in having their needs recognized, obtaining necessary information about the condition and sources of support, dealing with poorly coordinated services, and dealing with often unsympathetic and poorly informed professionals. One parent explained:

> The medical side should be a bit more informed about the illness so they can inform us about it, but I mean we've come across doctors, nurses ... and they've turned round and said, 'Well I don't know anything about sickle cell.' So straight away, I mean I doubt them straight away. I think, 'Well why are they caring for my child if they don't know anything about it?' (Atkin et al 2000: 114).

The next example comes from research with people with learning difficulties. Atkinson (1997), along with others, has been developing an auto/biographical approach that 'has the capacity to combine the political document with the historical – to reflect the lives which have been lived, but to see beyond the individuals to a wider view of learning disability. Auto/biography contains many voices and tells stories at different levels' (Atkinson 1997: 22). Individual life stories were recounted and shared in a group context. Nine participants, age-range 57–77 years, met on 30 occasions. One of the themes was 'tales of hospital life' and the following is a short extract in which Margaret tells her story of running away:

> The sister would keep on at me, saying my work wasn't done properly. She was being horrible. I'd scrubbed the ward and she said I had to do it over again. I said, 'Well I aren't going to do it over again!' I told the doctor. He come round and he wanted to know what I was doing on the stairs again. I said, 'I've been told I've got to do it again, it wasn't done properly.'
>
> I planned it with the other girl, we planned it together. She was fed up. She was doing the dayroom and dining room, cleaning and polishing. Then I was put on it, as well as scrubbing. We planned to get into Bedford, walk across the fields (Atkinson 1997: 91).

The following two examples are from therapy research. Martlew (1996), a physiotherapist, evaluated on-site physiotherapy in a day hospice providing care for patients with terminal illness, using 'client-centred action research'. She concluded that the learning experience was:

> greater because this study was conducted by a practitioner–researcher doing her own action research [and that] this study has confirmed the benefit of taking time to listen sensitively – both for the professionals, to gain greater insight into patient problems, hopefully leading to more appropriate and therefore effective intervention; and for patients who feel supported and understood (Martlew 1996: 564).

Blanche (1996), an occupational therapist, explored the effect of cultural differences on the delivery of health care services through a life story approach with the mother of a disabled child. She used a 'cooperative story-making' approach which rejects the ideology of 'observed versus observer' and sees both the interviewer and the informer as building the story together. Blanche concludes that:

> clinicians need to acknowledge the client's and their own culture as well as the perceptions, expectations, values, and beliefs that are inherent in each … Stereotyping persons and treating them as homogeneous ethnic or racial groups saves time but is not effective. Listening to a client's life story may give us the information we need to place our services within the complexity of his or her life (Blanche 1996: 274–275).

The final example is a more fully developed example of participatory research in that the participants were involved in the decision-making process throughout the research. The project was controlled, conducted and reported, with support, by the Bristol Self-Advocacy Research Group, a group of four people with learning difficulties (Palmer et al 1999). Their responses to the experience of conducting research were positive:

> We've all really enjoyed the research visits, meeting new people and making new friends.

I was looking at my photographs yesterday when I was at home, and all the different places I've been. And I've got the photographs in my photograph album at home. I'm quite proud of what I did. And you feel very important. People say: 'You do do a lot.' They're quite impressed with what I do. I've achieved a lot – too much (Palmer et al 1999: 34).

The themes covered are: what is disability? cutting out all the labels; jobs and work; the staff who support us; transport; and self-advocacy – what does it mean? For example, under the theme of support, they write about being forced to be independent:

Staff people always think that we all want to be more and more independent. This can be wrong, because they expect us to do too many things ourselves. It should be our choice, not theirs.

If you're married, you've got to give and take. One person does one thing, and people help each other out. It's the same in any house – I don't want staff to keep on forcing me to be independent. How would they feel? (Palmer et al 1999: 42).

20.5 PHYSIOTHERAPY RESEARCH: TOWARDS A PARTICIPATORY APPROACH

Research of any kind may seem somewhat removed from the everyday pressures of the practising physiotherapist, although most will have had considerable exposure to research ideas and practice during their undergraduate education. Physiotherapists are, however, in an ideal position to involve disabled people in research. Unlike many health professionals, physiotherapists frequently spend considerable time with their patients and clients and are in a position to get to know them as people. Sensitive, empowering research can give invaluable insights into patients' and clients' complex experiences of illness, disability and impairment, which may, in turn, have the potential to improve physiotherapy practice as well as patient and client satisfaction. Many patients and clients live with disability and impairment on a daily basis and the knowledge and experience they have gained should not be underestimated, however young they may be.

Over the last 20 years, physiotherapy education in the UK has moved into the university sector and has broadened its scope from a narrow biomedical perspective to one that includes a consideration of psychological, sociological and cultural aspects of health care. It is now recognized that physiotherapy draws on a wide range of diverse disciplines to inform its practice. This is reflected in research textbooks for therapists where a large number of methodologies and approaches are explained (see, for example, Seale & Barnard 1998, Sim & Wright 2000, French et al 2001).

This diversity is not, however, reflected in physiotherapy journals, where a biomedical approach is still paramount, leading to a concentration of articles based upon experimental research with little if any involvement by research 'subjects'. We undertook a brief content analysis of the peer-reviewed articles in the UK journal *Physiotherapy* from January 1999 to December 2001. This revealed that, with regard to research studies of patients and clients, the experimental method was three times more common than the summed total of qualitative and survey methods. Qualitative and survey methods which focused on health care professionals (where, for example, their opinions and feelings were sought) were over three times as common as those which focused on the opinions and feelings of patients and clients. Twelve case studies and five studies using a documentary method were published during this period. All of these studies showed a strong biomedical and quantitative orientation. Psychological, social and cultural perspectives were minor compared with the biomedical perspective, while the perspective of the disabled people's movement was entirely absent. This indicates the dominance of biomedical knowledge within physiotherapy, derived from experimental research, and the marginalizing of other sources of knowledge, including the direct voice of disabled people themselves.

The Chartered Society of Physiotherapy regards knowledge of research as an essential characteristic of newly qualified physiotherapists (Chartered Society of Physiotherapy 2002a). It argues further that graduating physiotherapists should deliver services based upon the best available evidence and that they need to be competent in:

- Initiating and enacting change
- Promoting equality
- Seeking evidence and applying new knowledge
- Responding to changing demands
- Working in partnership with patients and clients
- Making paramount patient/client experience.

Research that involves and empowers patients and clients in a meaningful rather than a tokenistic way would be one means of achieving these goals. This is unlikely to happen, however, unless the study of disability and the voices of disabled people are given space within the physiotherapy curriculum. Disabled people have spoken out about the ways their perceptions of disability frequently clash with those of health professionals, and non-disabled people in general, and how the neglect of their perspective has created inappropriate policy and practice. The following quotations illustrate these points:

> I just can't imagine becoming hearing, I'd need a psychiatrist, I'd need a speech therapist, I'd need some new friends, I'd lose all my old friends, I'd lose my job. I wouldn't be here lecturing. It really hits people that a deaf person doesn't want to become hearing. I am what I am (Phillipe, cited in Shakespeare et al 1996: 184).

> I do not wish for a cure for Aspergers Syndrome. What I wish for is a cure for the common ill that makes people compare themselves to a normal that is measured in terms of perfect and absolute standards, most of which are impossible for anyone to reach (Holliday-Willey 1999: 96).

20.6 CONCLUSION

With the implementation and the strengthening of the Disability Discrimination Act 1995 in the UK, and the growing philosophy of working with patients and clients in partnership and collaboration, a move towards participatory and emancipatory research in physiotherapy is becoming urgent. Brothers et al (2002) believe that health professionals need to consult with disabled customers, disabled staff and disability organizations in order to prevent discrimination and to comply with the Act.

Disabled people are being empowered by the disabled people's movement. The question is: can research by physiotherapists be part of that empowerment?

References

Abad V, Boyce E 1979 Issues in psychiatric evaluations of Puerto Ricans: a sociocultural perspective. Journal of Operational Psychiatry 10:28–29

Abberley P 1992 Counting us out: a discussion of the OPCS disability surveys. Disability, Handicap and Society 7: 139–155

Abberley P 1996 Work, utopia and impairment. In: Barton L (ed) Disability and society: emerging issues and insights. Longman, London, pp 61–79

Abbott J, Dodd M, Gee L, Webb K 2001 Ways of coping with cystic fibrosis: implications for treatment adherence. Disability and Rehabilitation 23:315–324

Adams N 1997 The psychophysiology of low back pain. Churchill Livingstone, Edinburgh

Adams N, Sim J 1998 An overview of fibromyalgia syndrome: mechanisms, differential diagnosis and treatment approaches. Physiotherapy 84: 304–318

Adams N, Ravey J, Taylor D 1996 Psychological models of chronic pain and implications for practice. Physiotherapy 82:124–129

Adamson C 1997 Existential and clinical uncertainty in the medical encounter: an idiographic account of an illness trajectory defined by inflammatory bowel disease and avascular necrosis. Sociology of Health and Illness 19: 131–159

Adamson B J, Nordholm L A 1994 A comparison of Australian and Swedish physiotherapists' view of professional practice. Physiotherapy Theory and Practice 10:161–169

Ader R 1980 Psychosomatic and psychoimmunologic research. Psychosomatic Medicine 42:307–321

Admani K 1993a Special needs of elderly Muslims. In: Hopkins A, Bahl V (eds) Access to health care for people from black and ethnic minorities. Royal College of Physicians, London, pp 99–104

Admani K 1993b Black and ethnic minority doctors in the National Health Service. In: Hopkins A, Bahl V (eds) Access to health care for people from black and ethnic minorities. Royal College of Physicians, London, pp 195–198

Admi H 1996 Growing up with a chronic health condition: a model of an ordinary lifestyle. Qualitative Health Research 6:163–183

Affleck G, Tennen H, Pfeiffer C, Fifield J 1987 Appraisals of control and predictability in adapting to a chronic disease. Journal of Personality and Social Psychology 53: 273–279

Affleck G, Urrows S, Tennen H, Higgins P 1992 Daily coping with pain from rheumatoid arthritis. Pain 51:221–229

AGILE-Thames 2002 Elder rehabilitation: core learning objectives for physiotherapy students during clinical placements. Physiotherapy 88:158–166

Ahles T A, Yunus M B, Gaulier B, Riley S D, Masi A T 1986 The use of contemporary MMPI norms in the study of chronic pain patients. Pain 24:159–163

Ahmad W I U 1989 Policies, pills and political will: a critique of policies to improve the health status of ethnic minorities. Lancet 1:148–150

Ahmad W I U 1993 Race and health in contemporary Britain. Open University Press, Buckingham

Ahmad W I U 2000 Ethnicity, disability and chronic illness. Open University Press, Buckingham

Ahmad W I U, Atkin K, Chamba R 2000 Causing havoc among their children: parental and professional perspectives on consanguinity and childhood disability. In: Ahmad W I U (ed) Ethnicity, disability and chronic illness. Open University Press, Buckingham, pp 28–44

Ainsworth M D S 1964 Patterns of attachment behaviour shown by the infant in interaction with his mother. Merrill-Palmer Quarterly 10:51–58

Alcock C, Payne S, Sullivan M 2000 Introducing social policy. Prentice Hall, Harlow

Alderson P 1990 Choosing for children: parents' consent to surgery. Oxford University Press, Oxford

Alderson P 1993 Children's consent to surgery. Open University Press, Buckingham

Aldrich S, Eccleston C 2000 Making sense of everyday pain. Social Science and Medicine 50:1631–1641

Allen I, Bourke Dowling S, Williams S 1997 A leading role for midwives? Evaluation of midwifery group practice development projects. Policy Studies Institute, London

Allmark P 1995 Can there be an ethics of care? Journal of Medical Ethics 21:19–24

Alsop A 2000 Continuing professional development. Blackwell Science, Oxford

American Psychiatric Association 1994 Diagnostic and statistical manual of mental disorders, 4th edn, DSM-IV. American Psychiatric Association, Washington

Anderson T 1992 Reflections on reflecting with families. In: McNamee S, Gergen K J (eds) Therapy as social construction. Sage Publications, London, pp 54–69

Anderson H 1997 Conversation, language, and possibilities: a postmodern approach to therapy. Basic Books, New York

Andrasik F, Holroyd K A 1980 A test of specific and non-specific effects in the biofeedback treatment of tension headache. Journal of Consulting and Clinical Psychology 48:575–586

Andrews M M, Boyle J S 1995 Transcultural concepts in nursing care, 2nd edn. J B Lippincott, Philadelphia

Andrews J, Rolph S 2000 Scrub, scrub, scrub … Bad times and good times: some of the jobs I've had in my life. In: Atkinson D, McCarthy M, Walmsley J, Cooper M, Rolph S, Aspis S, Barette P, Coventry M, Ferris G (eds) Good times, bad times: women with learning difficulties telling their stories. British Institute of Learning Disabilities, Kidderminster, pp 35–42

Anionwu E, Atkin K 2001 The politics of sickle cell and thalassaemia. Open University Press, Buckingham

Annandale A 1998 The sociology of health and medicine: a critical introduction. Polity Press, Cambridge

Antonovsky A 1990 Pathways leading to successful coping and health. In: Rosenbaum M (ed) Learned resourcefulness: on coping skills, self-control and adaptive behavior. Springer, New York, pp 31–63

Antonovsky A 1993 The sense of coherence as a determinant of health. In: Beattie A, Gott M, Jones L J, Sidell M (eds) Health and wellbeing: a reader. Macmillan, Basingstoke, pp 202–211

Aristotle 1986 The Nicomachean ethics. Translated by D Ross. Oxford University Press, Oxford

Armstrong D 1994 An outline of sociology as applied to medicine, 4th edn. Butterworth-Heinemann, Oxford

Armstrong D 2002 Clinical autonomy, individual and collective: the problem of changing doctors' behaviour. Social Science and Medicine 55:1771–1777

Armstrong F, Barton L 1999 Disability, human rights and education. Open University Press, Buckingham

Arntz A, Schmidt J M A 1989 Perceived control and the experience of pain. In: Steptoe A, Appels A (eds) Stress, personal control and health. Wiley, Chichester, pp 131–162

Åsbring P 2001 Chronic illness – a disruption in life: identity-transformation among women with chronic fatigue syndrome and fibromyalgia. Journal of Advanced Nursing 34:312–319

Åsbring P, Närvänen A-L 2002 Women's experiences of stigma in relation to chronic fatigue syndrome and fibromyalgia. Qualitative Health Research 12:148–160

Astin J A, Beckner W, Soeken K, Hochberg M C, Berman B 2002 Psychological interventions for rheumatoid arthritis: a meta-analysis of randomized controlled trials. Arthritis and Rheumatism 47:291–302

Astington J W 1994 The child's discovery of the mind. Fontana, London

Astington J W, Harris P L, Olson D R 1988 Developing theories of the mind. Cambridge University Press, Cambridge

Atkin K 1996 Race and social policy. In: Lunt N, Coyle D (eds) Welfare and policy. Taylor and Francis, Basingstoke, pp 141–158

Atkin K 1998 Ageing in a multi-racial Britain: demography, policy and practice. In: Bernard M, Phillips J (eds) The social policy of old age: moving into the 21st century. Centre for Policy on Ageing, London, pp 163–181

Atkin K, Rollings J 1996 Looking after their own? Family caregiving in Asian and Afro-Caribbean communities. In: Ahmad W I U, Atkin K (eds) Race and community care. Open University Press, Buckingham, pp 73–86

Atkin K, Ahmad W I U, Anionwu E 1998 Screening and counselling for sickle cell disorders and thalassaemia: the experience of parents and health professionals. Social Science and Medicine 47:1639–1651

Atkin K, Ahmad W I U, Anionwu E 2000 Service support to families caring for a child with a sickle cell disorder or beta thalassaemia major: parents' perspectives. In: Ahmad W I U (ed) Ethnicity, disability and chronic illness. Open University Press, Buckingham, pp 103–122

Atkin K, Ahmad W I U, Jones L 2002 Being deaf and being other things: young Asian deaf people negotiating identities. Sociology of Health and Illness 24:21–45

Atkinson D 1997 An auto/biographical approach to learning disability research. Ashgate, Aldershot

Atkinson D 1999 An old story. In: Swain J, French S (eds) Therapy and learning difficulties: advocacy, participation and partnership. Butterworth-Heinemann, Oxford, pp 11–21

Atkinson D, McCarthy M, Walmsley J, Cooper M, Rolph S, Aspis S, Barette P, Coventry M, Ferris G 2000 (eds) Good times, bad times: women with learning difficulties telling their stories. British Institute of Learning Disabilities, Kidderminster

Audit Commission 1993 What seems to be the matter: communication between hospital and patients. National Health Service Report no. 12. HMSO, London

Ayres A J 1973 Sensory integration and learning disorders. Western Psychological Services, Los Angeles

Ayres A J 1978 Southern California sensory integration tests. Western Psychological Services, Los Angeles

Ayres A J 1989 Sensory integration and praxis test. Western Psychological Services, Los Angeles

Azmitia M, Hesser J 1993 Why siblings are important agents of cognitive development: a comparison of siblings and peers. Child Development 64:430–444

Bacon N M K, Bacon S F, Atkinson J H, Slater M A, Patterson T L, Grant I, Garfin D R 1994 Somatization symptoms in chronic low back pain patients. Psychosomatic Medicine 56:118–127

Bahl V 1993 Access to health care for black and ethnic minority elderly people: general principles. In: Hopkins A, Bahl V (eds) Access to health care for people from black and ethnic minorities. Royal College of Physicians, London, pp 93–97

Bailey D M, Schwartzberg S L 1995 Ethical and legal dilemmas in occupational therapy. W B Saunders, Philadelphia

Bailey K, Wilkinson S 1998 Patients' views on nurses' communication skills: a pilot study. International Journal of Palliative Nursing 4:300–305

Baistow K 1994 Liberation and regulation: some paradoxes of empowerment. Critical Social Policy 42:34–46

Bajekal M 2001 Use of health services and prescribed medicines in health survey for England, 1999. The health of minority ethnic groups. Department of Health, London. http://www.official-documents.co.uk/document/doh/survey99/hse99-11.htm

Balfour C 1993 Physiotherapists and smoking cessation. Physiotherapy 79:247–250

Bandura A 1977 Self-efficacy: toward a unifying theory of behavioral change. Psychological Review 84: 191–215

Bandura A, O'Leary A, Barr-Taylor C, Gauthier J, Gossard D 1987 Perceived self-efficacy and pain control: opioid and nonopioid mechanisms. Journal of Personality and Social Psychology 53:563–571

Bandura A, Cioffi D, Taylor C B, Brouillard H E 1988 Perceived self-efficacy in coping with cognitive stressors and opioid activation. Journal of Personality and Social Psychology 55:479–488

Banks S M, Kerns R D 1996 Explaining high rates of depression in chronic pain: a diathesis stress framework. Psychological Bulletin 199:95–110

Barclay J 1994 In good hands: the history of the Chartered Society of Physiotherapy, 1894–1994. Butterworth-Heinemann, Oxford

Barker R H 1958 Thomas Middleton. Greenwood Press, Westport

Barker P 1989 Reflections on the philosophy of caring in mental health. International Journal of Nursing Studies 26:131–141

Barlow J H, Cullen L A, Foster N E, Harrison K, Wade M 1999 Does arthritis influence perceived ability to fulfill a parenting role? Perceptions of mothers, fathers and grandparents. Patient Education and Counseling 37:141–151

Barnes C 1991 Disabled people in Britain and discrimination: a case for anti-discrimination legislation. Hurst Company, London

Barnes C 1992 Qualitative research: valuable or irrelevant? Disability and Society 7:115–124

Barnes C 2001 'Emancipatory' disability research: project or process? Public lecture for the Strathclyde Centre for Disability Research, University of Glasgow. www.le(eds).ac.uk/disability-studies/archiveuk/index

Barnes C 2003 What a difference a decade makes: reflections on doing 'emancipatory' disability research. Disability and Society 18:3–17

Barnes C, Mercer G (eds) 1996 Exploring the divide: illness and disability. Disability Press, Leeds

Barnes C, Mercer M, Shakespeare T 1999 Exploring disability: a sociological introduction. Polity Press, London

Barnes M, Bowl R 2001 Taking over the asylum: empowerment and mental health. Palgrave, Houndmills

Barnitt R 1998 Ethical dilemmas in occupational therapy and physical therapy: a survey of practitioners in the UK National Health Service. Journal of Medical Ethics 24:193–199

Barnitt R, Fulton C 1994 Patient agreement to treatment: a framework for therapists. British Journal of Therapy and Rehabilitation 1:121–127

Barnitt R, Partridge C 1997 Ethical reasoning in physical therapy and occupational therapy. Physiotherapy Research International 2:178–192

Barnitt R, Pomeroy V 1995 An holistic approach to rehabilitation. British Journal of Therapy and Rehabilitation 2:87–92

Baron-Cohen S, Swettenham J 1997 Theory of mind in autism: its relationship to executive function and central coherence. In: Cohen D J, Volkmar F R (eds) Handbook of autism and pervasive developmental disorders, 2nd edn. John Wiley, New York, pp 880–893

Baron-Cohen S, Tager-Flusberg H, Cohen D J 1993 Understanding other minds: perspectives from autism. Oxford University Press, Oxford

Barr H 2002 Interprofessional education today, yesterday and tomorrow: a review. UK Centre for Advancement of Interprofessional Education, London

Barton L 1998 Developing an emancipatory research agenda: possibilities and dilemmas. In: Clough P, Barton L (eds) Articulating with difficulty: research voices in inclusive education. Paul Chapman, London, pp 29–39

Barton L 2001 Disability politics and the struggle for change. David Fulton Publishers, London

Barton L, Tomlinson S 1984 Special education and social interests. Croom Helm, London

Bartrop R W, Luckhurst E, Lazarus L, Kiloh L G, Penny R 1977 Depressed lymphocyte function after bereavement. Lancet 1:834–836

Basnett I 2001 Health care professionals and their attitudes towards decisions affecting disabled people. In: Albrecht G L, Seelman K D, Bury M (eds) Handbook of disability studies. Sage Publications, London, pp 450–467

Baszanger I 1989 Pain: its experience and treatments. Social Science and Medicine 29:425–434

Baszanger I 1997 Deciphering chronic pain. In: Strauss A, Corbin J (eds) Grounded theory in practice. Sage Publications, Thousand Oaks, pp 1–34

Bates M, Rankin-Hill L, Sanchez-Ayendez M 1997 The effects of the cultural context of health care on treatment of and response to chronic pain. Social Science and Medicine 45:1433–1448

Baumann A O, Deber R B, Silverman B E, Mallette C M 1998 Who cares? Who cures? The ongoing debate in the provision of health care. Journal of Advanced Nursing 28:1040–1045

Baxter C 1988 The black nurse: an endangered species. National Extension College for Training in Health and Race, London

Baxter C, Poonia K, Ward L, Nadirshaw Z 1990 Double discrimination: issues and services for people with learning difficulties from black and ethnic minority communities. King's Fund Centre/Commission for Racial Equality, London

Bayley N 1969 Manual for the Bayley scales of infant development. Psychological Corporation, New York

BBC 1998 Rising life expectancy strains health budgets. BBC News Online: Health [accessed 27.05.01]. http://news1.thdo.bbc.co.uk/low/english/health/newsid_221000/221694.stm

Beard R 1969 An outline of Piaget's developmental psychology. Routledge and Kegan Paul, London

Beattie A 1993 The changing boundaries of health. In: Beattie A, Gott M, Jones L, Sidell M (eds) Health and wellbeing: a reader. Macmillan, London, pp 260–271

Beattie A, Gott M, Jones L, Sidell M 1993 Health and wellbeing: a reader. Macmillan, London

Beauchamp T L, Childress J F 1994 Principles of biomedical ethics, 4th edn. Oxford University Press, New York

Beauchamp T L, Childress J F 2001 Principles of biomedical ethics, 5th edn. Oxford University Press, New York

Becher T 1996 The learning professions. Studies in Higher Education 21:43–55

Beck A T, Ward C H, Mendelson M, Mock J, Erbaugh J 1961 An inventory for measuring depression. Archives of General Psychiatry 4:561–571

Beck A T, Kovacs M, Weissman A 1979 Assessment of suicidal intention: the scale for suicide ideation. Journal of Consulting and Clinical Psychology 47:343–352

Beck A T, Steer R A, Kovacs M, Garrison B 1985 Hopelessness and eventual suicide: a 10-year prospective study of patients hospitalized with suicidal ideation. American Journal of Psychiatry 142:559–563

Bedford S 1993 The developing child. In: Eckersley P M (ed) Elements of paediatric physiotherapy. Churchill Livingstone, Edinburgh, pp 35–60

Beevers G, Beevers M 1993 Hypertension: impact upon black and minority ethnic people. In: Hopkins A, Bahl V (eds) Access to health care for people from black and ethnic minorities. Royal College of Physicians, London, pp 123–130

Belsky J 1986 Infant day care: a cause for concern? Zero to Three 6:1–9

Belsky J 2001 Emanuel Miller lecture. Developmental risks still associated with early child care. Journal of Child Psychology and Psychiatry 42:845–859

Bendelow G 1993 Pain perceptions, emotions and gender. Sociology of Health and Illness 15:273–294

Bendelow G A, Williams S J 1995 Transcending the dualisms: towards a sociology of pain. Sociology of Health and Illness 17:139–165

Bendelow G A, Williams S J 1996 The end of the road? Lay views on a pain-relief clinic. Social Science and Medicine 43:1127–1136

Benjamin M, Curtis J 1986 Ethics in nursing, 2nd edn. Oxford University Press, New York

Bennett P 1993 Counselling for heart disease. British Psychological Society, Leicester

Bennett R M, Campbell S, Burckhardt C 1991 A multidiciplinary approach to fibromyalgia management. Journal of Musculoskeletal Medicine 8:21–32

Bennett P, Mayfield T, Norman P, Lowe R, Morgan M 1999 Affective and social-cognitive predictors of behavioural change following first myocardial infarction. British Journal of Health Psychology 4:247–256

Benzeval M, Judge K, Whitehead M 1995 Tackling inequalities in health: an agenda for action. King's Fund, London

Beresford P, Croft S 1995 It's our problem too! Challenging the exclusion of poor people from poverty discourse. Critical Social Policy 44/45:75–95

Bernstein D A, Borkovec T D 1973 Progressive relaxation training: a manual for the helping professions. Research Press, Champaign

Bernstein D A, Given B A 1984 Progressive relaxation: abbreviated methods. In: Woolfolk R L, Lehrer P M (eds) Principles and practice of stress management. Guilford Press, New York, pp 43–69

Bevan S, Buchan J, Heyday S 1989 Women in hospital pharmacy. Institute of Manpower Studies, University of Sussex, Brighton

Beveridge Report 1942 Social insurance and allied services. Cmd. 6404. HMSO, London

Bewley B, Bewley T H 1975 Hospital doctors' career structure and misuse of medical womanpower. Lancet 2:270–272

Bhakta P, Katbamna S, Parker G 2000 South Asian carers' experiences of primary care teams. In: Ahmad W I U (ed) Ethnicity, disability and chronic illness. Open University Press, Buckingham, pp 123–139

Bhopal R S, White M 1993 Health promotion for ethnic minorities: past, present and future. In: Ahmad W I U (ed) 'Race' and health in contemporary Britain. Open University Press, Buckingham, pp 137–166

Bimrose J 1998 Increasing multicultural competence. In: Bayne R, Nicolson P, Horton I (eds) Counselling and communication skills for medical and health practitioners. British Psychological Society, Leicester, pp 88–102

Birren J E 1959 Handbook of aging and the individual: psychological and biological aspects. University of Chicago Press, Chicago

Blaikie A 1999 Ageing and popular culture. Cambridge University Press, Cambridge

Blanche E I 1996 Alma: coping with culture, poverty, and disability. American Journal of Occupational Therapy 50:265–276

Blaxter M 1985 Self definition of health status and consulting rates in primary care. Quarterly Journal of Social Affairs 1:131–171

Blumer D, Heilbronn M 1982 Chronic pain as a variant of depressive disease. Journal of Nervous and Mental Disease 170:381–414

Blumer D, Heilbronn M 1984 'Chronic pain as a variant of depressive disease' – a rejoinder. Journal of Nervous and Mental Disease 172:405–407

Boden M A 1985 Piaget. Fontana, London

Bok S 1978 Lying: moral choice in public and private life. Harvester Press, Hassocks

Bond J, Bond S 1994 Sociology and health care: an introduction for nurses and other health care professionals, 2nd edn. Churchill Livingstone, Edinburgh

Bornstein M H, Tamis-LeMonda C S, Tal J, Ludemann P, Toda S, Rahn C W, Pêcheux M G, Azuma H, Vardi D 1992 Maternal responsiveness to infants in three societies: the United States, France, and Japan. Child Development 63:808–821

Bottery M 1998 Professionals and policy: management strategy in a competitive world. Cassell, London

Bowlby J 1971 Attachment and loss. Vol. 1: Attachment. Penguin, Harmondsworth

Bowlby J 1980 Attachment and loss. Vol. 3: Loss, sadness and depression. Hogarth Press, London

Bowlby J 1982 Attachment and loss: retrospect and prospect. American Journal of Orthopsychiatry 52:664–678

Bradshaw A 1996 Yes! There is an ethics of care: an answer for Peter Allmark. Journal of Medical Ethics 22:8–12

Braye S 2000 Participation and involvement in social care: an overview. In: Kemshall H, Littlechild R (eds) User involvement and participation in social care. Jessica Kingsley, London, pp 9–28

Braye S, Preston-Shoot M 1995 Empowering practice in social care. Open University Press, Buckingham

Brechin A 1993 Sharing. In: Shakespeare P, Atkinson D, French S (eds) Reflections on research in practice. Open University Press, Buckingham, pp 70–82

Brechin A, Liddiard P, Swain J 1988 Handicap in a social world. Hodder and Stoughton, Sevenoaks

British Medical Journal 1976 Women in medicine (editorial). British Medical Journal 1:56

British Medical Journal 1977 One hundred years ago (taken from British Medical Journal 1877). British Medical Journal 2:1149

Britten N 2000 Qualitative interviews in health care research. In: Pope C, Mays N (eds) Qualitative research in health care, 2nd edn. B M J Books, London, pp 11–19

Brothers M, Scullion P, Eathorne V 2002 Rights of access to services for disabled people. British Journal of Therapy and Rehabilitation 9:232–236

Brown G, Nicassio P, Wallston K 1989a Pain coping strategies and depression in rheumatoid arthritis. Journal of Clinical and Consulting Psychology 57:652–657

Brown G, Wallston K, Nicassio P 1989b Social support and depression in rheumatoid arthritis: a one-year prospective study. Journal of Applied Social Psychology 19:1164–1181

Bruininks R H 1978 Bruininks–Oseretsky test of motor proficiency: examiner's manual. American Guidance Services, Circle Pines

Bruner J S 1975 The ontogenesis of speech acts. Journal of Child Language 2:1–19

Bruner J 1995 Meaning and self in cultural perspective. In: Bakhurst D, Sypnowich C (eds) The social self. Sage Publications, London, pp 18–29

Bruner J S, Jolly A, Sylva K 1976 Play – its role in development and evolution. Penguin, Harmondsworth

Buchan J 2000 Workforce planning: pressure is on. Health Service Journal 11(Dec 7):26–27

Buchan J, Pike G 1989 PAMS into the 1990s – professions allied to medicine: the wider labour market context. IMS Report no. 175. Institute of Manpower Studies, University of Sussex, Brighton

Buchanan A 1981 Medical paternalism. In: Cohen M, Nagel T, Scanlon T (eds) Medicine and moral philosophy. Princeton University Press, Princeton, pp 214–234

Buchanan A E, Brock D W 1989 Deciding for others: the ethics of surrogate decision making. Cambridge University Press, Cambridge

Burchardt T 2000 Enduring economic exclusion: disabled people, income and work. Joseph Rowntree Foundation, York

Burish T G, Carey M P, Wallston K A, Stein M J, Jamison R N, Naramore Lyles J 1984 Health locus of control and chronic disease: an external orientation may be advantageous. Journal of Social and Clinical Psychology 2:326–332

Burkitt A 1986 Health, health education and the physiotherapist. Physiotherapy 72:2–4

Burnard P 1992 Effective communication skills for health professionals. Chapman and Hall, London

Burnard P 1999 Counselling skills for health professionals. Stanley Thornes, Cheltenham

Burr V 1995 An introduction to social constructionism. Routledge, London

Burrage M 1990 Introduction: the professions in sociology and history. In: Burrage M, Torstendahl R (eds) Professions in theory and history. Sage Publications, London, pp 1–23

Burton A K, Tillotson K M, Main C J, Hollis S 1995 Psychosocial predictors of outcome in acute and subchronic low back trouble. Spine 20:722–728

Bury M 1982 Chronic illness as biographical disruption. Sociology of Health and Illness 4:167–182

Bury M 1997 Health and illness in a changing society. Routledge, London

Butler R N, Lewis M I 1973 Ageing and mental health. C V Mosby, St Louis

Butt J 1994 Same service or equal service. HMSO, London

Butt J, Mirza K 1996 Social care and black communities. HMSO, London

Byrne A, Morton J, Salmon P 2001 Defending against patients' pain: a qualitative analysis of nurses' responses to children's postoperative pain. Journal of Psychosomatic Research 50:69–76

Bytheway B 1995 Ageism. Open University Press, Buckingham

Cain 1998 The limits of confidentiality. Nursing Ethics 5:158–165

California Supreme Court 1994 Tarosoff *v.* Regents of the University of California. In: Beauchamp T L, Walters L (eds) Contemporary issues in bioethics, 4th edn. Wadsworth, Belmont, pp 174–178

Callahan J C 1988 Basics and background. In: Callahan J C (ed) Ethical issues in professional life. Oxford University Press, New York, pp 3–25

Calvillo E R, Flaskerud J H 1993 Evaluation of the pain response by Mexican American and Anglo American women and their nurses. Journal of Advanced Nursing 18:451–459

Cameron E, Badger F, Evers H, Atkin K 1989 Black old women and health carers. In: Jefferys M (ed) Growing old in the twentieth century. Routledge, London, pp 230–248

Campbell K 1970 Body and mind. Macmillan, London

Campbell J, Oliver M 1996 Disability politics: Understanding our past, changing our future. Routledge, London

Campling J 1981 Images of ourselves: women with disabilities talking. Routledge and Kegan Paul, London

Capilouto G J 2000 Rehabilitation settings. In: Kumar S (ed) Multidisciplinary approach to rehabilitation. Butterworth-Heinemann, Boston, pp 1–27

Caplan A L 1988 Informed consent and provider–patient relationships in rehabilitation medicine. Archives of Physical Medicine and Rehabilitation 69:312–317

Caplan G 1990 Stress and mental health. Community Mental Health Journal 26:27–48

Cardol M, De Jong B A, Ward C D 2002 On autonomy and participation in rehabilitation. Disability and Rehabilitation 24:970–974

Carey M P, Burish T G 1987 Providing relaxation training to cancer chemotherapy patients: a comparison of three methods. Journal of Consulting and Clinical Psychology 55:732–737

Carnelley K B, Wortman C B, Kessler R C 1999 The impact of widowhood on depression: findings from a prospective study. Psychological Medicine 29:1111–1123

Carson M G, Mitchell G J 1998 The experience of living with persistent pain. Journal of Advanced Nursing 28: 1242–1248

Carver V, Liddiard P 1978 An ageing population. Hodder and Stoughton, Sevenoaks

Carver C S, Scheier M F, Weintraub J K 1989 Assessing coping strategies: a theoretically based approach. Journal of Personality and Social Psychology 56:267–283

Cashmore E, Tronya B 1990 Introduction to race relations. Falmer Press, Brighton

Cassell E J 1978 The healer's art: a new approach to the doctor–patient relationship. Penguin, Harmondsworth

Cassell E J 1985 Talking with patients. Vol. 2: Clinical techniques. MIT Press, Cambridge

Cattell P 1940 The measurement of intelligence of infants and young children. Psychological Corporation, New York

Chalmers J, Muir R 2003 Patient privacy and confidentiality. British Medical Journal 326:725

Chamba R, Ahmad W I U, Hirst M, Lawton D, Beresford B 1999 On the edge: a national survey of minority ethnic parents caring for a severely disabled child. Policy Press, Bristol

Chambers R 1986 Normal professionalism, new paradigms and developments. Institute of Development Studies Discussion Paper no. 227. University of Sussex, Brighton

Chambers R 1997 Whose reality counts: putting the first last. Intermediate Technology Publications, London

Chang J T, Szczyglinski J A, King S A 2000 A case of malingering: feigning a painful disorder in the presence of true medical illness. Pain Medicine 1:280–282

Chaplin J 1999 Feminist counselling in action, 2nd edn. Sage Publications, London

Chapman C R 1995 The affective dimension of pain: a model. In: Bromm B, Desmedt J E (eds) Advances in pain research and therapy. Vol. 2: Pain and the brain: from nociception to cognition. Raven Press, New York, pp 283–302

Chapman C R, Turner J A 1986 Psychological control of acute pain in medical settings. Journal of Pain and Symptom Management 1:9–20

Charmaz K 1991 Good days, bad days: the self in chronic illness and time. Rutgers University Press, New Brunswick

Charmaz K 1994 Identity dilemmas of chronically ill men. Sociological Quarterly 35:269–288

Charmaz K 1999a From the 'sick role' to stories of self: understanding the self in illness. In: Contrada R, Ashmore R (eds) Self, social identity and physical health. Oxford University Press, Oxford, pp 209–239

Charmaz K 1999b Stories of suffering: subjective tales and research narratives. Qualitative Health Research 9:362–382

Chartered Society of Physiotherapy 1979a The Chartered Society's policy on degree courses. Physiotherapy 65:353–354

Chartered Society of Physiotherapy 1979b Reply of the Chartered Society of Physiotherapy to the DHSS draft document on the planning for graduates in the remedial professions in Great Britain. Chartered Society of Physiotherapy, London

Chartered Society of Physiotherapy 1984 How to become a chartered physiotherapist. Chartered Society of Physiotherapy, London

Chartered Society of Physiotherapy 1988 Health education workshop: a venture in collaboration. Physiotherapy 74:602–606

Chartered Society of Physiotherapy 2000 The CPD process. Information Paper no. 30. Chartered Society of Physiotherapy, London

Chartered Society of Physiotherapy 2002a Curriculum framework for qualifying programmes in physiotherapy. Chartered Society of Physiotherapy, London

Chartered Society of Physiotherapy 2002b Rules of professional conduct, 2nd edn. Chartered Society of Physiotherapy, London

Chaudbury A 1990 Problems for parents – experiences of Tower Hamlets. In: Orton C (ed) Asian children and special needs: a report for ACE. Advisory Centre for Education, London, pp 9–10

Chaves J F, Brown J M 1987 Spontaneous coping strategies for pain. Journal of Behavioral Medicine 10:263–276

Cherkin D C, Deyo R A, Street J H, Barlow W 1996 Predicting poor outcome for back pain seen in primary care using patients' own criteria. Spine 21:2900–2907

Cherry C 1957 On human communication. MIT Press, Cambridge

Childress J F 1982 Who should decide? Paternalism in health care. Oxford University Press, New York

Chomsky N 1959 Review of verbal behaviour by B F Skinner. Language 35:26–58

Chomsky N 1965 Aspects of theory of syntax. MIT Press, Cambridge

Ciccone D S, Grzesiak R C 1984 Cognitive dimensions of chronic pain. Social Science and Medicine 19:1339–1345

Cioni G, Paolicelli P B, Sorti C, Vinter A 1993 Sensori-motor development in cerebral-palsied infants assessed with the Uzgiris–Hunt scales. Developmental Medicine and Child Neurology 35:1055–1066

Clampitt P G 1990 Communicating for managerial effectiveness. Sage Publications, Newbury Park

Clapton J, Kendall E 2002 Autonomy and participation in rehabilitation: time for a new paradigm? Disability and Rehabilitation 24:987–991

Clare A 2000 On men: masculinity in crisis. Chatto and Windus, London

Clarke B M 2000 The impact of suffering in physiotherapy practice: cost containment issues. Physiotherapy Canada 52:25–32

Clarke A D B, Clarke A M 1974 The changing concept of intelligence: a selective historical review. In: Clarke A D B, Clarke A M (eds) Mental deficiency: the changing outlook, 2nd edn. Methuen, London, pp 143–163

Clarke J, Cochrane A 1998 The social construction of social problems. In: Saraga E (ed) Embodying the social: constructions of difference. Routledge, London, pp 3–42

Clarke-Stewart K 1989 Infant day care: maligned or malignant? American Psychologist 44:266–273

Closs A 1998 Quality of life of children and young people with serious medical conditions. In: Robinson C, Stalker K (eds) Growing up with disability. Jessica Kingsley, London, pp 111–127

Closs S J, Briggs M 2002 Patients' verbal descriptions of pain and discomfort following orthopaedic surgery. International Journal of Nursing Studies 39:563–572

Clouder D L 2000a Reflective practice in physiotherapy education: a critical conversation. Studies in Higher Education 25:211–223

Clouder D L 2000b Reflective practice: realising its potential. Physiotherapy 86:517–522

Coates R 1990 Ethics and physiotherapy. Australian Journal of Physiotherapy 36:84–87

Coburn D, Willis E 2000 The medical profession: knowledge, power, and autonomy. In: Albrecht G L, Fitzpatrick R, Scrimshaw S C (eds) Handbook of social studies in health and medicine. Sage Publications, London, pp 377–393

Cohen S, Rodriguez M S 1995 Pathways linking affective disturbances and physical disorders. Health Psychology 14:374–380

Cole T R, Winkler M G 1994 The Oxford book of ageing: reflections on the journey of life. Oxford University Press, Oxford

Collier J 1989 The health conspiracy. Century Hutchinson, London

Collins G A, Cohen M J, Naliboff B D, Schandler S L 1982 Comparative analysis of paraspinal and frontalis EMG, heart rate and skin conductance in chronic low back pain patients and normals to various postures and stresses. Scandinavian Journal of Rehabilitation Medicine 14:39–46

Commission for Racial Equality 1988 Racial equality in social service departments. Commission for Racial Equality, London

Condie E 1991 A therapeutic approach to physical disability. Physiotherapy 77:72–77

Confederation of Indian Organisations 1987 Double bind: to be disabled and Asian. Confederation of Indian Organisations, London

Cooper L 1997 Myalgic encephalomyelitis and the medical encounter. Sociology of Health and Illness 19:186–207

Cooper M C 1991 Principle-oriented ethics and the ethic of care: a creative tension. Advances in Nursing Science 14:22–31

Cooper M, Rowan J 1999 Introduction: self-plurality – the one and the many. In: Rowan J, Cooper M (eds) The plural self: multiplicity in everyday life. Sage Publications, London, pp 1–9

Copp G 1998 A review of current theories of death and dying. Journal of Advanced Nursing 28:382–390

Corbett J 1996 Bad-mouthing: the language of special needs. Falmer Press, London

Corey M S, Corey G 1987 Groups: process and practice, 3rd edn. Brooks/Cole, Monterey

Corey M S, Corey G 1993 Becoming a helper, 2nd edn. Brooks/Cole, Pacific Grove

Corker M 1994 Counselling – the deaf challenge. Jessica Kingsley, London

Corker M 1996 Deaf transitions: images and origins of deaf families, deaf communities and deaf identities. Jessica Kingsley, London

Cornwell A, Jewkes R 1995 What is participatory research? Social Science and Medicine 41:1667–1676

Corr C A, Corr D M 1986 Developing a philosophy for caring. In: Downie P A (ed) Cash's textbook of neurology for physiotherapists, 4th edn. Faber and Faber, London, pp 21–32

Costa P T Jr, McCrae R R 1985 Hypochondriasis, neuroticism, and aging. When are somatic complaints unfounded? American Psychologist 40:19–28

Council J R, Ahern D K, Follick M J, Kline C L 1988 Expectancies and functional impairment in chronic low back pain. Pain 33:323–331

Coutts L C, Hardy L K 1985 Teaching for health: the nurse as health educator. Churchill Livingstone, Edinburgh

Coy J A 1989 Autonomy-based informed consent: ethical implications for patient noncompliance. Physical Therapy 69:826–833

Craig K D 1999 Emotions and psychobiology. In: Wall P D, Melzack R (eds) Textbook of pain, 4th edn. Churchill Livingstone, Edinburgh, pp 331–343

Craig K D, Hill M L, McMurtry B 1999 Detecting deception and malingering. In: Block A R, Kremer E F, Fernandez E (eds) Handbook of chronic pain syndromes. Lawrence Erlbaum, Hillsdale, pp 41–58

Cratty B J 1974 Motor activity and the education of retardates. Lea and Febiger, Philadelphia

Crisson J E, Keefe F J 1988 The relationship of locus of control to pain coping strategies and psychological distress in chronic pain patients. Pain 35:147–154

Crombez G, Eccleston C, Baeyens F, Eelen P 1998a When somatic information threatens, catastrophic thinking enhances attentional interference. Pain 75:187–198

Crombez G, Vervaet L, Lysens R, Baeyens F, Eelen P 1998b Avoidance and confrontation of painful, back-straining movements in chronic back pain patients. Behavior Modification 22:62–77

Crombez G, Eccleston C, Baeyens F, Eelen P 1998c Attentional disruption is enhanced by the threat of pain. Behaviour Research and Therapy 36:195–204

Crombez G, Vlaeyen J W S, Heuts P H T G, Lysens R 1999 Fear of pain is more disabling than pain itself. Evidence of the role of pain-related fear in chronic back pain disability. Pain 80:329–340

Crombez G, Hermans D, Adriaensen H 2000 The emotional Stroop task and chronic pain: what is threatening for chronic pain sufferers? European Journal of Pain 4:37–44

Cross S, Sim J 2000 Confidentiality within physiotherapy: perceptions and attitudes of clinical practitioners. Journal of Medical Ethics 26:447–453

Crossley M L 2000 Introducing narrative psychology: self, trauma and the construction of meaning. Open University Press, Buckingham

Crow L 1996 Including all of our lives: renewing the social model of disability. In: Morris J (ed) Encounters with strangers: feminism and disability. Women's Press, London, pp 206–226

Cruickshank W M 1967 The brain-injured child in home, school and community. Syracuse University Press, New York

Culley L 1996 A critique of multiculturalism in health care: the challenge for nurse education. Journal of Advanced Nursing 23:564–570

Cunningham C, Davis H 1985 Working with parents: frameworks for collaboration. Open University Press, Milton Keynes

Cunningham A J, Lockwood G A, Cunningham J A 1981 A relationship between perceived self-efficacy and quality of life in cancer patients. Patient Education and Counselling 17:71–78

Currer C, Stacey M 1986 Concepts of health, illness and disease: a comparative perspective. Berg, Leamington Spa

Currier D P 1984 Elements of research in physical therapy, 2nd edn. Williams and Wilkins, Baltimore

Dahlgren G, Whitehead M 1991 Policies and strategies to promote social equity in health. Institute for Future Studies, Stockholm

Dallos R 1997 Interacting stories: narratives, family beliefs and therapy. Karnac Books, London

Dalrymple J, Burke B 1995 Anti-oppressive practice: social care and the law. Open University Press, Buckingham

Dalton P 1994 Counselling people with communication problems. Sage Publications, London

Daniels H 1993 Charting the agenda: educational activity after Vygotsky. Routledge, London

Daniels H 1996 An introduction to Vygotsky. Routledge, London

Danton W G, May J R, Lynn E J 1984 Psychological and physiological effects of relaxation and nitrous oxide training. Psychological Reports 55:311–322

Darr A 1997 Consanguineous marriage and genetics: a model for genetic health service delivery. In: Clarke A, Parson E (eds) Culture, kinship and genes. Macmillan, London, pp 83–96

Darr A, Bharj K 1999 Addressing cultural diversity in health care: the challenge facing nursing. In: Atkin K, Thompson C, Lunt N (eds) Evaluating community nursing. Baillière Tindall, London, pp 23–44

Das J P, Gindis B 1995 Lev Vygotsky and contemporary educational psychology. Lawrence Erlbaum Associates, Hillsdale

Dauphinee D, Norcini J 1999 Assessing health care professions in the new millennium. Advances in Health Science Education 4:3–7

Davey B 1999 Solving economic, social and environmental problems together: an empowerment strategy for losers. In: Barnes M, Warren L (eds) Alliances and partnerships in empowerment. Polity Press, Bristol, pp 37–51

Davey B 2001 Health in transition. In: Davey B (ed) Birth to old age: health in transition. Open University, Buckingham, pp 273–283

Davey B, Gray A, Seale C 1995 Health and disease: a reader, 2nd edn. Open University Press, Buckingham

Davidhizar R, Giger J 1998 Patients' use of denial: coping with the unacceptable. Nursing Standard 12:44–46

Davis K 1993a The crafting of good clients. In: Swain J, Finkelstein V, French S, Oliver M (eds) Disabling barriers – enabling environments. Sage Publications, London, pp 197–200

Davis K 1993b On the movement. In: Swain J, Finkelstein V, French S, Oliver M (eds) Disabling barriers – enabling environments. Sage Publications, London, pp 285–292

Dawson C 2000 Independent successes: implementing direct payments. Joseph Rowntree Foundation, York

Day A 1991 Remarkable survivors: insights into successful aging among women. Urban Institute, Washington

de Koning K, Martin M 1996 Participatory research in health: setting the context. In: de Koning K, Martin M (eds) Participatory research in health: issues and experiences. Zed Books, London, pp 1–18

De Souza L H, Frank A O 2002 Subjective pain experience of people with chronic back pain. Physiotherapy Research International 5:207–219

Deci E L 1980 The psychology of self determination. Lexington Books, Lexington

DeMayo R A 1997 Patient sexual behaviour and sexual harassment: a national survey of physical therapists. Physical Therapy 77:739–744

Dennett D C 1981 Brainstorms: philosophical essays on mind and psychology. Harvester Press, Brighton

Department of Health 1991 The health of the nation: a consultative document for health in England. HMSO, London

Department of Health 1995 Variations in health, what can the Department of Health and the NHS do? Report of the Variations Sub-Group of the Chief Medical Officer's Health of the Nation Working Group. HMSO, London

Department of Health 1997 The new NHS: modern – dependable. HMSO, London

Department of Health 1998a Independent inquiry into inequalities in health (Acheson Report). HMSO, London

Department of Health 1998b A first class service – quality in the new NHS. HMSO, London

Department of Health 1999 Saving lives: our healthier nation. HMSO, London

Department of Health 2000a The NHS plan – a plan for investment, a plan for reform. HMSO, London

Department of Health 2000b Meeting the challenge. Department of Health, London

Department of Health 2001a National service framework for older people: modern standards and service models. Department of Health, London

Department of Health 2001b National survey of NHS patients in general practice 1988. Department of Health, London, http://www.doh.gov.uk/public/nhssurveyrs.htm

Department of Health 2001c The national health inequalities targets. Department of Health, London [accessed 14.05.01]. http://www.doh.gov.uk/healthinequalities

Department of Health 2001d Public health. Department of Health, London [accessed 23.05.01]. http://www.doh.gov.uk/HPSSS/TBL_A1.HTM and http://www.doh.gov.uk/HPSSS/TBL_A2.HTM

Department of Health 2002 Tackling health inequalities – summary of the 2002 Cross–Cutting review. Department of Health, London

Department of Health and Social Security 1980 Inequalities in health, report of a working group (Black Report). Department of Health and Social Security, London

DePoy E, Gitlin L N 1998 Introduction to research: understanding and applying multiple strategies, 2nd edn. Mosby, St Louis

Derber C, Magrass Y 2001 Attention for sale: the hidden privileges of class. In: Branaman A (ed) Self and society. Blackwell, Malen, pp 321–332

Derogatis L R 1983 The SCL–90–R manual II. Administration, scoring and procedures manual. Johns Hopkins University Press, Baltimore

Derryberry D, Tucker D M 1992 Neural mechanisms of emotion. Journal of Consulting and Clinical Psychology 60:329–338

Descartes R 1985 The philosophical writings of Descartes, vol. 1. Translated by J Cottingham, R Stoothoff, D Murdoch. Cambridge University Press, Cambridge

Descartes R 1989 Selected philosophical writings. Translated by J Cottingham, R Stoothoff, D Murdoch. Cambridge University Press, Cambridge

DeVellis B M 1993 Depression in rheumatological diseases. Baillière's Clinical Rheumatology 7:241–258

Diamond J 1999 C: Because cowards get cancer too. Vermilion, London

Dimmock A F 1993 Cruel legacy: an introduction to the record of deaf people in history. Scottish Workshop Publications, Edinburgh

Dionne C, Koepsell T D, Von Korff M, Deyo R A, Barlow W I, Checkoway H 1995 Formal education and back-related disability: in search of an explanation. Spine 20: 2721–2730

Dolce J J, Crocker M F, Moletteire C, Doleys D M 1986a Exercise quotas, anticipatory concern and self-efficacy expectancies in chronic pain: a preliminary report. Pain 24:365–372

Dolce J J, Doleys D M, Raczynski J M, Lossie J, Poole L, Smith M 1986b The role of self-efficacy expectancies in the prediction of pain tolerance. Pain 27:261–272

Domholdt E 2000 Physical therapy research: principles and applications, 2nd edn. W B Saunders, Philadelphia

Donaldson M 1978 Children's minds. Fontana, London

Donati S, Ward C 1999 Contexts for working in partnership. In: Swain J, French S (eds) Therapy and learning difficulties: advocacy, participation and partnership. Butterworth-Heinemann, Oxford, pp 244–254

Donovan J L, Blake D R 2000 Qualitative study of interpretation of reassurance among patients attending rheumatology clinics: 'Just a touch of arthritis, doctor?' British Medical Journal 320:541–544

Dowling S, Martin R, Doyal L, Cameron A, Lloyd S 1996 Nurses taking on juniors doctors' work: a confusion of accountability. British Medical Journal 312:1211–1214

Downie R S 1980 Ethics, morals and moral philosophy. Journal of Medical Ethics 6:33–34

Downie R S 1988 Health promotion and health education. Journal of Philosophy of Education 22:3–11

Downie R S, Telfer E 1969 Respect for persons. George Allen and Unwin, London

Downie R S, Telfer E 1980 Caring and curing: a philosophy of medicine and social work. Methuen, London

Dowswell T, Hewison J, Millar B 1997 Joining the learning society and working in the NHS: some issues. Journal of Educational Policy 12:539–550

Doyal L 1991 The political economy of health. Pluto Press, London

Drake R F 1996 A critique of the role of the traditional charities. In: Barton L (ed) Disability and society: emerging issues and insights. Longman, London, pp 147–166

Drewery W, Winslade J 1997 The theoretical story of narrative therapy. In: Monk G, Winslade J, Crocket K, Epston D (eds) Narrative therapy in practice: the archaeology of hope. Jossey-Bass, San Francisco, pp 32–52

Drummond A E R, Walker M F 1995 A randomised controlled trial of leisure rehabilitation after stroke. Clinical Rehabilitation 9:283–290

Duncan G 2000 Mind–body dualism and the biopsychosocial model of pain: what did Descartes really say? Journal of Medicine and Philosophy 25:485–513

Dunn L M, Dunn L M, Whetton C, Pintilie D 1982 British picture vocabulary scale. NFER-Nelson, Windsor

Dunst C J 1980 A clinical and educational manual for use with the Uzgiris and Hunt scales of infant psychological development. University Park Press, Baltimore

Dworkin G 1972 Paternalism. Monist 56:64–84

Dyer A R 1985 Ethics, advertising and the definition of a profession. Journal of Medical Ethics 11:72–78

Dyer C 1996 Gynaecologist acquitted in hysterectomy case. British Medical Journal 312:11–12

Earll L, Johnston M, Mitchell E 1993 Coping with motor neurone disease: an analysis using self-regulation theory. Palliative Medicine 7(Suppl. 2):21–30

Eccleston C, Crombez G, Aldrich S, Stannard C 1997 Attention and somatic awareness in chronic pain. Pain 72:209–215

Eckersley P M 1993 Elements of paediatric physiotherapy. Churchill Livingstone, Edinburgh

Edelmann R J 1992 Anxiety: theory, research and intervention in clinical and health psychology. Wiley, New York

Edmonds B 1988 The certificate of health education: a personal perspective. Physiotherapy Practice 4:26–29

Edwards L, Pearce S, Collett B-J, Pugh R 1992 Selective memory for sensory and affective information in chronic pain and depression. British Journal of Clinical Psychology 31:239–248

Egan G 1990 The skilled helper: a systematic approach to effective helping, 4th edn. Brooks/Cole, Monterey

Eisenbruch M 1990 The cultural bereavement interview: a new clinical research approach for refugees. Psychiatric Clinics of North America 13:715–735

Elder G H Jr, Caspi A 1990 Studying lives in a changing society: sociological and personological exploration. In: Rabin A I (ed) Studying persons and lives: the Henry A Murray lectures in personality. Springer, New York, pp 201–247

Ellin J S 1982 Special professional morality and the duty of veracity. Business and Professional Ethics Journal 1:75–90

Ellis K 1993 Squaring the circle: user and carer participation in needs assessment. Joseph Rowntree Foundation, London

Ellis-Hill C S, Horn S 2000 Change in identity and self-concept: a new theoretical approach to recovery following a stroke. Clinical Rehabilitation 14:279–287

Ellis-Hill C, Payne S, Ward C 2000 Self-body split: issues of identity in physical recovery following stroke. Disability and Rehabilitation 22:725–733

Ellos W J 1990 Ethical practice in clinical medicine. Routledge, London

Emtner M, Hedin A, Stalenheim G 1998 Asthmatic patients' views of a comprehensive asthma rehabilitation programme: a three year follow-up. Physiotherapy Research International 3:175–193

Encandela J A 1993 Social science and the study of pain since Zborowski: a need for a new agenda. Social Science and Medicine 36:783–791

Endler N S, Parker J D A, Summerfeldt L J 1998 Coping with health problems: developing a reliable and valid multidimensional measure. Psychological Assessment 10: 195–205

Endler N S, Kocovski N L, Macrodimitris S D 2001 Coping, efficacy and perceived control in acute versus chronic illnesses. Personality and Individual Differences 30: 617–625

Engel G 1959 Psychogenic pain and the pain prone patient. American Journal of Medicine 26:899–918

Engel J M 1992 Relaxation training: a self-help approach for children with headaches. American Journal of Occupational Therapy 46:591–596

Engel J M, Rapoff M A 1990 Biofeedback assisted relaxation training for adult and pediatric headache disorders. Occupational Therapy Journal of Research 10:283–299

Engel J M, Rapoff M A, Pressman A R 1994 The durability of relaxation training in pediatric headache management. Occupational Therapy Journal of Research 14:183–190

Engelhardt H T Jr 1996 The foundations of bioethics, 2nd edn. Oxford University Press, New York

Enkin M, Keirse M J, Chalmers I 1990 A guide to effective care in pregnancy and childbirth. Oxford University Press, Oxford

Epping-Jordan J E, Wahlgren D R, Williams R A, Pruitt S D, Atkinson J H, Slater M A, Patterson T L, Webster J S 1998 Transition to chronic pain in men with low back pain: predictive relationships among pain intensity, disability, and depressive symptoms. Health Psychology 17: 421–427

Erhardt R P 1982 The Erhardt developmental prehension assessment (EDPA). Therapy Skill Builders, Tucson

Erhardt R P 1992 Eye–hand coordination. In: Case-Smith J, Pehoski C (eds) Development of hand skills in the child. American Occupational Therapy Association, Rockville, pp 13–33

Erikson E 1982 The life cycle completed – a review. Norton, New York

Estes C 1979 The ageing enterprise. Jossey-Bass, San Francisco

Estes C 1999 Critical economy and the new political economy of aging. In: Minkler M, Estes C (eds) Critical gerontology: perspectives from political and moral economy. New York, Baywood, Amityville, pp 17–35

Estes C, Binney E A 1989 The biomedicalization of aging: dangers and dilemmas. Gerontologist 29:587–596

Etzioni A 1964 Modern organizations. Prentice Hall, New Jersey

Etzioni A 1969 Preface. In: Etzioni A (ed) The semi-professions and their organization. Free Press, New York, pp v–xviii

Everitt A, Hardiker P, Littlewood J, Mullender A 1992 Applied research for better practice. Macmillan, London

Evetts J 1999 Professionalisation and professionalism: issues for interprofessional care. Journal of Interprofessional Care 13:119–128

Ewles L, Simnett I 1999 Promoting health: a practical guide, 4th edn. Baillière Tindall, Edinburgh

Exline J J, Dorrity K, Wortman C B 1996 Coping with bereavement: a research review for clinicians.

In: Worden J W (ed) Dealing with grief. John Wiley, New York, pp 3–19

Exner C E 1992 In-hand manipulation skills. In: Case-Smith J, Pehoski C (eds) Development of hand skills in the child. American Occupational Therapy Association, Rockville, pp 32–41

Exton-Smith A N 1955 Medical problems of old age. John Wright, Bristol

Eysenck H J 1967 The biological basis of personality. C C Thomas, Springfield

Eysenck M 1998 Psychology, an integrated approach. Longman, London

Eysenck H J, Eysenck S B G 1975 Manual of the Eysenck personality questionnaire. Hodder and Stoughton, London

Fabrega H J, Tyma S 1976 Language and cultural influences in the description of pain. British Journal of Medical Psychology 49:349–371

Fagerhaugh S, Strauss A 1977 Politics of pain management: staff–patient interaction. Addison-Wesley, Reading

Fairhurst E 1998 Suffering, emotion and pain: towards a sociological understanding. In: Carter B (ed) Perspectives on pain: mapping the territory. Arnold, London, pp 127–141

Farkas S, Duffet S, Johnson J 2000 Necessary compromises: how parents, employers and children's advocates view child care today. Public Agenda, New York

Farooqi A 1993 How can family practice improve access to health care for black and ethnic minority patients? In: Hopkins A, Bahl V (eds) Access to health care for people from black and ethnic minorities. Royal College of Physicians, London, pp 57–62

Farrant W, Russell J 1986 The politics of health information: 'Beating heart disease' as a case study of Health Education Council Publications. Bedford Way Papers no. 28. Institute of Education, University of London, London

Farver J A, Wimbarti S 1995 Indonesian children's play with their mothers and older siblings. Child Development 66:1493–1503

Fatchett A 1994 Politics, policy and nursing. Baillière Tindall, London

Fawcett B 2000 Feminist perspectives on disability. Prentice Hall, London

Fealy G M 1995 Professional caring: the moral dimension. Journal of Advanced Nursing 22:1135–1140

Felton B, Revenson T, Hinrichsen G 1984 Stress and coping in the explanation of psychological adjustment among chronically ill adults. Social Science and Medicine 18:889–898

Fernandez E 1986 A classification system of cognitive coping strategies for pain. Pain 26:141–151

Fernandez E, Turk D C 1989 The utility of cognitive coping strategies for altering pain perceptions: a meta-analysis. Pain 38:123–135

Fernandez E, Turk D C 1995 The scope and significance of anger in the experience of chronic pain. Pain 61:165–175

Field D 1976 The social dimension of illness. In: Tuckett D (ed) An introduction to medical sociology. Tavistock, London, pp 334–366

Field L, Adams N 2001 Pain management: 2. The use of psychological approaches to pain. British Journal of Nursing 10:971–974

Fieldhouse R and Associates 1996 A history of modern British adult education. National Institute of Adult Continuing Education, Leicester

Fields H L 1987 Pain. McGraw-Hill, New York

Finch J 2000 Interprofessional education and team working: a view from the educational provider. British Medical Journal 321:1138–1140

Finkelstein V 1981 To deny or not to deny disability. In: Brechin A, Liddiard P, Swain J (eds) Handicap in a social world. Hodder and Stoughton, Sevenoaks, pp 34–36

Finkelstein V 1993 Disability: a social challenge or an administrative responsibility? In: Swain J, Finkelstein V, French S, Oliver M (eds) Disabling barriers – enabling environments. Sage Publications, London, pp 34–43

Finkelstein V 1998 Emancipating disability studies. In: Shakespeare T (ed) The disability reader: social science perspectives. Cassell, London, pp 28–49

Finkelstein V, French S 1993 Towards a psychology of disability. In: Swain J, Finkelstein V, French S, Oliver M (eds) Disabling barriers – enabling environments. Sage Publications, London, pp 26–33

Finkelstein V, Stuart O 1996 Developing new services. In: Hales G (ed) Beyond disability: towards an enabling society. Sage Publications, London, pp 170–187

Fitzpatrick R 1991 Surveys of patient satisfaction: I. Important general considerations. British Medical Journal 302:887–889

Flavell J H 1963 The developmental psychology of Jean Piaget. Van Nostrand, New York

Flavell J H, Everett B A, Croft K, Flavell E R 1981 Young children's knowledge about visual perception: further evidence for the Level 1–Level 2 distinction. Developmental Psychology 17:99–103

Flew A 1983 A dictionary of philosophy, 2nd edn. Pan Books, London

Flor H, Haag G, Turk D C, Koehler H 1983 Efficacy of EMG biofeedback, pseudotherapy and conventional medical treatment for chronic rheumatic back pain. Pain 17:21–31

Flor H, Birbaumer N, Schulte W, Roos R 1991 Stress related electromyographic responses in patients with chronic temporomandibular pain. Pain 46:145–152

Flor H, Behle D J, Birbaumer N 1993 Assessment of pain-related cognitions in chronic pain patients. Behaviour Research and Therapy 31:63–73

Floyd A 1979 Cognitive development in the school years: a reader. Croom Helm, London

Fodor J 1983 The modularity of the mind. MIT Press, Cambridge

Folkman S, Lazarus R S, Dunkel-Schetter C, DeLongis A, Gruen R J 1986a Dynamics of a stressful encounter: cognitive appraisal, coping, and encounter outcomes. Journal of Personality and Social Psychology 50: 992–1003

Folkman S, Lazarus R S, Gruen R J, DeLongis A 1986b Appraisal, coping, health status and psychological symptoms. Journal of Personality and Social Psychology 50:571–579

Fordyce W E 1976 Behavioral methods for chronic pain and illness. C V Mosby, St Louis

Fordyce W E 1986 Learning processes in pain. In: Sternbach RA (ed) The psychology of pain. Raven Press, New York, pp 49–66

Fordyce W E 1988 Pain and suffering: a reappraisal. American Psychologist 43:276–283

Fordyce W E 1995 Back pain in the workplace: management of disability in nonspecific conditions. IASP Press, Seattle

Fordyce W E 1997 On the nature of illness and disability: an editorial. Clinical Orthopaedics and Related Research 336:47–51

Foster P 1995 Women and the health care industry. Open University Press, Buckingham

Foucault M 1980 Power/knowledge: selected interviews and other writings, 1972–77. Harvester Press, Brighton

Francis B, Humphreys J 2000 Professional education as a structural barrier to lifelong learning in the NHS. Journal of Educational Policy 15:281–290

Frank A W 1995 The wounded storyteller: body, illness, and ethics. University of Chicago Press, Chicago

Frank A 2001 Can we research suffering? Qualitative Health Research 11:353–362

Frank A O, Maguire G P 1988 Disabling diseases: physical, environmental and psychosocial management. Butterworth-Heinemann, Oxford

Frawley W 1997 Vygotsky and cognitive science. Harvard University Press, Cambridge

Freedman J, Combs G 1996 Narrative therapy: the social construction of preferred realities. Norton, New York

Freidson E 1970 The profession of medicine: a study of the sociology of applied knowledge. Aldine, New York

Freidson E 1994 Professionalism reborn: theory, prophecy and policy. University of Chicago Press, Chicago

French S 1992 Health care in a multi-ethnic society. Physiotherapy 78:174–180

French S 1993 Can you see the rainbow? The roots of denial. In: Swain J, Finkelstein V, French S, Oliver M (eds) Disabling barriers – enabling environments. Sage Publications, London, pp 69–77

French S 1994a On equal terms: working with disabled people. Butterworth-Heinemann, Oxford

French S 1994b Researching disability. In: French S (ed) On equal terms: working with disabled people. Butterworth-Heinemann, Oxford, pp 136–147

French S 1994c The disabled role. In: French S (ed) On equal terms: working with disabled people. Butterworth-Heinemann, Oxford, pp 47–60

French S 1996a Out of sight out of mind: the experience and effect of a special residential school. In: Morris J (ed) Encounters with strangers: feminism and disability. The Women's Press, London, pp 17–47

French S 1996b Simulation exercises in disability awareness training: a critique. In: Hales G (ed) Beyond disability: towards an enabling society. Sage Publications, London, pp 114–123

French S 1997 Ageism. In: French S (ed) Physiotherapy: a psychosocial approach, 2nd edn. Butterworth-Heinemann, Oxford, pp 73–85

French S 2001 Disabled people and employment: a study of the working lives of visually impaired physiotherapists. Ashgate, Aldershot

French S, Swain J 1997 Changing disability research: participatory and emancipatory research with disabled people. Physiotherapy 83:26–32

French S, Swain J 2000 Personal perceptions on the experience of exclusion. In: Moore M (ed) Insider perspectives on inclusion: raising voices, raising issues. Philip Armstrong Publications, Sheffield, pp 18–35

French S, Swain J 2001 The relationship between disabled people and health and welfare professionals. In: Albrecht G, Seelman K D, Bury M (eds) Handbook of disability studies. Sage Publications, London, pp 734–753

French S, Reynolds F, Swain J 2001 Practical research: a guide for therapists, 2nd edn. Butterworth-Heinemann, Oxford

Freund P E S, McGuire M B, Podhurst L S 2003 Health, illness and the social body: a critical sociology, 4th edn. Prentice-Hall, Upper Saddle River

Friedan B 1993 The fountain of age. Simon and Schuster, New York

Friedman-Campbell M, Hart C A 1984 Theoretical strategies and nursing interventions to promote psychological adaptation to spinal cord injuries and disability. Journal of Neurosurgical Nursing 16:335–342

Frith U 1989 Autism – explaining the enigma. Blackwell, Oxford

Frostig M 1966 Marianne Frostig developmental test of visual perception. Consulting Psychologists Press, Palo Alto

Fulcher J, Scott J 1999 Sociology. Oxford University Press, Oxford

Fuss D 1989 Essentially speaking: feminism, nature and difference. Routledge, London

Galler R 1993 The myth of the perfect body. In: Beattie A, Gott M, Jones L, Sidell M (eds) Health and wellbeing: a reader. Macmillan, London, pp 152–157

Gamsa A 1990 Is emotional disturbance a precipitator or a consequence of chronic pain? Pain 42:183–195

Gamsa A 1994 The role of psychological factors in pain: 1. A half century of study. Pain 57:5–15

Gardiner B M 1980 Psychological aspects of rheumatoid arthritis. Psychological Medicine 10:159–163

Garfield F B, Garfield J M 2000 Clinical judgement and clinical practice guidelines. International Journal of Technology Assessment in Healthcare 16:1050–1060

Garland Thomson R 1997 Feminist theory, the body and the disabled figure. In: Davis J L (ed) The disability studies reader. Routledge, London, pp 279–292

Gaston-Johansson F, Ohly K V, Fall-Dickson J M, Nanda J P, Kennedy M J 1999 Pain, psychological distress and health status in patients with breast cancer scheduled for autotransplantation. Oncology Nursing Forum 26: 1337–1345

Gatchel R J, Epker J T 1999 Psychosocial predictors of chronic pain and response to treatment. In: Gatchel R J, Turk D C (eds) Psychological factors in pain: critical perspectives. Guilford Press, New York, pp 412–434

Gatchel R J, Turk D C 1996 Psychological approaches to pain management: a practitioner's handbook. Guilford Press, New York

Gatchel R J, Turk D C 1999 Psychosocial factors in pain: critical perspectives. Guilford Press, New York

Gatchel R J, Weisberg J N 2000 Personality characteristics of patients with pain. American Psychological Association, Washington

Gatchel R J, Polatin P B, Kinney R K 1995a Predicting outcome of chronic back pain using clinical predictors of psychopathology: a prospective analysis. Health Psychology 14:415–420

Gatchel R J, Polatin P B, Mayer T G 1995b The dominant role of psychosocial risk factors in the development of chronic low back pain disability. Spine 20:2702–2709

Gaussen T 1984 Developmental milestones or conceptual millstones? Some practical and theoretical limitations in infant assessment procedures. Child: Care, Health and Development 10:99–115

Gaussen T 1985 Beyond the milestone model – a system framework for alternative infant assessment procedures. Child: Care, Health and Development 11:131–150

Gauthier C C 1997 Teaching the virtues: justifications and recommendations. Cambridge Quarterly of Healthcare Ethics 6:339–346

Geisser M E, Robinson M E, Keefe F J, Weiner M L 1994 Catastrophizing, depression and the sensory, affective and evaluative aspects of chronic pain. Pain 59:79–83

Gergen K J 1999 An invitation to social construction. Sage Publications, London

Gerhardt U 1989 Ideas about illness: an intellectual and political history of medical sociology. New York University Press, New York

Gerrish K, Husband C, MacKenzie J 1996 Nursing for a multi-ethnic society. Open University Press, Buckingham

Gert B, Culver C M 1981 Paternalistic behavior. In: Cohen M, Nagel T, Scanlon T (eds) Medicine and moral philosophy. Princeton University Press, Princeton, pp 201–213

Gert B, Culver C M, Clouser K D 1997 Bioethics: a return to fundamentals. Oxford University Press, New York

Gesell A, Amatruda C S 1947 Developmental diagnosis. Hoeber/Hamish Hamilton, New York

Gesser B 1985 Utbildning, jamlikhet, arebetsdelning. Lund: Arkiv. cited in: Selander S 1990 Associative strategies in the process of professionalization: professional strategies and the scientification of occupations. In: Burrage M, Torstendahl R (eds) Professions in theory and history. Sage Publications, London, pp 139–150

Gianakos I 2002 Predictors of coping with work stress: the influences of sex, gender role, social desirability and locus of control. Sex Roles 46:149–158

Giddens A 1979 Central problems in social theory. Macmillan, London

Giddens A 1989 Sociology. Polity Press, Cambridge

Gilleard C, Higgs P 2000 Cultures of ageing: self, citizen and the body. Prentice Hall, Harlow

Gillespie J E, Jackson A 2000 MRI and CT of the brain. Arnold, London

Gillman M, Swain J, Heyman B 1997 Life history or 'case' history: the objectification of people with learning difficulties through the tyranny of professional discourses. Disability and Society 12:675–693

Gillon R 1985a 'It's all too subjective': scepticism about the possibility of use of philosophical medical ethics. British Medical Journal 290:1574–1575

Gillon R 1985b Confidentiality. British Medical Journal 291: 1634–1636

Gillon R, Lloyd A 1994 Principles of health care ethics. John Wiley, Chichester

Glaser B G, Strauss A L 1971 Status passage. Routledge and Kegan Paul, London

Glasgow D 1980 The black underclass. Jossey Bass, London

Glazer-Waldman H R, Hart J P, LeVeau B F 1989 Health beliefs and health behaviors of physical therapists. Physical Therapy 69:204–210

Glenton C 2002 Developing patient-centred information for back pain sufferers. Health Expectations 5: 319–329

Glenton C 2003 Chronic back pain sufferers – striving for the sick role. Social Science and Medicine 57:2243–2252

Glossop E S, Goldenberg E, Smith D S, Williams I M 1982 Patient compliance in back and neck pain. Physiotherapy 68:225–226

Goffman I 1968 Stigma: notes on the management of spoiled identity. Penguin Books, Harmondsworth

Goldberg D P 1978 Manual of the general health questionnaire. NFER-Nelson, Windsor

Goldie L 1982 The ethics of telling the patient. Journal of Medical Ethics 8:128–133

Gomm R 1993 Issues of power in health and welfare. In: Walmsley J, Reynolds J, Shakespeare P, Woolfe R (eds) Health, welfare and practice: reflecting on roles and relationships. Sage Publications, London, pp 131–138

Goodlad S 1984 Introduction. In: Goodlad S (ed) Education for the professions. Quis custodiet? SRHE and NFER-Nelson, Surrey, pp 3–16

Goodyear-Smith F, Buetow S 2001 Power in the doctor–patient relationship. Health Care Analysis 9:449–462

Gordon D 1988 Tenacious assumptions in western medicine. In: Loch M, Gordon D (eds) Biomedicine examined. Kluwer, Dordrecht, pp 19–56

Gormley K J 1996 Altruism: a framework for caring and providing care. International Journal of Nursing Studies 33:581–588

Grace V M 1998 Mind/body dualism in medicine: the case of chronic pelvic pain without organic pathology: a critical review of the literature. International Journal of Health Services 28:127–151

Gracely R H 1999 Pain measurement. Acta Anaesthesiologica Scandinavica 43:897–908

Gracely R H, Dubner R 1981 Pain assessment in humans: a reply to Hall. Pain 11:109–120

Graham H 1984 Women, health and the family. Wheatsheaf, Brighton

Graham H 1987 Women's poverty and caring. In: Glendinning C, Millar J (eds) Women and poverty in Britain. Wheatsheaf, Brighton

Graham H 1990 Behaving well: women's health behaviour in context. In: Roberts H (ed) Women's health counts. Routledge, London, pp 195–219

Graham H 2001 The health variations programme and the public health agenda. Health Variations 7:2–3

Gray A 2001a The decline of infectious diseases: the case of England. In: Gray A (ed) World health and disease. Open University Press, Buckingham, pp 105–130

Gray A 2001b Mortality and morbidity: causes and determinants. In: Gray A (ed) World health and disease. Open University Press, Buckingham, pp 34–61

Gray A 2001c Contemporary patterns of disease in the United Kingdom. In: Gray A (ed) World health and disease. Open University Press. Buckingham, pp 178–222

Gray A 2001d World patterns of mortality. In: Gray A (ed) World health and disease. Open University Press, Buckingham, pp 14–33

Gray A 2001e The world transformed: population and the rise of industrial society. In: Gray A (ed) World health and disease. Open University Press, Buckingham, pp 81–104

Gray A 2001f Health in a world of wealth and poverty. In: Gray A (ed) World health and disease. Open University Press, Buckingham, pp 131–157

Green J 1989a Death with dignity: Islam. Nursing Times 85(5):56–57

Green J 1989b Death with dignity: Hinduism. Nursing Times 85(6):50–51

Green J 1989c Death with dignity: Sikhism. Nursing Times 85(7):56–57

Green J 1989d Death with dignity: Judaism. Nursing Times 85(8):64–65

Green J 2001 Children and accidents. In: Davey B (ed) Birth to old age: health in transition. Open University Press, Buckingham, pp 103–124

Green A S, Waterfield J 1997 Admissions and progression trends in physiotherapy. Physiotherapy 83:472–479

Green C R, Wheeler J R C, LaPorta F, Marchant B, Guerrero E 2002 How well is chronic pain managed? Who does it well? Pain Medicine 3:56–65

Greenberg M S, Alloy L B 1989 Depression vs anxiety: processing of self- and other-referent information. Cognition and Emotion 3:207–223

Greene L C, Hardy J D 1958 Spatial summation of pain. Journal of Applied Physiology 13:457–464

Greenhalgh S 2001 Under the medical gaze: facts and fictions of chronic pain. University of California Press, Berkeley

Griffin A P 1983 A philosophical analysis of caring in nursing. Journal of Advanced Nursing 8:289–295

Griffiths R 1954 The abilities of babies: a study in mental measurement. University of London Press, London

Griffiths P 1987 Creating a learning environment. Physiotherapy 73:328–331

Grimmer K, Beard M, Bell A, Chipchase L, Edwards E, Fulton I, Gill T 2000 On the constructs of quality physiotherapy. Australian Journal of Physiotherapy 46:3–7

Grimsley M, Bhat A 1988 Health. In: Bhat A, Carrhill P, Ohri S (eds) Britain's black population: a new perspective, 2nd edn. Gower, Aldershot

Grindle N, Dallat J 2000 Nurse education: from casualty to scapegoat? Teaching in Higher Education 5:205–218

Griswold W 1994 Cultures and societies in a changing world. Pine Forge Press, Thousand Oaks

Grzesiak R C, Perrine K R 1987 Psychological aspects of chronic pain. In: Wu W H, Smith L G (eds) Pain management: assessment and treatment of chronic and acute syndromes. Human Sciences Press, New York, pp 44–69

Guccione A A 1980 Ethical issues in physical therapy practice: a survey of physical therapists in New England. Physical Therapy 60:1264–1272

Guzman J, Esmail R, Karjalainen K, Malmivaara A, Irvin E, Bombardier C 2001 Multidisciplinary rehabilitation for chronic low back pain: systematic review. British Medical Journal 322:1511–1516

Haas J 1993 Ethical considerations of goal setting for patient care in rehabilitation medicine. American Journal of Physical Medicine and Rehabilitation 74(Suppl.):S16–S20

Hafsteindottir T, Grypdonck M 1997 Being a stroke patient: a review of the literature. Journal of Advanced Nursing 26:580–588

Hagestad G O, Dannefer D 2001 Concepts and theories of aging: beyond microfication in social science approaches. In: Binstock R H, George L K (eds) Handbook of aging and the social sciences. Academic Press, San Diego, pp 3–21

Hales G (ed) 1996 Beyond disability: towards an enabling society. Sage Publications, London

Haley S M 1992 Pediatric evaluation of disability inventory (PEDI): development, standardization and administration manual. New England Medical Center Hospitals and PEDI Research Group, Boston

Hammond A 1998 The use of self-management strategies by people with rheumatoid arthritis. Clinical Rehabilitation 12:81–87

Hanford L 1994 Nursing and the concept of care: an appraisal of Noddings' theory. In: Hunt G (ed) Ethical issues in nursing. Routledge, London, pp 181–197

Happé F G E 1995 The role of age and verbal ability in the theory of mind task performance of subjects with autism. Child Development 66:843–855

Harding V, Williams A C de C 1995 Extending physiotherapy skills using a psychological approach: cognitive-behavioural management of chronic pain. Physiotherapy 81:681–688

Hardy J, Wolff H, Goodell H 1952 Pain sensations and reactions. Williams and Wilkins, Baltimore

Hargreaves S 1987 The relevance of non-verbal skills in physiotherapy. Physiotherapy 73:685–688

Harkapaa K, Jarvikoski A, Mellin G, Hurri H, Luoma J 1991 Health locus of control beliefs and psychological distress as predictors for treatment outcome in low back pain patients: results of a 3-month follow-up of a controlled intervention study. Pain 46:35–41

Harré R 1990 Health as an aesthetic concept. Cogito 4:35–40

Harré R 1998 The singular self: an introduction to the psychology of personhood. Sage Publications, London

Harrison S, Ahmad W I U 2000 Medical autonomy and the UK state 1975 to 2025. Sociology 34:129–146

Harrison S, Pollitt C 1994 Controlling health professionals: the future of work and organisation within the NHS. Open University Press, Buckingham

Hartley P 1993 Parents and children. In: Eckersley P M (ed) Elements of paediatric physiotherapy. Churchill Livingstone, Edinburgh, pp 447–457

Hartley P 1999 Interpersonal communication, 2nd edn. Routledge, London

Haskell S H, Barrett K, Taylor H 1977 The education of motor and neurologically handicapped children. Croom Helm, London

Hasler J C 1985 Communications and relationships in general medical practice. Physiotherapy 71:435–436

Hasler F 1993 Developments in the disabled people's movement. In: Swain J, Finkelstein V, French S, Oliver M (eds) Disabling barriers – enabling environments. Sage Publications, London, pp 285–292

Hathaway S R, McKinley J C 1951 The Minnesota multiphasic personality inventory. Psychological Corporation, New York

Hawley D J, Wolfe F 1993 Depression is not more common in rheumatoid arthritis: a 10 year longitudinal study of 6153 patients with rheumatic disease. Journal of Rheumatology 20:2025–2031

Hayne C R 1988 The preventive role of physiotherapy in the National Health Service and Industry. Physiotherapy 74:2–3

Haythornthwaite J A, Sieber W J, Kerns R D 1991 Depression and the chronic pain experience. Pain 46:177–184

Hazell K 1960 Social and medical problems of the elderly. Hutchinson, London

Heckman T, Somlai A, Kalichman S, Franzoi S, Kelly J 1998 Psychosocial differences between urban and rural people living with HIV/AIDS. Journal of Rural Health 14:138–145

Hegge M, Fischer C 2000 Grief responses of senior and elderly widows: practice implications. Journal of Gerontological Nursing 26:35–43

Heinz W 1999 Lifelong learning: learning for life? Some cross-national observations. In: Coffield F (ed) Why's the beer always stronger up north? Studies of Lifelong Learning in Europe. Policy Press, Bristol, pp 13–20

Hellström O, Bullington J, Karlsson G, Lindqvist P, Mattson B 1999 A phenomenological study of fibromyalgia: patient perspectives. Scandinavian Journal of Primary Health Care 17:11–16

Helman C G 2001 Culture, health, and illness, 4th edn. Butterworth-Heinemann, Oxford

Hennekens C H, Buring J E 1987 Epidemiology in medicine. Lippincott, Williams and Wilkins, Philadelphia

Henriksen M 1994 A reflective look at the use of comforting touch on infants receiving high dependency care in the neonatal unit, and the importance of parental participation. Unpublished dissertation, University of Northumbria, Newcastle

Henriksson C M 1995a Living with continuous muscular pain – patient perspectives: II. Strategies for daily life. Scandinavian Journal of Caring Sciences 9:77–86

Henriksson C M 1995b Living with continuous muscular pain – patient perspectives: I. Encounters and consequences. Scandinavian Journal of Caring Sciences 9:67–76

Hepworth M 2000 Stories of ageing. Open University Press, Buckingham

Herman E, Baptiste S 1990 Group therapy: a cognitive behavioural model. In: Tunks E, Bellissimo A, Roy R (eds) Chronic pain: psychosocial factors in rehabilitation, 2nd edn. Krieger, Melbourne, pp 212–228

Hervey G R 1984 The functions of pain. In: Holden A V, Winlow W (eds) The neurobiology of pain. Manchester University Press, Manchester, pp 399–407

Hesse H 1976 On old age. In: Hesse H (ed) My belief: essays on life and art. Jonathan Cape, London, pp 269–271

Hewison A, Sim J 1998 Managing interprofessional working: using codes of ethics as a foundation. Journal of Interprofessional Care 12:309–321

Hicks C M 1988 Practical research methods for physiotherapists. Churchill Livingstone, Edinburgh

Higgs R 1994 Truth-telling, lying and the doctor–patient relationship. In: Gillon R, Lloyd A (eds) Principles of health care ethics. John Wiley, Chichester, pp 499–509

Higgs J, Titchen A 1995 The nature, generation and verification of knowledge. Physiotherapy 81:521–530

Higgs J, Titchen A 2000 Knowledge and reasoning. In: Higgs J, Jones M (eds) Clinical reasoning in the health professions, 2nd edn. Butterworth-Heinemann, Oxford, pp 23–32

Higgs J, Refshauge K, Ellis E 2001 Portrait of the physiotherapy profession. Journal of Interprofessional Care 15:79–98

Hilbert R A 1984 The acultural dimensions of chronic pain: flawed reality construction and the problem of meaning. Social Problems 31:365–378

Hill M 1994 They are not our brothers: the disability movement and the black disability movement. In: Begum N, Hill M, Stevens A (eds) Reflections: views of black disabled people of their lives and community care. Central Council for Education and Training in Social Work, London, pp 68–80

Hill H E, Kornetsky H, Flanary H G, Wikler A 1952 Studies of anxiety with anticipation of pain. Archives of Neurological Psychiatry 67:612–617

Hills R 1995 The role of the physiotherapist in health education (abstract of higher degree thesis). Physiotherapy 81:270

Hilton R W 1995 Fragmentation within interprofessional work: a result of isolationism in healthcare professional education and the preparation of students to function only in the confines of their disciplines. Journal of Interprofessional Care 9:33–40

Hoehn T P, Baumeister A A 1994 A critique of the application of sensory integration therapy to children with learning difficulties. Journal of Learning Disabilities 27:338–350

Hogg J 1987 Early development and Piagetian tests. In: Hogg J, Raynes N V (eds) Assessment in mental handicap: a guide to assessment practices, tests and checklists. Croom Helm, London, pp 45–80

Holahan C J, Moos R H, Schaefer J A 1996 Coping, stress resistance, and growth: conceptualizing adaptive functioning. In: Zeidner M, Endler N S (eds) Handbook of coping: theory, research, applications. Wiley, New York, pp 24–43

Holahan C J, Moos R H, Holahan C K, Cronkite R A, Randall P K 2001 Drinking to cope, emotional distress and alcohol use and abuse: a ten-year model. Journal of Studies on Alcohol 62:190–198

Holden G 1988 Why are people from ethnic minorities losing out? Disability Now (August):8–9

Holliday-Willey L 1999 Pretending to be normal: living with Asperger's syndrome. Jessica Kingsley, London

Holman A, Bewley C 2000 Funding freedom 2000: people with learning difficulties using direct payments. Values into Action, London

Holt K S 1991 Child development: diagnosis and assessment. Butterworth-Heinemann, Oxford

Honkasalo M-L 2000 Chronic pain as a posture towards the world. Scandinavian Journal of Psychology 41: 197–208

Hopkins A 1993 Envoi. In: Hopkins A, Bahl V (eds) Access to health care for people from black and ethnic minorities. Royal College of Physicians, London, pp 201–205

Horton I, Bayne R 1998 Counselling and communication in health care. In: Bayne R, Nicolson P, Horton, I (eds) Counselling and communication skills for medical and health practitioners. British Psychological Society, Leicester, pp 3–21

Hough A 1987 Communication in health care. Physiotherapy 73:56–59

Hough A 2001 Physiotherapy in respiratory care: an evidence-based approach to respiratory and cardiac management, 3rd edn. Nelson Thornes, Cheltenham

Houle C O 1980 Continuing learning in the professions. Jossey Bass, San Francisco

Howell T H 1953 Our advancing years: an essay on the modern problems of old age. Phoenix House, London

Howell S L 1994 A theoretical model for caring for women with chronic nonmalignant pain. Qualitative Health Research 4:94–122

Hughes M 1975 Ego-centrism in pre-school children. Unpublished doctoral dissertation, Edinburgh University, Edinburgh

Hughes G 1998 A suitable case for treatment? Constructions of disability. In: Saraga E (ed) Embodying the social: constructions of difference. Routledge, London, pp 43–90

Hughes B, Paterson K 1997 The social model of disability and the disappearing body: towards a sociology of impairment. Disability and Society 12:225–240

Hugman R 1991 Power in caring professions. Macmillan, London

Humphries S, Gordon P 1992 Out of sight: the experience of disability, 1900–1950. Northcote House, Plymouth

Huntley A, White A R, Ernst E 2002 Relaxation therapies for asthma: a systematic review. Thorax 57:127–131

Hurst R 2000 To revise or not to revise. Disability and Society 15:1083–1087

Hydén L-C, Peolsson M 2002 Pain gestures: the orchestration of speech and body gestures. Health 6:325–345

Hydén L-C, Sachs L 1998 Suffering, hope and diagnosis: on the negotiation of chronic fatigue syndrome. Health 2:175–193

Hyland T 1987 Value-free? Education and Health 5:89

Hyland T 1988 Values and health education: a critique of individualism. Educational Studies 14:23–31

Iezzoni L 1998 What should I say? Communication around disability. Annals of Internal Medicine 129:661–665

Illich I 1976 Limits to medicine: medical nemesis: the expropriation of health. Penguin, Harmondsworth

Illich I 1997 Disabling professions. In: Illich I, Zola IK, McKnight J, Caplan J, Shaiken H (eds) Disabling professions. Marion Boyars, London, pp 11–39

Illingworth R S 1987 The development of the infant and young child: normal and abnormal. Churchill Livingstone, Edinburgh

Imara M 1983 Growing through grief. In: Corr C A, Corr D M (eds) Hospice care: principles and practice. Faber and Faber, London, pp 249–265

Imrie R, Ramey D W 2000 The evidence for evidence based medicine. Complementary Therapies in Medicine 8:123–126

Ingstad B, Reynolds Whyte S 1995 Disability and culture. University of California Press, Los Angeles

International Association for the Study of Pain 1986 Classification of chronic pain: descriptions of chronic pain syndromes and definitions of pain terms. Pain 27(Suppl.):S1–S225

Irvine D 1997 Professionalism and self regulation in a changing world. The performance of doctors, part 1. British Medical Journal 314:1540–1543

Jackson J A 1970 Professions and professionalization – editorial introduction. In: Jackson J A (ed) Professions and professionalization. Cambridge University Press, Cambridge, pp 1–16

Jackson D A 1987 Where is the physiotherapy profession going? Physiotherapy 73:590–591

Jackson A 1999 The book of life: one man's search for the wisdom of age. Gollancz, London

Jackson J 2001 Truth, trust and medicine. Routledge, London

Jackson M, Quaal C 1991 Effects of multiple sclerosis on occupational and career patterns. Axon 13:16–22

Jacobson E 1938 Progressive relaxation: a physiological and clinical investigation of muscular states and their significance in psychology and medical practice. University of Chicago Press, Midway Reprint 1974, London

Jacobson B, Smith A, Whitehead M 1991 The nation's health: a strategy for the 1990s. King Edward's Hospital Fund, London

Jaggi A, Bithell C 1995 Relationships between physiotherapists' level of contact, cultural awareness and communication with Bangladeshi patients in two health authorities. Physiotherapy 81:330–337

Jarrold C, Boucher J, Smith P 1993 Symbolic play in autism: a review. Journal of Autism and Developmental Disorders 23:281–307

Jefree D, McConkey R 1976 An observational scheme for recording children's imaginative doll play. Journal of Child Psychology and Psychiatry and Allied Disciplines 17:189–197

Jelsma J, de Weerdt W, de Cock P 2002 Disability adjusted life years (DALYs) and rehabilitation. Disability and Rehabilitation 24:378–382

Jenkins R 1996 Social identity. Routledge, London

Jensen L, Allen M 1994 A synthesis of qualitative research on wellness–illness. Qualitative Health Research 4:349–369

Jensen M P, Karoly P 1992 Pain-specific beliefs, perceived symptom severity, and adjustment to chronic pain. Clinical Journal of Pain 8:123–130

Jensen M P, Turner J A, Romano J M 1991a Self-efficacy and outcome expectancies: relationship to chronic pain coping strategies and adjustment. Pain 44:263–269

Jensen M P, Turner J A, Romano J M, Karoly P 1991b Coping with chronic pain: a critical review of the literature. Pain 47:249–283

Jensen M P, Karoly P, Romano J M, Lawler B K 1994a Relationship of pain-specific beliefs to chronic pain adjustment. Pain 57:301–309

Jensen M P, Turner J A, Romano J M 1994b Correlates of improvement in multidisciplinary treatment of chronic pain. Journal of Consulting and Clinical Psychology 62:172–179

Jewson N D 1993 The disappearance of the sick man from medical cosmology, 1770–1870. In: Beattie A, Gott M, Jones L, Sidell M (eds) Health and wellbeing: a reader. Macmillan Press, London, pp 44–54

Jeyasingham M 1992 Acting for health: ethnic minorities and the community health movement. In: Ahmad W I U (ed) The politics of race and health. Race Relations Research Unit, Bradford University, Bradford, pp 143–157

Jobling M H 1987 Cognitive styles: some implications for teaching and learning. Physiotherapy 73:335–338

Johansson E, Hamberg K, Lindgren G, Westman G 1999 The meanings of pain. Social Science and Medicine 48:1791–1802

Johnes M 2000 Aberfan and the management of trauma. Disasters 24:1–17

Johns C 1994 The Burford NDU model: caring in practice. Blackwell Science, Oxford

Johnson T J 1972 Professions and power. Macmillan, London

Johnson J E 1973 The effects of accurate expectations about sensations on the sensory and distress components of pain. Journal of Personality and Social Psychology 27:261–275

Johnson A G 1990 Pathways in medical ethics. Edward Arnold, London

Johnson M 1997 Developmental cognitive neuroscience: an introduction. Blackwell, Oxford

Johnson J, Slater R 1993 Ageing and later life. Sage Publications, London

Johnstone M-J 1994 Bioethics: a nursing perspective, 2nd edn. W B Saunders/Baillière Tindall, Sydney

Jolly M, Brykczynska G 1992 Nursing care: the challenge to change. Edward Arnold, London

Jones M 1972 A Developmental schedule based on Piaget's sensori-motor writings: an examination of the schedule's potential value as an instrument for assessing severe and profoundly subnormal children. Unpublished MSc thesis, University of London, London

Jones J H 1988 The importance of children's funerals in the mourning process. Bereavement Care 7:34–37

Jones L J 1994 The social context of health and health work. Macmillan Press, London

Jones G E 1995 Enhancing provision for children with autism: what can we learn from current approaches and practice? Unpublished manuscript, University of Birmingham, Birmingham

Jones L 2000a What is health? In: Katz J, Peberdy A, Douglas J (eds) Promoting health: knowledge and practice, 2nd edn. Open University in association with Palgrave, Houndmills, pp 18–36

Jones L 2000b Behavioural and environmental influences on health. In: Katz J, Peberdy A, Douglas J (eds) Promoting health: knowledge and practice, 2nd edn. Open University in association with Palgrave, Houndmills, pp 37–57

Jones L, Douglas J 2000 The rise of health promotion. In: Katz J, Peberdy A, Douglas J (eds) Promoting health: knowledge and practice, 2nd edn. Open University in association with Palgrave, Houndmills, pp 58–79

Jordan S 2000 Educational input and patient outcomes: exploring the gap. Journal of Advanced Nursing 31:461–471

Jorgensen P 2000 Concepts of body and health in physiotherapy: the meaning of the social/cultural aspects of life. Physiotherapy Theory and Practice 16:105–115

Kagawa-Singer M 1998 The cultural context of death rituals and mourning practice. Oncology Nursing Forum 25:1752–1756

Kahn J 1976 Utility of the Uzgiris and Hunt scales of sensori-motor development with severely and profoundly retarded children. American Journal of Mental Deficiency 80:663–665

Kaivanto K K, Estlander A M, Moneta G B, Vanharanta H 1995 Isokinetic performance in low-back pain patients – the predictive power of the self-efficacy scale. Journal of Occupational Rehabilitation 5:87–99

Karl G T 1987 A new look at grief. Journal of Advanced Nursing 12:641–645

Karmiloff-Smith A 2001 Why babies' brains are not Swiss army knives. In: Rose H, Rose S (eds) Alas poor Darwin: arguments against evolutionary psychology. Vantage, London, pp 144–156

Katz J 2000 What counts as evidence in health information? In: Katz J, Peberdy A, Douglas J (eds) Promoting health: knowledge and practice, 2nd edn. Open University in association with Palgrave, Houndmills, pp 198–220

Keefe F J, Lefebvre J 1994 Pain behaviour concepts: controversies, current status and future directions. In: Gebhart G F, Hammond D L, Jensen T S (eds) Proceedings of the 7th World Congress on Pain. Progress in pain research and management, vol. 2. IASP Press, Seattle, pp 127–148

Keefe F J, Brown G K, Wallston K A, Caldwell D S 1989 Coping with rheumatoid arthritis pain: catastrophizing as a maladaptive strategy. Pain 37:51–56

Keefe F J, Caldwell D S, Williams D A, Gil K M, Mitchell D, Robertson C, Martinez S, Nunley J, Beckham J C, Crisson J E, Helms M 1990a Pain coping skills training in the management of osteoarthritic knee pain: a comparative study. Behavior Therapy 21:49–62

Keefe F J, Crisson J, Urban B J, Williams D A 1990b Analyzing chronic low back pain: the relative contribution of pain coping strategies. Pain 40:293–301

Keefe F J, Dunsmore J, Burnett R 1992 Behavioral and cognitive-behavioral approaches to chronic pain: recent advances and future directions. Journal of Consulting and Clinical Psychology 60:528–536

Keefe F J, Kashikar-Zuck S, Robinson E, Salley A, Beaupre P, Caldwell D, Baucom D, Haythornthwaite J 1997 Pain coping strategies that predict patients' and spouses ratings' of patients' self-efficacy. Pain 73:191–199

Keith L 1994 Mustn't grumble: writing by disabled women. Women's Press, London

Keith L, Morris J 1995 Easy targets: a disability rights perspective on the 'children as carers' debate. Critical Social Policy 44/45:36–57

Kennedy I 1981 The unmasking of medicine. George Allen and Unwin, London

Kent G 1986 Effects of pre-appointment inquiries on dental patients' post-appointment ratings of pain. British Journal of Medical Psychology 59:97–100

Keogh E, Ellery D, Hunt C, Hannent I 2000 Selective attentional bias for pain-related stimuli amongst pain fearful individuals. Pain 91:91–100

Kephart N C 1971 The slow learner in the classroom, 2nd edn. Merrill, Columbus

Kerlinger F N 1986 Foundations of behavioral research, 3rd edn. Harcourt Brace Jovanovich, Fort Worth

Kersten P 2002 Autonomy: the be all and end all in rehabilitation. Disability and Rehabilitation 24:993–995

Kiernan C C 1974 Behaviour modification. In: Clarke A M, Clarke A D B (eds) Mental deficiency: the changing outlook, 2nd edn. Methuen, London, pp 729–803

Kingston P 1998 Older people and 'falls': a randomised control trial of health visitor intervention. Unpublished PhD thesis, Keele University, Keele

Kingston P 1999 Ageism in history. Nursing Times Clinical Monographs no. 28. Nursing Times, London

Kingston P 2000 Falls in later life: status passage and preferred identities as a new orientation. Health 4:216–234

Kiple K 1996 The history of disease. In: Porter R (ed) Cambridge illustrated history of medicine. Cambridge University Press, Cambridge, pp 16–51

Kirkwood T 1999 Time of our lives. Weidenfield and Nicholson, London

Kirkwood T 2001 Reith lectures. http://www.bbc.co.uk/radio4/reith2001/

Kitzinger S 1984 The experience of childbirth, 5th edn. Penguin, Harmondsworth

Klaber-Moffett J A, Richardson P H 1995 The influence of psychological variables on the development and perception of musculoskeletal pain. Physiotherapy Theory and Practice 11:3–11

Kleinman A 1988 The illness narratives: suffering, healing and the human condition. Basic Books, New York

Kleinman A, Brodwin P E, Good B J, DelVecchio Good M-J 1992 Pain as human experience: an introduction. In: Delvecchio Good M-J, Brodwin P E, Good B J, Kleinman A (eds) Pain as human experience: an anthropological perspective. University of California Press, Berkeley, pp 1–28

Kline P 1994 An easy guide to factor analysis. Routledge, London

Kogan M 2000 Lifelong learning in the UK. European Journal of Education 35:341–359

Kores R C, Murphy W D, Rosenthal T L, Elias D B, North W C 1990 Predicting outcome of chronic pain treatment via a modified self-efficacy scale. Behaviour Research and Therapy 28:165–169

Kori S H, Miller R P, Todd D D 1990 Kinesiophobia: a new view of chronic pain behavior. Pain Management 3:35–43

Kotarba J A 1983a Chronic pain: its social dimensions. Sage Publications, Beverley Hills

Kotarba J A 1983b Perceptions of death, belief systems and the process of coping with chronic pain. Social Science and Medicine 17:681–689

Kotarba J A, Seidel J V 1984 Managing the problem pain patient: compliance or social control? Social Science and Medicine 19:1393–1400

Kottow M H 1986 Medical confidentiality: an intransigent and absolute obligation. Journal of Medical Ethics 12:117–122

Kottow M H 1994 Stringent and predictable medical confidentiality. In: Gillon R, Lloyd A (eds) Principles of health care ethics. John Wiley, Chichester, pp 471–478

Kouyanou K, Pither C E, Rabe-Hesketh S, Wessely S 1998 A comparative study of iatrogenesis, medication abuse and psychiatric comorbidity in chronic pain patients with and without medically explained symptoms. Pain 76:417–426

Krahe B 1992 Personality and social psychology: towards a synthesis. Sage Publications, London

Kroll D 1990 Equal access to care. Nursing Times 86(23):72–73

Kubler-Ross F 1969 On death and dying. Tavistock Publications, London

Kugelmann R 1999 Complaining about chronic pain. Social Science and Medicine 49:1663–1676

Kuhse H 1995 Clinical ethics and nursing: 'yes' to caring, but 'no' to a female ethics of care. Bioethics 9:207–219

Kumar V 1993 Poverty and inequality in the UK: the effects on children. National Children's Bureau, London

Kumar S 2000 Preface. In: Kumar S (ed) Multidisciplinary approach to rehabilitation. Butterworth-Heinemann, Boston, pp xi–xlv

Kurtz Z 1993 Better health for black and ethnic minority children and young people. In: Hopkins A, Bahl V (eds) Access to health care for people from black and ethnic minorities. Royal College of Physicians, London, p 63–78

Kyler-Hutchison P 1988 Ethical reasoning and informed consent in occupational therapy. American Journal of Occupational Therapy 42:283–287

Lackner S, Goldenberg S, Arrizza G, Tjosvold I 1994 The contingency of social support. Qualitative Health Research 4:224–243

Lackner J, Carosella A, Feuerstein M 1996 Pain expectancies as determinants of disability in patients with chronic low back disorders. Journal of Consulting and Clinical Psychology 64:212–220

Ladd P 1990 Language oppression and hearing impairment. In: Disability – changing practice (k665x) (Book of readings of the disability equality pack). Open University, Milton Keynes, pp 9–14

Lalonde M 1974 A new perspective on the health of Canadians. Ministry of Supply and Services, Ottowa

Lansbury G 2000 Chronic pain management: a qualitative study of elderly people's preferred coping strategies and barriers to management. Disability and Rehabilitation 22:2–14

Largo R H, Howard J A 1979a Developmental progression in play behaviour of children between nine and thirty months: I. Spontaneous play and imitation. Developmental Medicine and Child Neurology 21:299–310

Largo R H, Howard J A 1979b Developmental progression in play behaviour of children between nine and thirty months: II. Spontaneous play and language development. Developmental Medicine and Child Neurology 21:492–503

Larivière C, Gagnon D, Loisel P 2000 The comparison of trunk muscles EMG activation between subjects with and without chronic low back pain during flexion–extension and lateral bending tasks. Journal of Electromyographic Kinesiology 10:79–91

Larue F, Fontaine A, Colleau S M 1997 Underestimation and undertreatment of pain in HIV disease: multicentre study. British Medical Journal 314:23–28

Lavin M A, Ruebling I, Banks R, Block L, Counte M, Furman G, Miller P, Reese C, Viehmann V, Holt J 2001 Interdisciplinary health professional education: a historical review. Advances in Health Sciences Education 6:25–47

Law I 1996 Racism, ethnicity and social policy. Harvester Wheatsheaf, Brighton

Lazarus R, Folkman S 1984 Stress, appraisal and coping. Springer, New York

Le Fanu J 1999 The rise and fall of modern medicine. Little, Brown, London

Leathley M 1988 Physiotherapists and health education: report of a survey. Physiotherapy 74:218–220

Leathley M, Stone S 1986 Shared concerns: reflections on some health education issues which are common to four of the professions allied to medicine. Physiotherapy 72:12–13

Leder D 1990 The absent body. University of Chicago Press, Chicago

Lee M C, Essoka G 1998 Patients' perception of pain: comparison between Korean-American and Euro-American obstetric patients. Journal of Cultural Diversity 5:29–37

Lefcourt H, Davidson-Katz K 1991 The role of humor and the self. In: Snyder C, Forsyth D (eds) Handbook of social and clinical psychology: the health perspective. Pergamon Press, New York, pp 41–56

Lengua L, Stormshak E 2000 Gender, gender roles and personality: gender differences in the prediction of coping and psychological symptoms. Sex Roles 43:787–820

Lennane K J, Lennane R J 1973 Alleged psychogenic disorders in women – a possible manifestation of sexual prejudice. New England Journal of Medicine 288:288–292

Leon D, Walt G 2001 Poverty, inequality and health in international perspective: a divided world? In: Leon D, Walt G (eds) Poverty, inequality, and health: an international perspective. Oxford University Press, Oxford, pp 1–16

Lesser H 1991 The patient's right to information. In: Brazier M, Lobjoit M (eds) Protecting the vulnerable: autonomy and consent in health care. Routledge, London, pp 150–160

Lethem J, Slade P D, Troup J D G, Bentley G 1983 Outline of a fear-avoidance model of exaggerated pain perception. Behaviour Research and Therapy 21:401–408

Levenson J L 1992 Psychosocial interventions in chronic medical illness: an overview of outcome research. General Hospital Psychiatry 14(Suppl. 6):S43–S49

Leventhal H, Everhart D 1979 Emotion, pain and physical illness. In: Izard C A (ed) Emotions in personality and psychopathology. Plenum Press, New York, pp 263–299

Leventhal H, Mosbach P A 1983 The perceptual-motor theory of emotion. In: Cacioppo J T, Petty R E (eds) Social psychophysiology – a sourcebook. Guilford Press, New York, pp 353–388

Leventhal H, Leventhal E A, Schaefer P M 1990 Vigilant coping and health behavior. In: Ory M, Abeles R, Lipman P (eds) Aging, health and behavior. Johns Hopkins Press, Baltimore, pp 109–140

Leventhal H, Benyamini Y, Brownlee S, Diefenbach M, Leventhal E A, Patrik Miller L, Robitaille C 1997 Illness representations: theoretical foundations. In: Petrie K,

Weinman J (eds) Perceptions of health and illness: current research and applications. Harwood Academic Publishers, Singapore, pp 19–46

Leventhal H, Idler E, Leventhal E 1999 The impact of chronic illness on the self system. In: Contrada R, Ashmore R (eds) Self, social identity and physical health. Oxford University Press, Oxford, pp 185–208

Levick P 1992 The Janus face nature of community care legislation: an opportunity for radical possibilities. Critical Social Policy 12:75–92

Levine R, Reicher S 1996 Making sense of symptoms: self-categorisation and the meaning of illness and injury. British Journal of Social Psychology 35:245–256

Lewis C S 1961 A grief observed. Faber and Faber, London

Lewis C B 2002 Aging: the health-care challenge. an interdisciplinary approach to assessment and rehabilitative management of the elderly, 4th edn. F A Davis, Philadelphia

Ley P 1988 Communicating with patients: improving communication, satisfaction and compliance. Croom Helm, London

Liabo K, Curtis K, McNeish D, Roberts H 2002 Consulting children and young people about health services in Camden and Islington. Camden and Islington Health Authority, London

Lilley M 1983 Preventive medicine and the benefit of exercise programmes for the sedentary worker. Physiotherapy 69:8–10

Lillrank A 2003 Back pain and the resolution of diagnostic uncertainty in illness narratives. Social Science and Medicine 57:1045–1054

Lindemann E 1944 Symptomatology and management of acute grief. American Journal of Psychiatry 101:141–148

Linton S 1982 A critical review of behavioural treatment for chronic benign pain other than headache. British Journal of Clinical Psychology 21:311–337

Linton S 1998 Claiming disability: knowledge and identity. New York University Press, New York

Linton S J 2000 A review of psychological risk factors in back and neck pain. Spine 25:1148–1156

Linton S J, Buer N 1995 Working despite pain: factors associated with work attendance versus dysfunction. International Journal of Behavioral Medicine 2:252–262

Linton S J, Gotestam K G 1984 A controlled study of the effects of applied relaxation and applied relaxation plus operant procedures in the regulation of chronic pain. British Journal of Clinical Psychology 23:291–299

Linton S J, Ryberg M 2001 A cognitive behavioural group intervention as prevention for persistent neck and back pain in a non-patient population: a randomized controlled trial. Pain 90:75–82

Lipsky M 1980 Street level bureaucracy: dilemmas of the individual in public service. Russell Sage Foundation, New York

Lipton J A, Marbach J J 1984 Ethnicity and the pain experience. Social Science and Medicine 19:1279–1298

Lloyd N 1999 BJTR and interdisciplinary practice: moving forward. British Journal of Therapy and Rehabilitation 6:573

Lloyd M, Preston-Shoot M, Temple B, Wuu R 1996 Whose project is it anyway? Sharing and shaping the research and development agenda. Disability and Society 11:301–315

Locker D 1983 Disability and disadvantage: the consequences of chronic illness. Tavistock, London

Loewy E H 1989 Textbook of medical ethics. Plenum Publishing, New York

Loewy E H 1997 Developing habits and knowing what habits to develop: a look at the role of virtue in ethics. Cambridge Quarterly of Healthcare Ethics 6:347–355

Lonsdale S 1990 Women and disability: the experience of physical disability among women. Macmillan, London

Lorig K, Castain R L, Ung E, Shoor S, Holman H R 1989 Development and evaluation of a scale to measure perceived self-efficacy in people with arthritis. Arthritis and Rheumatism 32:37–44

Love A W, Peck C L 1987 The MMPI and psychological factors in chronic low back pain: a review. Pain 28:1–12

Lowe M, Costello A J 1988 Manual for the symbolic play test. NFER, Windsor

Ludmerer K M 1999 Instilling professionalism in medical education. Journal of the American Medical Association 282:881–882

Lundmark P, Branholm I 1996 Relationship between occupation and life satisfaction in people with multiple sclerosis. Disability and Rehabilitation 18:449–453

Lupton D 1994 Medicine as culture. Sage Publications, London

Luthe W 1969 Autogenic therapy, vols 1–6. Grune and Stratton, New York

Lyne P A 1985 Health education and the professions allied to medicine. Physiotherapy Practice 1:46–47

Lyne P A 1986 The professions allied to medicine – their potential contribution to health education. Physiotherapy 72:8–10

Lyne P A, Phillipson C 1986 The barriers to health education. Physiotherapy 72:10–12

McAteer M F 1989 Some aspects of grief in physiotherapy. Physiotherapy 75:55–58

McAteer M F 1992 Reactions to terminal illness. Physiotherapy 76:9–12

McAteer M F 1993 The concept of the bodymind in physiotherapy. Physiotherapy Ireland 14:3–5

McCain G A, Bell D A, Mai F M, Halliday P D 1988 A controlled study of the effects of a supervised cardiovascular fitness program of the manifestations of primary fibromyalgia. Arthritis and Rheumatism 31:1135–1141

McCallin A 2001 Interdisciplinary practice – a matter of team work: an integrated literature review. Journal of Clinical Nursing 10:419–428

McComas J, Hebert C, Giacomin C, Kaplan D, Dulberg C 1993 Experiences of student and practicing physical therapists with inappropriate patient sexual behaviour. Physical Therapy 73:769–770

McConkey R 1985 Working with parents: a practical guide for teachers and therapists. Croom Helm, London

McConkey R, Martin H 1980 The development of pretend play in Down's syndrome infants: a longitudinal study. St Michael's House, Dublin

McConway K 1994 The web of explanations. In: McConway K (ed) Studying health and disease. Open University Press, Buckingham, pp 127–131

McCracken L M, Zayfert C, Gross R T 1992 The pain anxiety symptoms scale: development and validation of a scale to measure fear of pain. Pain 50:63–67

McCubbin J A, Kaufmann P G, Nemeroff C B 1991 Stress, neuropeptides and systemic disease. Academic Press, San Diego

McCune-Nicholich L 1977 Beyond sensori-motor intelligence: assessment of symbolic maturity through analysis of pretend play. Merrill-Palmer Quarterly 23:88–99

MacDonald L 1988 The experience of stigma: living with rectal cancer. In: Anderson R, Bury M (eds) Living with chronic illness: the experience of patients and their families. Unwin, London, pp 177–202

McDonald M V, Pasik S D, Dugan W, Rosenfeld B, Theobald D E, Edgerton S 1999 Nurses' recognition of depression in their patients with cancer. Oncology Nursing Forum 26:593–599

Macfarlane A 1990 Official statistics and women's health and illness. In: Roberts H (ed) Women's health counts. Routledge, London, pp 18–62

Macfarlane A J, Mugford M 2000 Birth counts: statistics of pregnancy and childbirth: 1, 2nd edn. Stationery Office, London

Macfarlane A J, Mugford M, Henderson J, Furtado A, Stevens J, Dunn A 2000 Birth counts: statistics of pregnancy and childbirth: 2, 2nd edn. Stationery Office, London

McGaghie W C, Mytko J J, Brown W N, Cameron J R 2002 Altruism and compassion in the health professions: a search for clarity and precision. Medical Teacher 24: 374–378

McGinn C 1982 The character of mind. Oxford University Press, Oxford

McGuire F, Boyd R 1993 The role of humor in enhancing the quality of later life. In: Kelly J (ed) Activity and aging: staying involved in later life. Sage Publications, Newbury Park, pp 164–173

McIlwaine G, Rosenberg K, Rooney I 1989 The health of mid-life inner city women. Journal of Psychosomatic Obstetrics and Gynaecology 10(Suppl. 1):102

McIntosh J M 1989 Women – the captive audience. Physiotherapy 75:10–13

MacIntyre A 1985 After virtue: a study in moral theory, 2nd edn. Duckworth, London

McKay E A, Ryan S 1995 Clinical reasoning through story telling: examining a student's case story on fieldwork placement. British Journal of Occupational Therapy 58: 234–238

McKeown T 1984 The medical contribution. In: Black N, Boswell D, Gray A, Murphy S, Popay J (eds) Health and disease: a reader. Open University Press, Buckingham, pp 107–114

McKnight J 1995 The careless society. Basic Books, New York

McLeod J 1998a An introduction to counselling, 2nd edn. Open University Press, Buckingham

McLeod J 1998b Listening to stories about illness and health: applying the lessons of narrative psychology. In: Bayne R, Nicolson P, Horton I (eds) Counselling and communication skills for medical and health practitioners. British Psychological Society, Leicester, pp 51–64

McLeod J 1999 Counselling as a social process. Counselling 10:217–222

McMahon C E 1975 Harvey on the soul: a unique episode in the history of psycho-physiological thought. Journal of the History of the Behavioral Sciences 11:276–283

McMurdo M E T 2000 A healthy old age: realistic or futile goal? British Medical Journal 321:1149–1151

MacPherson K I 1989 A new perspective on nursing and caring in a corporate context. Advances in Nursing Science 11:32–39

McPherson K 1997 Variations in hospital treatment rates for common conditions. In: McPherson A, Waller D (eds) Women's health, 4th edn. Oxford University Press, Oxford, pp 60–68

McPherson A, Waller D 1997 Women's health, 4th edn. Oxford University Press, Oxford

Maes S, Leventhal H, De Ridder D 1996 Coping with chronic illness. In: Zeidner M, Endler N (eds) Handbook of coping: theory, research, applications. Wiley, New York, pp 221–251

Main C J 2000 Assessment of social, economic and occupational factors. In: Main C J, Spanswick C C (eds) Pain management – an interdisciplinary approach. Churchill Livingstone, Edinburgh, pp 223–232

Main C J, Spanswick C C 1995 Personality assessment and the Minnesota multiphasic personality inventory: 50 years on. Do we still need our security blanket? Pain Forum 4:90–96

Main C, Waddell G 1991 A comparison of cognitive measures in low back pain: statistical structure and clinical validity at initial assessment. Pain 46:287–298

Main C J, Wood P L, Hollis S, Spanswick C C, Waddell G 1992 The distress and risk assessment method: a simple patient classification to identify distress and evaluate the risk of poor outcome. Spine 17:42–51

Maniadakis N, Gray A 2000 The economic burden of back pain in the UK. Pain 84:95–103

Manne S, Zautra A 1989 Spouse criticism and support: their association with coping and psychological adjustment among women with rheumatoid arthritis. Journal of Personality and Social Psychology 56:608–617

Mannerkorpi K, Kroksmark T, Ekdahl C 1999 How patients with fibromyalgia experience their symptoms in everyday life. Physiotherapy Research International 4: 110–122

Marks A 1999 Really useful knowledge: the new vocationalism in higher education and its consequences for mature students. British Journal of Educational Studies 47:157–169

Marmot M 2001 A social view of health and disease. In: Heller T, Muston R, Sidell M, Lloyd C (eds) Working for health. Sage Publications, London, pp 55–68

Marshall K, Walsh D M 1994 Health of mother and child: striking the balance. Physiotherapy 80:767–771

Martin L, Nutting A, MacIntosh B R, Edworthy S M, Butterwick D, Cook J 1996 An exercise program in the treatment of fibromyalgia. Journal of Rheumatology 23: 1050–1053

Martlew B 1996 What do you let the patient tell you? Physiotherapy 82:558–565

Mason V 1989 Women's experience of maternity care: a survey manual. HMSO, London

Mason M 1992 Internalised oppression. In: Rieser R, Mason M (eds) Disability equality in the classroom: a human rights issue, 2nd edn. Disability Equality in Education, London, pp 27–28

Mason D 2000 Race and ethnicity in modern Britain. Oxford University Press, Oxford

Mathews A, Steptoe A 1988 Essential psychology for medical practice. Churchill Livingstone, London

Mattingly C 1998 Healing dramas and clinical plots: the narrative structure of experience. Cambridge University Press, Cambridge

May D 2000 Becoming adult: school leaving, jobs and the transition to adult life. In: May D (ed) Transition and change in the lives of people with intellectual disabilities. Jessica Kingsley, London, pp 75–95

May C, Doyle H, Chew-Graham C 2002 Medical knowledge and the intractable patient: the case of chronic low back pain. Social Science and Medicine 48:523–534

Mayer R 1991 Living with amyotrophic lateral sclerosis. Loss, Grief and Care 4:23–30

Meager N, Buchan J, Rees C 1989 Job sharing in the NHS. Institute of Manpower Studies, University of Sussex, Brighton

Mearns D, Thorne B 1999 Person-centred counselling in action, 2nd edn. Sage Publications, London

Mearns D, Thorne B 2000 Person-centred therapy today: new frontiers in theory and practice. Sage Publications, London

Melia K 1989 Everyday nursing ethics. Macmillan, London

Meltzoff A N, Moore M K 1985 Cognitive foundations and social functions of imitation and intermodal representation in infancy. In: Mehler J, Fox R (eds) Neonate cognition: beyond the blooming buzzing confusion. Lawrence Erlbaum, Hillsdale, pp 139–156

Melzack R, Dennis S G 1980 Phylogenetic evolution of pain expression in animals. In: Kosterlitz H W, Terenius L Y (eds) Pain and society. Verlag Chemie, Weinheim

Melzack R, Katz J 2001 The McGill pain questionnaire: appraisal and current status. In: Turk D C, Melzack R (eds) Handbook of pain assessment, 2nd edn. Guilford Press, New York, pp 35–52

Melzack R, Wall P D 1965 Pain mechanisms: a new theory. Science 150:971–979

Melzack R, Wall P 1982 The challenge of pain, revised edn. Penguin Books, Harmondsworth

Melzack R, Wall P D 1988 The challenge of pain. Penguin Books, Harmondsworth

Melzack R, Guite S, Gonshor A 1980 Relief of dental pain by ice massage of the hand. Canadian Medical Association Journal 122:189–191

Mercado A, Carroll L J, Cassidy J D, Cote P 2000 Coping with neck and low back pain in the general population. Health Psychology 19:333–338

Merleau-Ponty M 1996 Phenomenology of perception, 10th edn. Routledge and Kegan Paul, London

Merry T 2002 Learning and being in person-centred counselling, 2nd edn. PCCS Books, Ross-on-Wye

Merskey H 1980 Some features of the history of the idea of pain. Pain 9:3–8

Miell D, Croghan R 1996 Examining the wider context of social relationships. In: Miell D, Dallos R (eds) Social interaction and personal relationships. Sage Publications, London, pp 267–318

Milani-Comparetti A, Gidoni E A 1967 Routine developmental examination in normal and retarded children. Developmental Medicine and Child Neurology 9:631–638

Miller P A, Geddes E L, Edey L E 1996 Loss, grief and the therapeutic relationship. Physiotherapy Canada 48: 240–243

Mills D 1994 Variability in cerebral organization during primary language acquisition. In: Dawson G, Fischer K (eds) Human behaviour and the developing brain. Guilford Press, New York, pp 427–455

Minardi H A, Riley M J 1997 Communication in health care: a skills-based approach. Butterworth-Heinemann, Oxford

Mirvis D M 1993 Physicians' autonomy – the relation between public and professional expectations. New England Journal of Medicine 328:1346–1349

Mitchell P 1992 The psychology of childhood. Falmer Press, London

Modood T, Betthould R, Lakey J, Nazroo J, Smith J, Virdde S, Beishon S 1997 Ethnic minorities in Britain. Social Policy Studies Institute, London

Mohr D, Dick L, Russo D, Pinn J, Boudewyn A C, Likosky W, Goodkin D E 1999 The psychosocial impact of multiple sclerosis: exploring the patient's perspective. Health Psychology 18:376–382

Moore M 2000 (ed) Insider perspectives on inclusion. Philip Armstrong Publications, Sheffield

Moore M, Beazley S, Maelzer J 1998a Researching disability issues. Open University Press, Buckingham

Moore R, Brodsgaard I, Mao T K, Miller M L, Dworkin S F 1998b Acute pain and use of local anesthesia: tooth drilling and childbirth labor pain beliefs among Anglo-Americans, Chinese, and Scandinavians. Anesthesia Progress 45:29–37

Moos R, Schaefer J 1984 The crisis of physical illness: an overview and conceptual approach. In: Moos R (ed) Coping with physical illness: 2. New perspectives. Plenum, New York, pp 3–25

Morgan M, Calnan M, Manning N 1988 Sociological approaches to health and medicine. Routledge, London

Morley S, Eccleston C, Williams A 1999 Systematic review and meta-analysis of randomized controlled trials of cognitive behaviour therapy and behaviour therapy for chronic pain in adults, excluding headache. Pain 80:1–13

Morris J 1989 Able lives: women's experience of paralysis. Women's Press, London

Morris D B 1991a The culture of pain. University of California Press, Berkeley

Morris J 1991b Pride against prejudice: transforming attitudes to disability. Women's Press, London

Morris J 1993 Prejudice. In: Swain J, Finkelstein V, French S, Oliver M (eds) Disabling barriers – enabling environments. Sage Publications, London, pp 101–106

Morris J 1995 Pride against prejudice: 'lives not worth living'. In: Davey B, Gray A, Seale C (eds) Health and disease: a reader, 2nd edn. Open University Press, Buckingham, pp 107–110

Morris J 1996 Encounters with strangers: feminism and disability. Women's Press, London

Morrison P 1989 Nursing and caring: a personal construct theory study of some nurses' self-perceptions. Journal of Advanced Nursing 14:421–426

Muir D 1989 Look after yourself. Nursing Times 85(36):59–61

Mullins L L, Cote M P, Fuemmeler B F, Jean V M, Beatty W W, Paul R H 2001 Illness intrusiveness, uncertainty, and distress in individuals with multiple sclerosis. Rehabilitation Psychology 46:139–153

Munro K, Elder-Woodward K 1992 Independent living. Churchill Livingstone, Edinburgh

Murphy F A, Hunt F C 1997 Early pregnancy loss: men have feelings too. British Journal of Midwifery 5:87–90

Murray R 1998 Communicating about ethical dilemmas: a medical humanities approach. In: Bayne R, Nicolson P, Horton I (eds) Counselling and communication skills for medical and health practitioners. British Psychological Society, Leicester, pp 189–203

Murray-Parkes C 1972 Components of the reaction to loss of a limb, spouse or home. Journal of Psychosomatic Research 16:343–349

Murray-Parkes C 1975 Bereavement. Penguin, Harmondsworth

Murray-Parkes C 1985 Bereavement. British Journal of Psychiatry 146:11–17

Na Y M, Kim M Y, Kim Y K, Ha Y R, Yoon D S 2000 Exercise therapy effect on natural killer cell cytotoxic activity stomach cancer patients after curative surgery. Archives of Physical Medicine and Rehabilitation 81:777–779

National Children's Homes Action for Children 1998 Fact file. National Children's Homes, London

Nayak S, Shiflett S C, Eshun S, Levine F M 2000 Culture and gender effects in pain beliefs and the prediction of pain tolerance. Cross-Cultural Research 34:135–151

Nazroo J 1998 The health of Britain's ethnic minorities. Policy Studies Institute, London

Newbeck I 1986 The whole works. Nursing Times 82:48–49

Newbeck I, Rowe D 1986 Going the whole way. Nursing Times 82:24–25

Newman G 1997 Physiotherapy recruitment and retention: a crisis. British Journal of Therapy and Rehabilitation 4: 355–356

Newman G 2001 Can the NHS hold onto new PAM graduates? British Journal of Therapy and Rehabilitation 10:365

NICHD Early Child Care Research Network 1997 The effects of infant child care on infant–mother attachment security. Child Development 68:860–879

NICHD Early Child Care Research Network 1999 Child care and mother child interaction in the first three years of life. Developmental Psychology 35:1399–1413

NICHD Early Child Care Research Network 2000 The relation of child care to cognitive and language development. Child Development 71:958–978

Nicholas M K 1989 Self-efficacy and chronic pain. Paper presented to the British Psychological Society Annual Conference

Nicholson R H 1994 Limitations of the four principles. In: Gillon R, Lloyd A (eds) Principles of health care ethics. John Wiley, Chichester, pp 267–275

Nielson W R, Weir R 2001 Biopsychosocial approaches to the treatment of chronic pain. Clinical Journal of Pain 17: S114–S127

Nightingale D J, Cromby J 1999 Social constructionist psychology: a critical analysis of theory and practice. Open University Press, Buckingham

Nind M, Hewett D 1994 Access to communication. Fulton, London

Noddings N 1984 Caring: a feminine approach to ethics and moral education. University of California Press, Berkeley

Northouse P G, Northouse L L 1998 Health communication: strategies for health professionals, 3rd edn. Appleton and Lange, Norwalk

O'Brien J, Chantler C 2003 Confidentiality and the duties of care. Journal of Medical Ethics 29:36–40

O'Donohue J 1997 Anam cara: spiritual wisdom from the Celtic world. Bantam Books, London

O'Gorman S M 1998 Death and dying in contemporary society. Journal of Advanced Nursing 27:1127–1135

O'Hara P 1996 Pain management for health professionals. Chapman and Hall, London

O'Leary A, Brown S 1995 Self-efficacy and the physiological stress response. In: Maddux J E (ed) Self-efficacy, adaptation and adjustment: theory, research, and applications. Plenum Press, New York, pp 227–246

Oakley A 1981 From here to maternity. Penguin, Harmondsworth

Oakley J 1998 A virtue ethics approach. In: Kuhse H, Singer P (eds) A companion to bioethics. Blackwell, Oxford, pp 86–97

Office for National Statistics 2000 Labour market status for women with young children. Labour Market Trends 108:10

Ohnuki-Tierney E 1981 Illness and healing among the Sakhalin Ainu: a symbolic interpretation. Cambridge University Press, Cambridge

Olders H 1989 Mourning and grief as healing processes in psychotherapy. Canadian Journal of Psychiatry 34: 271–278

Oliver M 1983 Social work with disabled people. Macmillan, London

Oliver M 1990 The politics of disablement, Macmillan, London

Oliver M 1991 Disability and participation in the labour market. In: Brown P, Scase R (eds) Poor work. Open University Press, Milton Keynes, pp 132–145

Oliver M 1992 Changing the social relations of research production. Disability, Handicap and Society 7:101–115

Oliver M 1993a Re-defining disability: a challenge to research. In: Swain J, Finkelstein V, French S, Oliver M (eds) Disabling barriers – enabling environments. Sage Publications, London, pp 61–67

Oliver M 1993b Disability and dependency: a creation of industrial societies? In: Swain J, Finkelstein V, French S, Oliver M (eds) Disabling barriers – enabling environments. Sage Publications, London, pp 49–60

Oliver M 1996a Understanding disability: from theory to practice. Macmillan, London

Oliver M 1996b Defining impairment and disability: issues at stake. In: Barnes C, Mercer M (eds) Exploring the divide: illness and disability. Disability Press, Leeds, pp 39–54

Oliver M 1997 Emancipatory research: realistic goal or impossible dream? In: Barnes C, Mercer G (eds) Doing disability research. Disability Press, Leeds, pp 15–31

Oliver M, Barnes C 1998 Disabled people and social policy: from exclusion to inclusion. Longman, London

Oliver M, Sapey B 1999 Social work with disabled people, 2nd edn. Macmillan, London

Onuoha A R A 1981 A degree course is the answer. Physiotherapy 67:70

Orem D E 1991 Nursing: concepts of practice, 4th edn. Mosby, London

Ortner D, Theobald G 1993 Diseases in the pre-Roman world. In: Kiple K (ed) The Cambridge world history of human disease. Cambridge University Press, Cambridge, pp 247–261

Osborn M, Smith J A 1998 The personal experience of chronic benign lower back pain: an interpretive phenomenological analysis. British Journal of Health Psychology 3:65–83

Owen D 1993 Ethnic minorities in Britain: age and gender structure. University of Warwick National Ethnic Minority Data Archive, 1991 Census Statistical Paper no. 2. University of Warwick, Coventry

Pain Society 1997 Desirable criteria for pain management programmes: report of a working party of the Pain Society of Great Britain and Ireland. Pain Society, London

Pakenham K 1999 Adjustment to multiple sclerosis: application of a stress and coping model. Health Psychology 18:383–392

Palmer N, Peacock C, Turner F, Vasey B, Williams V 1999 Telling people what you think. In: Swain J, French S (eds) Therapy and learning difficulties: advocacy, participation and partnership. Butterworth-Heinemann, Oxford, pp 33–47

Parr S, Byng S, Gilpin S, Ireland C 1997 Talking about aphasia. Open University Press, Buckingham

Parry A W 1991 Physiotherapy and methods of enquiry: conflict and reconciliation. Physiotherapy 77:435–438

Parry A W 1995 Ginger Rogers did everything Fred Astaire did backwards and in high heels. Physiotherapy 81: 310–319

Parsons T 1951 The social system. Routledge and Kegan Paul, London

Parsons T 1968 Professions. In: Sills D L (ed) International encyclopedia of the social sciences. Macmillan Press and Free Press, New York, pp 536–547

Payne R 1989 Glad to be yourself: a course of practical relaxation and health education talks. Physiotherapy 75:8–9

Payne M 2000 Narrative therapy: an introduction for counsellors. Sage Publications, London

Payne P 2001 Food, health and disease: a case study. In: Gray A (ed) World health and disease. Open University Press, Buckingham, pp 259–317

Pearce W B 1994 Interpersonal communication: making social worlds. HarperCollins, New York

Pearce J, Morley S 1989 An experimental investigation of the construct validity of the McGill pain questionnaire. Pain 39:115–121

Pearce S A, Isherwood S, Hrouda D, Richardson P H, Erskine A, Skinner J 1990 Memory and pain: test of mood congruity and state dependent learning in induced and clinical pain. Pain 42:187–193

Peat M 1981 Physiotherapy: art or science? Physiotherapy Canada 33:170–176

Peat G M, Moores L, Goldinghay S, Hunter M 2001 Pain management program follow-ups: a national survey of current practice in the United Kingdom. Journal of Pain and Symptom Management 21:218–226

Pellegrino E D 1979 Toward a reconstruction of medical morality: the primacy of the act of profession and the fact of illness. Journal of Medicine and Philosophy 4: 32–56

Pellegrino E D, Thomasma D C 1988 For the patient's good: the restoration of beneficence in health care. Oxford University Press, New York

Pellegrino E D, Thomasma D C 1993 The virtues in medical practice. Oxford University Press, New York

Pelling M, Berridge V, Harrison M, Weindling P 1993 The era of public health, 1848 to 1918. In: Webster C (ed) Caring for health: history and diversity. Open University Press, Buckingham, pp 63–86

Peolsson M, Säljö R, Sätterlung Larsson U 2000 Experiencing and knowing pain – patients' perspectives. Advances in Physiotherapy 2:146–155

Perkins R, Barnett P, Powell M 2000 Corporate governance of public health services: lessons from New Zealand for the state sector. Australian Health Review 23:9–21

Perner J, Leekham S R, Winner M 1987 Three-year-olds' difficulty with false belief: the case for a conceptual deficit. British Journal of Developmental Psychology 5:125–137

Petrie K, Buick D, Weinman J, Booth R 1999 Positive effects of illness reported by myocardial infarction and breast cancer patients. Journal of Psychosomatic Research 47: 537–543

Petticrew M, Roberts H 2003 Evidence, hierarchies and typologies: horses for courses. Journal of Epidemiology and Community Health 57:527–529

Pfefferbaum B, Gurwitch R H, McDonald N B, Leftwich M J, Sconzo G M, Messenbaugh A K, Schultz R A 2000 Post traumatic stress among young children after the death of a friend or acquaintance in a terrorist bombing. Psychiatric Services 51:386–388

Pfeiffer D 2000 The devils are in the details: the ICIDH2 and the disability movement. Disability and Society 15: 1079–1082

Philips H 1988 Changing chronic pain experience. Pain 32: 165–307

Phillipson C 1982 Capitalism and the construction of old age. Macmillan, London

Phillipson C 1994 Modernity and post-modernity and the sociology of ageing: reformulating critical gerontology. Paper presented at XII World Congress of Sociology, Bielefeld, Germany

Phillipson C 1998 Reconstructing old age: new agendas in social theory and practice. Sage Publications, London

Piachaud D 1985 Round about fifty hours a week. Child Poverty Action Group, London

Piaget J 1951 Play, dreams and imitation in childhood. Routledge and Kegan Paul, London

Piaget J 1953 The origin of intelligence in the child. Routledge and Kegan Paul, London

Piaget J 1955 The child's construction of reality. Routledge and Kegan Paul, London

Pickles B, Compton A, Simpson J, Vandervoort A 1995 Physiotherapy with older people. W B Saunders, London

Piercy J M 1979 Physiotherapy education: what is the future? Physiotherapy 65:186–187

Pietroni P 1987 Holistic medicine: new lessons to be learned. Practitioner 231:1386–1390

Pincus T 1998 Assessing psychological factors in chronic pain – a new approach. Physical Therapy Reviews 3: 41–45

Pincus T, Morley S 2001 Cognitive processing bias in chronic pain: a review and integration. Psychological Bulletin 127:599–617

Pincus T, Williams A 1999 Models and measurements of depression in chronic pain. Journal of Psychosomatic Research 47:211–219

Pincus T, Callahan L F, Bradley L A, Vaughn W K, Wolfe F 1986 Elevated MMPI scores for hypochondriasis, depression, and hysteria in patients with rheumatoid arthritis reflect disease rather than psychological status. Arthritis and Rheumatism 29:1456–1466

Pincus T, Pearce S, McClelland A, Turner-Stokes L 1993 Self-referential selective memory in pain patients. British Journal of Clinical Psychology 32:365–374

Pincus T, Pearce S, McClelland A, Isenberg D 1995 Endorsement and memory bias of self-referential pain stimuli in depressed pain patients. British Journal of Clinical Psychology 34:267–277

Pincus T, Pearce S, Perrott A 1996 Pain patients' bias in the interpretation of ambiguous homophones. British Journal of Medical Psychology 69:259–266

Pincus T, Fraser L, Pearce S 1998 Do chronic pain patients 'Stroop' on pain stimuli? British Journal of Clinical Psychology 37:49–58

Pincus T, Burton A K, Vogel S, Field A P 2002 A systematic review of psychological factors as predictors of chronicity/disability in prospective cohorts of low back pain. Spine 27:E109–E120

Pinker S 1997 How the mind works. Norton, New York

Pither C, Nicholas M 1991 The identification of iatrogenic factors in the development of chronic pain syndromes: abnormal treatment behaviour? In: Bond M R, Charlton J R, Wolff C J (eds) Proceedings of the Sixth World Congress on Pain. Elsevier Science, Amsterdam, pp 429–434

Plowden B H 1967 Children and their primary schools: a report of the Central Advisory Council. Vol. 1: The report. HMSO, London

Plummer K 2001 Documents of life 2. An invitation to critical humanism. Sage Publications, London

Popay J 1991 Women's experience of ill health. In: Roberts H (ed) Women's health matters. Routledge, London, pp 99–120

Popper K 1972 Conjectures and reflections: the growth of scientific knowledge. Routledge and Kegan Paul, London

Porter R 1996 Introduction. In: Porter R (ed) Cambridge illustrated history of medicine. Cambridge University Press, Cambridge, pp 6–15

Potter C A, Whittaker C A 1997 Teaching the spontaneous use of semantic relations through multipointing to a child with autism and severe learning difficulties. Child Language Teaching and Therapy 132:177–193

Potter C A, Whittaker C A 2001 Enabling communication in children with autism. Jessica Kingsley, London

Potts M, Fido R 1991 A fit person to be removed: personal accounts of life in a mental deficiency institution. Northcote House, Plymouth

Pratt J W 1989 Towards a philosophy of physiotherapy. Physiotherapy 75:114–120

Prentice E D, Purtilo R B 1993 The use and protection of human and animal subjects. In: Bork C E (ed) Research in physical therapy. J B Lippincott, Philadelphia, pp 37–56

Price B 1996 Illness careers: the chronic illness experience. Journal of Advanced Nursing 24:275–279

Price D D 1999 Psychological mechanisms of pain and analgesia. Progress in Pain Research and Management, vol. 15. IASP Press, Seattle

Price D D, Harkins S W 1992a Psychological approaches to pain measurement and assessment. In: Turk D C, Melzack R (eds) Handbook of pain assessment. Guilford Press, New York, pp 111–134

Price D D, Harkins S W 1992b The affective-motivational dimension of pain: a two stage model. American Pain Society Journal 1:229–239

Priestley M 1999 Disability politics and community care. Jessica Kingsley, London

Prigerson H G, Maciejewski P K, Rosenheck R A 2000 Preliminary explorations of the harmful interactive effects of widowhood and martial harmony on health, health service use, and health care costs. Gerontologist 40:349–357

Purtilo R B 1977 The American Physical Therapy Association's code of ethics. Physical Therapy 57: 1001–1006

Purtilo R B 1984 Applying the principles of informed consent to patient care: legal and ethical considerations for physical therapy. Physical Therapy 64:934–937

Purtilo R 1986 Professional responsibility in physiotherapy: old dimensions and new directions. Physiotherapy 72: 579–583

Purtilo R B 1987 Codes of ethics in physiotherapy: a retrospective view and look ahead. Physiotherapy Practice 3:28–34

Quadagno J 1990 Generational equity and the politics of the welfare state. International Journal of Health Services 20: 631–649

Quigley D G, Schatz M S 1999 Men and women and their responses in spousal bereavement. Hospice Journal 14: 65–78

Rachels J 1993 The elements of moral philosophy, 2nd edn. McGraw-Hill, New York

Radloff L 1977 The CES-D scale: a self-report depression scale for research in the general population. Applied Psychological Measurement 1:385–401

Ramchandani D 1996 Pathological grief: two Victorian case studies. Psychiatry Quarterly 67:75–84

Raue P J, Goldfried M R 1997 The therapeutic alliance in psychodynamic-interpersonal and cognitive-behavioral therapy. Journal of Consulting and Clinical Psychology 65:582–587

Ray M A 1989 The theory of bureaucratic caring for nursing practice in the organizational culture. Nursing Administration Quarterly 13:31–42

Raymond M-C, Brown J B 2002 Experience of fibromyalgia: qualitative study. Canadian Family Physician 46: 1100–1106

Raz J 1986 The morality of freedom. Oxford University Press, Oxford

Read J 1988 The equal opportunities book. InterChange Books, London

Reason P, Heron J 1986 Research with people: the paradigm of co-operative experiential enquiry. Person-Centred Review 1:456–476

Reber A S 1985 The Penguin dictionary of psychology. Penguin Books, Harmondsworth

Reeve C 1999 Still me. Arrow Books, London

Reeves P, Merriam S, Courtenay B 1999 Adaptation to HIV infection: the development of coping strategies over time. Qualitative Health Research 9:344–361

Reid J, Ewan C, Lowy E 1991 Pilgrimage of pain: the illness experiences of women with repetition strain injury and the search for credibility. Social Science and Medicine 32: 601–612

Reimers S, Treacher A 1995 Introducing user-friendly family therapy. Routledge, London

Rennell T 2000 Last days of glory: the death of Queen Victoria. Viking, London

Rey R 1995 The history of pain. Harvard University Press, Cambridge

Reynolds F 1997 Coping with chronic illness and disability through creative needlecraft. British Journal of Occupational Therapy 60:352–356

Reynolds F 2001 Strategies for facilitating physical activity and wellbeing: a health promotion perspective. British Journal of Occupational Therapy 64: 330–336

Ribbens J 1994 Mothers and their children: a feminist sociology of childrearing. Sage Publications, London

Richardson B 1992 Professional education and professional practice today – do they match? Physiotherapy 78:23–26

Richardson B 1999a Professional development 1. Professional socialisation and professionalisation. Physiotherapy 85:461–467

Richardson B 1999b Professional development 2. Professional knowledge and situated learning in the workplace. Physiotherapy 85:467–474

Riches D 2000 The holistic person; or, the ideology of egalitarianism. Journal of the Royal Anthropological Institute 6:669–685

Rieser R 2001 The struggle for inclusion: the growth of a movement. In: Barton L (ed) Disability politics and the struggle for change. David Fulton Publishers, London, pp 132–148

Riikonen E, Smith G M 1997 Re-imagining therapy: living conversation and relational knowledge. Sage Publications, London

Ritchie J E 1989 Keeping Australians healthy: the challenge to physiotherapy practice posed by the concept of the new public health. Australian Journal of Physiotherapy 35:101–107

Ritchie J E 1999 Using qualitative research to enhance the evidence-based practice of health care providers. Australian Journal of Physiotherapy 45:251–256

Ritz T 2001 Relaxation therapy in adult asthma: is there new evidence for effectiveness? Behavior Modification 25: 640–666

Roberts P 1994 Theoretical models of physiotherapy. Physiotherapy 80:361–366

Roberts H, Smith S J, Bryce C 1995 Children at risk: safety as a social value. Open University Press, Buckingham

Robertson A 1991 The politics of Alzheimer's disease: a case study in apocalyptic demography. In: Minkler M, Estes C (eds) Critical perspectives on aging: the political and moral economy of growing old. Baywood, Amityville, pp 135–150

Robinson Y K 1986 Teaching adults: some issues in adult education for health education. Physiotherapy 72:49–52

Robinson I 1988 Multiple sclerosis. Routledge, London

Robinson M 2001 Communication and health in a multi-ethnic society. Policy Press, Bristol

Rocherson Y 1988 The Asian mother and baby campaign: the construction of ethnic minority health needs. Critical Social Policy 22:4–23

Rodmell S, Watt A 1986 The politics of health education: raising the issues. Routledge, London

Rogers C R 1961 On becoming a person. Houghton Mifflin, Boston

Rogers C R 1975 Empathic: an unappreciated way of being. Counselling Psychologist 5:2–10

Rogers C R 1978 Carl Rogers on person power: inner strength and its revolutionary impact. Constable, London

Rogers C R 1983 Freedom to learn for the 80s. Charles E Merrill, Colombus

Rogers C R, Stevens B 1967 Person to person: the problem of being human. Real People Press, Layfayette

Romano J M, Turner J A 1985 Chronic pain and depression: does the evidence support a relationship? Psychological Bulletin 97:18–34

Romano J, Turner J, Jensen M, Friedman L, Bulcroft R, Hops H, Wright S 1995 Chronic pain patient–spouse behavioral interactions predict patient disability. Pain 63:353–360

Rose H, Rose S 2001 Alas poor Darwin: arguments against evolutionary psychology. Vantage, London

Rosenberg M 2000 Life expectancy. About.com [accessed 27.05.01]. http://geography.about.com/science/geography/library/weekly/aa042000a.htm

Rosenblatt D 1977 Developmental trends in infant play. In: Tizard B, Harvey D (eds) Biology of play. Heinemann, London, pp 33–44

Rosentiel A K, Keefe F J 1983 The use of coping strategies in chronic low back pain patients: relationship to patient characteristics and current adjustment. Pain 17:33–44

Rosmus C, Johnston C C, Chan-Yip A, Yang F 2000 Pain response in Chinese and non-Chinese Canadian infants: is there a difference? Social Science and Medicine 51:175–184

Ross M M, Carswell A, Hing M, Hollingworth G, Dalziel W B 2001 Seniors' decision making about pain management. Journal of Advanced Nursing 35:442–451

Rozemond M 1995 Descartes's case for dualism. Journal of the History of Philosophy 33:29–63

Rozemond M 1999 Descartes on mind–body interaction: what's the problem? Journal of the History of Philosophy 37:435–467

Rungapadiachy D V 1999 Interpersonal communication and psychology for health care professionals: theory and practice. Butterworth-Heinemann, Oxford

Russell M 1998 Beyond ramps: disability at the end of the social contract. Common Courage Press, Monroe

Ryan S E 1999 Why narratives? In: Ryan S E, McKay E A (eds) Thinking and reasoning in therapy: narratives from practice. Stanley Thornes, Cheltenham, pp 1–15

Ryan T, Holman A 1998 Able and willing: supporting people with learning difficulties to use direct payments. Values into Action, London

Ryan S E, McKay E A 1999 Thinking and reasoning in therapy: narratives from practice. Stanley Thornes, Cheltenham

Ryan J, Thomas F 1987 The politics of mental handicap, 2nd edn. Free Association Books, London

Ryden M B, McCarthy P R, Lewis M L, Sherman C 1991 A behavioural comparison of the helping style of nursing students, psychotherapists, crisis interveners, and untrained individuals. Archives of Psychiatric Nursing 5:185–188

Ryle G 1973 The concept of mind. Penguin, Harmondsworth

Sackett D L, Straus S E, Richardson W S, Rosenberg W, Haynes R B 2000 Evidence based medicine: how to practice and teach EBM, 2nd edn. Churchill Livingstone, Edinburgh

Sailors P R 2001 Autonomy, benevolence and Alzheimer's disease. Cambridge Quarterly of Healthcare Ethics 10:184–193

Sanders S H 1985 Chronic pain: conceptualization and epidemiology. Annals of Behavioral Medicine 7:3–5

Sanders C, Donovan J, Dieppe P 2002 The significance and consequences of having painful and disabled joints in older age: co-existing accounts of normal and disrupted biographies. Sociology of Health and Illness 24:227–253

Santana M A, Dancy B L 2000 The stigma of being named 'AIDS carriers' on Haitian-American women. Health Care for Women International 21:161–171

Saraga E 1998a Embodying the social: constructions of difference. Routledge, London

Saraga E 1998b Abnormal, unnatural and immoral? The social construction of sexualities. In: Saraga E (ed) Embodying the social: constructions of difference. Routledge, London, pp 139–188

Saraga E 1998c Review. In: Saraga E (ed) Embodying the social: constructions of difference. Routledge, London, pp 189–206

Scambler G 2003 Sociology as applied to medicine, 5th edn. Saunders, London

Scarry E 1985 The body in pain: the making and unmaking of the world. Oxford University Press, New York

Schaefer K M 1995 Struggling to maintain balance: a study of women living with fibromyalgia. Journal of Advanced Nursing 21:95–102

Schaefer K M 1997 Health patterns of women with fibromyalgia. Journal of Advanced Nursing 26:565–571

Schaffer H R 1971 The growth of sociability. Penguin, Harmondsworth

Schaffer H R 1977 Studies in mother–infant interaction. Academic Press, London

Schafheute E I, Cantrill J A, Noyce P R 2001 Why is pain management suboptimal on surgical wards? Journal of Advanced Nursing 33:728–737

Scharloo M, Kaptein A 1997 Measurement of illness perceptions in patients with chronic somatic illness: a review. In: Petrie K, Weinman J (eds) Perceptions of health and illness: current research and applications. Harwood Academic Publishers, Singapore, pp 103–154

Scheper-Hughes N, Lock M 1987 The mindful body: a prolegomenon to future work in medical anthropology. Medical Anthropology Quarterly 1:6–41

Schleifer S J, Keller S E, Camerino M, Thornton J C, Stein M 1983 Suppression of lymphocyte stimulation following bereavement. Journal of the American Medical Association 250:374–377

Schön D A 1983 The reflective practitioner. Temple Smith, London

Schuldam C 1999 A review of the impact of pre-operative education on recovery from surgery. International Journal of Nursing Studies 36:171–177

Schultz J H, Luthe W 1969 Autogenic therapy 1. Autogenic methods. Grune and Stratton, New York

Schwartz C E, Daltroy L H 1999 Learning from unreliability: the importance of inconsistency in coping dynamics. Social Science and Medicine 48:619–631

Schwartz L, Kraft G 1999 The role of spouse responses to disability and family environment in multiple sclerosis.

American Journal of Physical Medicine and Rehabilitation 78:525–532

Schwartz C E, Sendor M 1999 Helping others helps oneself: response shift effects in peer support. Social Science and Medicine 48:1563–1575

Scofield G R 1993 Ethical considerations in rehabilitation medicine. Archives of Physical Medicine and Rehabilitation 74:341–346

Scott R W 1993 For the public good. In Practice 1:83–85

Scudds R A, Li L 1997 Fibromyalgia: a 'model' chronic pain syndrome. Physiotherapy Theory and Practice 13:81–88

Scudds R J, Scudds R A, Simmonds M J 2001 Pain in the physical therapy PT curriculum: a faculty survey. Physiotherapy Theory and Practice 17:239–256

Seale J, Barnard S 1998 Therapy research: processes and practicalities. Butterworth-Heinemann, Oxford

Seedhouse D 1986 Health: the foundations for achievement. Wiley, Chichester

Seedhouse D 1988 Ethics: the heart of health care. Wiley, Chichester

Seedhouse D 1994 Fortress NHS: a philosophical review of the National Health Service. Wiley, Chichester

Seedhouse D, Cribb A 1989 Changing ideas in health care. Wiley, Chichester

Seedhouse D, Lovett L 1992 Practical medical ethics. Wiley, Chichester

Selander S 1990 Associative strategies in the process of professionalization: professional strategies and scientification of occupations. In: Burrage M, Torstendahl R (eds) Professions in theory and history. Sage Publications, London, pp 115–138

Severeijens R, Vlaeyen J W, van den Hout M A, Weber W E 2001 Pain catastrophizing predicts pain intensity, disability, and psychological distress independent of the level of physical impairment. Clinical Journal of Pain 17: 165–172

Seymour W 1998 Remaking the body: rehabilitation and change. Routledge, London

Shakespeare T 1992 A reply to Liz Crow. Coalition (September):40–42

Shakespeare T 2000 Help. Venture Press, Birmingham

Shakespeare T, Watson N 1997 Defending the social model. Disability and Society 12:293–300

Shakespeare T, Gillespie-Sells K, Davies D 1996 The sexual politics of disability. Cassell, London

Shanas E, Townsend P, Wedderburn D, Friis H, Milhøj P, Stehouwer J 1968 Old people in three industrial societies. Routledge and Kegan Paul, London

Sharp I 1998 Gender issues and the prevention and treatment of coronary heart disease. In: Doyal L (ed) Women and health services. Open University Press, Buckingham, pp 100–112

Sharp T J 2001 Chronic pain: a reformulation of the cognitive-behavioural model. Behaviour Research and Therapy 39:787–800

Sharpe P 1990 An assessment of the cognitive abilities of multiply handicapped children: adaptations of the Uzgiris and Hunt scales and their use with children in Britain and Singapore. Child: Care, Health and Development 16:335–353

Sheahan M S, Brockway N F 1992 The high risk infant. In: Tecklin J (ed) Pediatric physical therapy, 2nd edn. J P Lippincott, Philadelphia, pp 56–81

Sheldon J H 1948 The social medicine of old age: report of an enquiry in Wolverhampton. Geoffrey Cumberlege and Oxford University Press, London

Sheldon F 1998 Bereavement. British Medical Journal 316: 456–458

Shepherd E, Rafferty A M, James V 1996 Prescribing the boundaries of nursing practice: professional regulations and nurse prescribing. Nursing Times Research 1: 465–478

Sheridan M D 1992 Spontaneous play in early childhood. NFER-Nelson, Windsor

Shinebourne E A, Bush A 1994 For paternalism in the doctor–patient relationship. In: Gillon R, Lloyd A (eds) Principles of health care ethics. John Wiley, Chichester, pp 399–408

Shore M 1986 The Health Education Council 'look after yourself programme'. Physiotherapy 71:14–16

Short S D 1986 Physiotherapy – a feminine profession. Australian Journal of Physiotherapy 32:241–243

Shuldham C 1999 A review of the impact of pre-operative education on recovery from surgery. International Journal of Nursing Studies 36:171–177

Sidell M 2001 Understanding chronic illness. In: Heller T, Muston R, Sidell M, Lloyd C (eds) Working for health. Sage Publications, London, pp 255–265

Siegler M 1999 Confidentiality in medicine – a decrepit concept. In: Kuhse H, Singer P (eds). Bioethics: an anthology. Blackwell, Oxford, pp 490–492

Siegrist H 1990 Professionalization as a process: patterns, progression and discontinuity. In: Burrage M, Torstendahl R (eds) Professions in theory and history. Sage Publications, London, pp 177–201

Siegrist J 2000 The social causation of health and illness. In: Albrecht G L, Fitzpatrick R, Scrimshaw S C (eds) Handbook of social studies in health and medicine. Sage Publications, London, pp 100–114

Sim J 1983 Ethical considerations in physiotherapy. Physiotherapy 69:119–120

Sim J 1985 Physiotherapy: a professional profile. Physiotherapy Practice 1:14–22

Sim J 1986a Informed consent: ethical implications for physiotherapy. Physiotherapy 72:584–587

Sim J 1986b Truthfulness in the therapeutic relationship. Physiotherapy Practice 2:121–127

Sim J 1990a Physical disability, stigma, and rehabilitation. Physiotherapy Canada 42:232–238

Sim J 1990b The concept of health. Physiotherapy 76: 423–428

Sim J 1993 Sports medicine: some ethical issues. British Journal of Sports Medicine 27:95–100

Sim J 1996a Client confidentiality: ethical issues in occupational therapy. British Journal of Occupational Therapy 59:56–61

Sim J 1996b Informed consent and manual therapy. Manual Therapy 2:104–106

Sim J 1997a Ethical decision making in therapy practice. Butterworth-Heinemann, Oxford

Sim J 1997b Confidentiality and HIV status. Physiotherapy 83:90–96

Sim J 1998 Respect for autonomy: issues in neurological rehabilitation. Clinical Rehabilitation 12:3–10

Sim J 2002 Interpersonal aspects of care: communication, counselling and health education. In: Pryor J A, Prasad A (eds) Physiotherapy for respiratory and cardiac conditions. Churchill Livingstone, Edinburgh, pp 281–299

Sim J, Adams N 1999 Physical and other non-pharmacological interventions for fibromyalgia. Baillière's Clinical Rheumatology 13:507–523

Sim J, Adams N 2003 Therapeutic approaches to fibromyalgia syndrome in the United Kingdom: a survey of occupational therapists and physical therapists. European Journal of Pain 7:173–180

Sim J, Richardson B 2004 The use and generation of practice knowledge in the context of regulating systems and moral frameworks. In: Higgs J, Richardson B, Abrandt Dahlgren M (eds) Developing practice knowledge for health professionals. Butterworth-Heinemann, Edinburgh, pp 127–146

Sim J, Waterfield J 1997 Validity, reliability and responsiveness in the assessment of pain. Physiotherapy Theory and Practice 13:223–237

Sim J, Wright C 2000 Research in health care: concepts, designs and methods. Stanley Thornes, Cheltenham

Simmonds M 2000 Degrees of sense. Physiotherapy Theory and Practice 16:55–56

Singleton J 1996a Justifications for ethical principles. In: Aitken V, Jellicoe H (eds) Behavioural sciences for health professionals. W B Saunders, London, pp 233–240

Singleton J 1996b Ethical issues, ethical principles and codes of conduct. In: Aitken V, Jellicoe H (eds) Behavioural sciences for health professionals. W B Saunders, London, pp 227–232

Skevington S M 1990 A standardised scale to measure beliefs about controlling pain BPCQ: a preliminary study. Psychology and Health 4:221–232

Skevington S M 1995 Psychology of pain. John Wiley, Chichester

Skinner B F 1957 Verbal behaviour. Appleton-Century-Crofts, New York

Skinner C M 1986 Talking to small groups: a specialised skill. Physiotherapy 72:535–538

Slack P 1985 Projecting the facts. Nursing Times (April 3): 24–27

Sloman R, Ahern M, Wright A 2001 Nurses' knowledge of pain in the elderly. Journal of Pain and Symptom Management 21:317–322

Sluijs E M 1991 Patient education in physiotherapy: towards a planned approach. Physiotherapy 77:503–508

Sluijs E M, Van der Zee J, Kok G J 1993 Differences between physical therapists in attention paid to patient education. Physiotherapy Theory and Practice 9:103–117

Smail D 1993 The origins of unhappiness: a new understanding of personal distress. Constable, London

Smith M 1998 Talking about pain. In: Carter B (ed) Perspectives on pain: mapping the territory. Arnold, London, pp 26–45

Smith M V 1989 Language and pain: private experience, cultural significance, and linguistic relativity. Unpublished PhD thesis, University of Cambridge, Cambridge

Smith S K 2000 Sensitive issues in life story research. In: Moch S D, Gates M F (eds) The researcher experience in qualitative research. Sage Publications, Thousand Oaks, pp 13–21

Smith W L, Duerksen D L 1980 Personality in the relief of chronic pain: predicting surgical outcome. In: Smith W L, Merskey H, Gross S C (eds) Pain: meaning and management. S P Medical and Scientific Books, New York, pp 119–126

Smith P, Jones O R 1987 The philosophy of mind: an introduction. Cambridge University Press, Cambridge

Smith J A, Harré R, Van Langenhove L 1995 Rethinking methods in psychology. Sage Publications, London

Smith L, Dockrell J, Tomlinson P 1997 Piaget, Vygotsky and beyond. Routledge, London

Smith S, Roberts P, Balmer S 2000 Role overlap and professional boundaries: future implications for physiotherapy and occupational therapy in the NHS. Physiotherapy 86:397–400

Smyth T R 1992 Impaired motor skill clumsiness in otherwise normal children: a review. Child: Care, Health, and Development 18:283–300

Söderberg S, Norberg A 1995 Metaphorical pain language among fibromyalgia patients. Scandinavian Journal of Caring Sciences 9:55–59

Söderberg S, Lundman B, Norberg A 1999 Struggling for dignity: the meaning of women's experiences of living with fibromyalgia. Qualitative Health Research 9: 575–587

Solomon P 2001 Congruence between health professionals' and patients' pain ratings: a review of the literature. Scandinavian Journal of Caring Sciences 15:174–180

Somers M 1994 The narrative construction of identity: a relational and network approach. Theory and Society 23: 606–649

Sorrells-Jones J 1997 The challenge of making it real: interdisciplinary practice in a 'seamless' organization. Nursing Administration Quarterly 21:20–30

Southon G, Braithwaite J 1998 The end of professionalism? Social Science and Medicine 46:23–28

Spielberger C D, Gorsuch D L, Lushene R E 1970 Manual for the state-trait anxiety inventory. Consulting Psychologists Press, Palo Alto

Spinhoven P, Linssen A C G 1991 Behavioral treatment of chronic low back pain I. Relation of coping strategy use to outcome. Pain 45:29–34

Spitzer R L, Gibbon M, Skodol A E, Williams J B W, First M B 1989 DSM-III-R casebook. American Psychological Press, Washington

Sprangers M A G, de Regt E B, Andries F, van Agt H M E, Bijl R V, de Boer J B, Foets M, Hoeymans N, Jacobs A E, Kempen G I J M, Miedema H S, Tijhuis M A R, de Haes H C J M 2000 Which chronic conditions are associated with better or poorer quality of life? Journal of Clinical Epidemiology 53:895–907

Squires A, Hastings M 2002 Rehabilitation of the older person: a handbook for the interdisciplinary team. Nelson Thornes, Cheltenham

Stachura K 1994 Professional dilemmas facing physiotherapists. Physiotherapy 80:357–360

Stalker K 1998 Some ethical and methodological issues in research with people with learning difficulties. Disability and Society 13:5–19

Standing S 1999 The practice of working in partnership. In: Swain J, French S (eds) Therapy and learning difficulties: advocacy, participation and partnership. Butterworth-Heinemann, Oxford, pp 255–260

Stanton A L, Danoff-Burg S, Cameron C L, Bishop M, Collins C A, Kirk S, Sworowski L A, Twillman R 2000 Emotionally expressive coping predicts psychological and physical adjustment to breast cancer. Journal of Consulting and Clinical Psychology 68:875–882

Stedman's medical dictionary 1976 Stedman's medical dictionary, 23rd edn. Williams and Wilkins, Baltimore

Steen E, Haugli L 2000 Generalised chronic musculoskeletal pain as a rational reaction to a life situation? Theoretical Medicine 21:581–599

Stenstrom C, Bergman B, Dahlgren L 1993 Everyday life with rheumatoid arthritis: a phenomenographic study. Physiotherapy Theory and Practice 9:235–245

Stetter F, Kupper S 2002 Autogenic training: a meta-analysis of clinical outcome studies. Applied Psychophysiology and Biofeedback 27:45–98

Stevens R 1996 The reflexive self: an experiential perspective. In: Stevens R (ed) Understanding the self. Sage Publications, London, pp 147–218

Stewart T, Shields C 1985 Grief in chronic illness: assessment and management. Archives of Physical Medicine and Rehabilitation 66:447–450

Stiker H 1999 A history of disability. University of Michigan Press, Ann Arbor

Stillwell W 1998 Questioning voices. Center for Studies of the Person, La Jolla

Stimson G V 1976 General practitioners, 'trouble' and types of patients. In: Stacey M (ed) The sociology of the NHS. Sociological Review Monograph no. 2. University of Keele, Keele, pp 43–60

Stott L H, Ball R S 1965 Evaluation of infant and preschool mental tests: review and evaluation. Monographs of the Society for Research in Child Development 30:4–42

Strauss A A, Lehtinen L E 1947 Psychopathology and education of the brain-injured child. Grune and Stratton, New York

Strawson P F 1984 Individuals: an essay in descriptive metaphysics. Methuen, London

Stroebe M S 1992 Coping with bereavement: a review of the grief work hypothesis. Omega 26:19–42

Stroebe M, Gergen M M, Gergen K J, Stroebe W 1992 Broken hearts or broken bonds: love and death in historical perspective. American Psychologist 47:1205–1212

Strong J 1996 Chronic pain: the occupational therapist's perspective. Churchill Livingstone, Edinburgh

Strong J, Unruh A M, Wright A, Baxter G D 2002 Pain: a textbook for therapists. Churchill Livingstone, Edinburgh

Stuart O 1993 Double oppression: an appropriate starting point? In: Swain J, Finkelstein V, French S, Oliver M (eds) Disabling barriers – enabling environments. Sage Publications, London, pp 93–100

Stuberg W A 1992 The Milani-Comparetti motor development screening test, 3rd edn. University of Nebraska Medical Centre, Omaha

Studd J 1989 Prophylactic oophorectomy. British Journal of Obstetrics and Gynaecology 96:506–509

Stuifbergen A, Rogers S 1997 Health promotion: an essential component of rehabilitation for persons with chronic disabling conditions. Advances in Nursing Science 19: 1–20

Sullivan M 1998 The problem of pain in the clinicopathological method. Clinical Journal of Pain 14: 197–201

Sullivan M J L, D'Eon J L 1990 Relationship between catastrophizing and depression in chronic pain patients. Journal of Abnormal Psychology 99:260–263

Sullivan M J L, Bishop S R, Pivak J 1985 The pain catastrophizing scale: development and validation. Psychological Assessment 7:524–532

Sullivan M J L, Reesor K, Mikail S, Fisher R 1992 The treatment of depression in chronic low back pain: review; and recommendations. Pain 50:5–13

Sullivan M J, Stanish W, Waite H, Sullivan M, Tripp D A 1998 Catastrophizing, pain and disability in patients with soft tissue injuries. Pain 77:253–260

Summerfield P 1996 The women's movement in Britain from the 1860s to the 1980s. In: Coslett T, Easton A, Summerfield P (eds) Women, power and resistance: an introduction to women's studies. Open University Press, Buckingham, pp 227–237

Sutherland A T 1981 Disabled we stand. Souvenir Press, London

Sutherland B, Jensen L 2000 Living with change: elderly women's perceptions of having a myocardial infarction. Qualitative Health Research 10:661–676

Swain J 1995 The use of counselling skills: a guide for therapists. Butterworth-Heinemann, Oxford

Swain J, French S 1998 Normality and disabling care. In: Brechin A, Walmley J, Katz J, Peace S (eds) Care matters: concepts, practice and research in health and social care. Sage Publications, London, pp 81–95

Swain J, French S 2000 Towards an affirmative model of disability. Disability and Society 15:169–182

Swain J, Lawrence P 1994 Learning about disability: changing attitudes or challenging understanding? In: French S (ed) On equal terms: working with disabled people. Butterworth-Heinemann, Oxford, pp 87–102

Swain J, Finkelstein V, French S, Oliver M 1993 Disabling barriers – enabling environments. Sage Publications, London

Swain J, Gillman M, French S 1998a Confronting disabling barriers: towards making organisations accessible. Venture Press, Birmingham

Swain J, Heyman B, Gillman M 1998b Public research, private concerns: ethical issues in the use of open-ended interviews with people who have learning difficulties. Disability and Society 13:21–36

Swain J, French S, Cameron C 2003a Controversial issues in a disabling society. Open University Press, Buckingham

Swain J, Griffiths C, Heyman B 2003b Towards a social model approach to counselling disabled clients. British Journal of Guidance and Counselling 31:137–153

Swain J, Clark J, French S, Parry K, Reynolds F 2004 Enabling relationships in health and social care: a guide for therapists. Butterworth-Heinemann, Edinburgh

Swimmer G I, Robinson M E, Geisser M E 1992 The relationship of MMPI cluster type, pain coping strategy and treatment outcome. Clinical Journal of Pain 8: 131–137

Swisher L L 2002 A retrospective analysis of ethics knowledge in physical therapy, 1970–2000 . Physical Therapy 82:692–706

Swisher L L, Krueger-Brophy C 1998 Legal and ethical issues in physical therapy. Butterworth-Heinemann, Boston

Switankowsky I 2000 Dualism and its importance for medicine. Theoretical Medicine 21:567–580

Syrjala K L, Donaldon G W, Davis M W, Kippes M E, Carr J E 1995 Relaxation and imagery and cognitive-behavioral training reduces pain during cancer treatment: a controlled clinical trial. Pain 63:189–198

Tan S Y 1982 Cognitive and cognitive behavioural methods for pain control: a selective review. Pain 12:201–228

Tannahill A 1985 What is health promotion? Health Education Journal 44:167–168

Tansley P, Panckhurst J 1981 Children with specific learning difficulties. NFER-Nelson, Windsor

Tarasuk V, Eakin J M 2002 The problem of legitimacy in the experience of work-related back injury. Qualitative Health Research 5:204–221

Taubes G 2001 The soft science of dietary fat. Science 291: 2536–2545

Taylor F W 1911 Scientific management. Harper, New York

Taylor D N, Lee C T 1991 Lack of correlation between frontalis electromyography and self-ratings of either frontalis tension or state anxiety. Perceptual and Motor Skills 72:1131–1134

Taylor S E, Lichtman R R, Wood J V 1984 Attributions, beliefs about control and adjustment to breast cancer. Journal of Personality and Social Psychology 46: 489–502

Teichler U 1999 Higher education policy and the world of work: changing conditions and challenges. Higher Education Policy 12:285–312

Teichman J 1974 The mind and the soul: an introduction to the philosophy of the mind. Routledge and Kegan Paul, London

Teo P 1990 Hysterectomy: a change of trend or a change of heart? In: Roberts H (ed) Women's health counts. Routledge, London, pp 113–146

Thomas C 1999 Female forms: experiencing and understanding disability. Open University Press, Buckingham

Thomas S P 2000 A phenomenologic study of chronic pain. Western Journal of Nursing Research 22:683–705

Thomas C 2001 Feminism and disability: the theoretical and significance of the personal and the experiential. In: Barton L (ed) Disability politics and the struggle for change. David Fulton Publishers, London, pp 48–58

Thomas E, Silman A, Croft P R, Papageorgiou A C, Jayson M I V, Macfarlane G J 1999 Predicting who develops low back pain in primary care: a prospective study. British Medical Journal 318:1662–1667

Thompson N 1998 Promoting equality: challenging discrimination and oppression in the human services. Macmillan, Houndmills

Thompson N 2001 Anti-discriminatory practice, 3rd edn. Macmillan, London

Thompson S, Kyle D 2000 The role of perceived control in coping with the losses associated with chronic illness. In: Harvey J, Miller E (eds) Loss and trauma: general and close relationship perspectives. Brunner-Routledge, Philadelphia, pp 131–145

Tibbitts C 1960 Handbook of social gerontology: societal aspects of aging. Chicago University Press, Chicago

Tiedemann D 1787 Beobachtungen uber die Entwicklung der Seelenfahrrifkeiten bei Kindern. Bonde, Alterburg

Toombs S K 1988 Illness and the paradigm of the lived body. Theoretical Medicine 9:201–226

Toombs S K 1993 The meaning of illness: a phenomenological account of the different perspectives of physician and patient. Kluwer Academic Publishers, Dordrecht

Tornstam L 1992 The quo vadis of gerontology: on the scientific paradigm of gerontology. Gerontologist 32: 318–326

Totton N 1999 The baby and the bathwater: professionalisation in psychotherapy and counselling. British Journal of Guidance and Counselling 27:313–325

Townsend P 1957 The family life of old people: an inquiry in East London. Routledge and Kegan Paul, London

Townsend P, Whitehead M, Davidson N 1992 Inequalities in health: the Black report and the health divide. Penguin, Harmondsworth

Triezenberg H L 1996 The identification of ethical issues in physical therapy practice. Physical Therapy 76: 1097–1106

Triezenberg H L 1997 Teaching ethics in physical therapy education: a Delphi study. Journal of Physical Therapy Education 11:16–22

Trigg R 1970 Pain and emotion. Clarendon Press, Oxford

Trollope A 1993 The fixed period. Oxford University Press, Oxford

Truchon M 2001 Determinants of chronic disability related to low back pain: towards an integrative biopsychosocial model. Disability and Rehabilitation 23:758–767

Truman C, Mertens D, Humphries B 2000 Research and inequality. UCL Press, London

Turk C D, Okifuji A 1999 Assessment of patients' reporting of pain: an integrated perspective. Lancet 353: 1784–1788

Turk D C, Okifuji A, Sinclair J D, Starz T W 1996 Pain, disability and physical functioning in subgroups of patients with fibromyalgia. Journal of Rheumatology 23: 1255–1262

Turner J A 1982 Comparison of group progressive relaxation training and cognitive behavioural group therapy for chronic low back pain. Journal of Consulting and Clinical Psychology 50:757–765

Turner B S 1984 The body and society: explorations in social theory. Basil Blackwell, Oxford

Turner B S 1988 Medical power and social knowledge. Sage Publications, London

Turner P, Whitfield T W A 1997 Physiotherapists' use of evidence based practice: a cross-national study. Physiotherapy Research International 1:17–29

Turner J A, Jensen M P, Romano J M 2000 Do beliefs, coping, and catastrophizing independently predict functioning in patients with chronic pain? Pain 85:115–125

Turner J A, Dworkin S F, Mancl L, Huggins K H, Truelove E L 2001 The role of beliefs, catastrophizing and coping in the functioning of patients with temporomandibular disorders. Pain 92:41–51

Twomey L 1986 Physiotherapy and health promotion. Physiotherapy Practice 2:153–154

Ubel P A, Zell M M, Miller D J, Fischer G S, Peters-Stefani D, Arnold R M 1995 Elevator talk: observational study of inappropriate comments in a public space. American Journal of Medicine 99:190–194

Union of the Physically Impaired Against Segregation 1976 Fundamental principles of disability. Union of the Physically Impaired Against Segregation, London

Uzgiris I, Hunt J McV 1987 Infant performance and experience: new findings with the ordinal scales of psychological development. University of Illinois Press, Chicago

Uzgiris I, Hunt J McV 1989 Assessment in infancy: ordinal scales of psychological development, 2nd edn. University of Illinois Press, Chicago

Vallance Owen A 1992 The health debate live. British Medical Journal, London

Van der Hart O 1988 An imaginary leave-taking ritual in mourning therapy. International Journal of Clinical and Experimental Hypnosis 36:63–69

Van Sant A F 1994 Motor development. In: Tecklin J (ed) Pediatric physical therapy, 2nd edn. J B Lippincott, Philadelphia, pp 10–29

Van Staden C W, Krüger C 2003 Incapacity to give informed consent owing to mental disorder. Journal of Medical Ethics 29:41–43

van Tulder M, Malmivaara A, Esmail R, Koes B 2000a Exercise therapy for low back pain: a systematic review within the framework of the Cochrane Collaboration back review group. Spine 25:2784–2796

van Tulder M W, Ostelo R, Vlaeyen J W, Linton S J, Morley S J, Assendelft W J 2000b Behavioral treatment for chronic low back pain: a systematic review within the framework of the Cochrane back review group. Spine 25: 2688–2699

Vasey S 1992 Disability culture: it's a way of life. In: Rieser R, Mason M (eds) Disability equality in the classroom: a human rights issue. Disability Equality in Education, London, pp 74–75

Veatch R M 1973 Generalization of expertise: scientific expertise and value judgments. Hastings Center Studies (May 1):29–40

Veatch R M 1981 A theory of medical ethics. Basic Books, New York

Veatch R M, Spicer C M 1994 Against paternalism in the doctor–patient relationship. In: Gillon R, Lloyd A (eds) Principles of health care ethics. John Wiley, Chichester, pp 409–419

Ventafridda V 1989 Continuing care: a major issue in cancer pain management. Pain 36:137–143

Verbrugge L M, Wingard D L 1987 Sex differentials in health and mortality. Women and Health 12:103–143

Vernon A 1996 Fighting two different battles: unity is preferable to enmity. Disability and Society 11:285–290

Vines P 1996 Informed consent: from paternal benevolence to trust mediated by truthfulness. Australian Journal of Physiotherapy 42:245–246

Visentin M, Trentin L, de Marco R, Zanolin E 2001 Knowledge and attitudes of Italian medical staff towards the approach and treatment of patients in pain. Journal of Pain and Symptom Management 22:925–930

Vlaeyen J W S, Linton S J 2000 Fear-avoidance and its consequences in chronic musculoskeletal pain: a state of the art. Pain 85:317–332

Vlaeyen J W, Geurts S M, Kole-Snijders A M, Schuerman J A, Groenman N H, van Eek H 1990 What do chronic pain patients think of their pain? Towards a pain cognition questionnaire. British Journal of Clinical Psychology 29: 383–394

Vlaeyen J W S, Kole-Snijders A M J, Boeren R G B, van Eek H 1995 Fear of movement/reinjury in chronic low back pain and its relation to behavioural performance. Pain 62: 363–372

Vlaeyen J W, de Jong J, Geilen M, Heuts P H, van Breukelen G 2002 The treatment of fear of movement/reinjury in chronic low back pain: further evidence on the effectiveness of exposure in vivo. Clinical Journal of Pain 8:251–261

Vousden M 1987 Racism in the wards. Nursing Times 83:918

Vygotsky L 1934 Thinking and speech: psychological investigations. Gosudarstvennoe Sotsial'no-Ekonomicheskoe Izdatel'stvo, Moscow

Vygotsky L 1978 Mind in society: the development of higher psychological processes. Harvard University Press, Cambridge

Vygotsky L 1981 The genesis of higher mental functions. In: Wertsch J V (ed) The concept of activity in Soviet psychology. Sharpe, Armonk, pp 134–143

Waddell G 1998 The back pain revolution. Churchill Livingstone, Edinburgh

Waddell G, Main C J 1984 Assessment of severity in low-back disorders. Spine 9:204–208

Waddell G, Turk D C 2001 Clinical assessment of low back pain. In: Turk D C, Melzack R (eds) Handbook of pain assessment, 2nd edn. Guilford Press, New York, pp 431–453

Waddell G, Waddell H 2000 A review of social influences on neck and back pain and disability. In: Nachemson A L,

Jonsson E (eds) Neck and back pain: the scientific evidence of causes, diagnosis, and treatment. Lippincott, Williams and Wilkins, Philadelphia, pp 13–55

Waddell G, Newton M, Henderson I, Somerville D, Main C 1993 A fear-avoidance beliefs questionnaire (FABQ) and the role of fear-avoidance beliefs in chronic low back pain and disability. Pain 52.157–168

Waddie N A 1996 Language and pain expression. Journal of Advanced Nursing 23:868–872

Wade J B, Dougherty L M, Hart R P, Cook D B 1992a Patterns of normal personality structure among chronic pain patients. Pain 48:37–43

Wade J B, Dougherty L M, Hart R P, Rafii A, Price D D 1992b A canonical correlation analysis of the influence of neuroticism and extraversion on chronic pain, suffering, and pain behaviour. Pain 51:67–73

Wade J B, Dougherty L M, Archer C R, Price D D 1996 Assessing stages of pain processing: a multivariate analytical approach. Pain 68:157–167

Wagstaff G F 1982 A small dose of common sense: communication, persuasion and physiotherapy. Physiotherapy 68:327–329

Walker R, Ahmad W I U 1994 Windows of opportunity in rotting frames: care providers' perspectives on community care. Critical Social Policy 40:46–49

Walker J, Holloway I, Sofaer B 1999 In the system: the lived experience of chronic back pain from the perspectives of those seeking help from pain clinics. Pain 80:621–628

Wall P D 1995 Overview of pain and its mechanisms. In: Shacklock M O (ed) Moving in on pain. Butterworth-Heinemann, Chatswood, p 13

Wall P 1999 Pain: the science of suffering. Weidenfeld and Nicolson, London

Wallston K A 1989 Assessment of control in health care settings. In: Steptoe A, Appels A (eds) Stress personal control and health. John Wiley, Chichester, pp 85–106

Wallston K A, Wallston B S, DeVellis R 1978 Development of multidimensional health locus of control (MHLC) scales. Health Education Monographs 6:161–170

Walmsley J 1993 Contradictions in caring: reciprocity and interdependence. Disability, Handicap and Society 8: 129–141

Walmsley J 2001 Normalisation, emancipatory research and inclusive research in learning disability. Disability and Society 16:187–205

Walsh M P 1995 Living after a death. Columba Press, Dublin

Walt G 2001 Health care in the developing world, 1974 to 2001. In: Webster C (ed) Caring for health: history and diversity. Open University, Buckingham, pp 253–294

Walter T 1999 On bereavement: the culture of grief. Open University Press, Buckingham

Waring E M, Weisz G M, Bailey S I 1976 Predictive factors in the treatment of low back pain by surgical intervention. In: Bonica J J, Albe-Fessard D (eds) Advances in pain research and therapy. Raven Press, New York, pp 939–942

Warnock M 1977 Schools of thought. Faber and Faber, London

Warren M D 1985 Promoting health and preventing disease and disability – an introduction to concepts,

opportunities and practice: a review, part I. Physiotherapy Practice 1:57–63

Warren M D 1986 Promoting health and preventing disease and disability – an introduction to concepts, opportunities and practice, part II. Physiotherapy Practice 2:3–10

Warren C D 1988 Review and synthesis of nine nursing studies on care and caring. Journal of the New York State Nurses Association 19:10–16

Watson M J 1988 New dimensions of human caring theory. Nursing Science Quarterly 1:175–181

Watson J, Ray M A 1988 The ethics of care and the ethics of cure: synthesis in chronicity. National League for Nursing, University of Colorado Publication Center for Human Caring, Colorado

Watts F N, McKenna F P, Sharrock R, Trezise L 1986 Colour naming of phobia related words. British Journal of Clinical Psychology 77:97–108

Webb P 1994a Teaching and learning about health and illness. In: Webb P (ed) Health promotion and patient education: a professional's guide. Chapman and Hall, London, pp 21–37

Webb P 1994b The sociology of health and illness. In: Webb P (ed) Health promotion and patient education: a professional's guide. Chapman and Hall, London, pp 3–20

Webster C 1994 Tuberculosis. In: Seale C, Pattinson S (eds) Medical knowledge: doubt and certainty. Open University Press, Buckingham, pp 36–59

Wechsler D 1974 Wechsler intelligence scale for children – revised. Psychological Corporation, New York

Weitzenkamp D, Gerhart K, Charlifue S, Whiteneck G, Glass C, Kennedy P 2000 Ranking the criteria for assessing quality of life after disability: evidence for priority shifting among long-term spinal cord injury survivors. British Journal of Health Psychology 5:57–70

Weller B 1991 Nursing in a multicultural world. Nursing Standard 5(30):31–32

Wendell S 1996 The rejected body: feminist philosophical reflections on disability. Routledge, London

Wendell S 1997 Towards a feminist theory of disability. In: Davis J L (ed) The disability studies reader. Routledge, London, pp 260–278

Werner H, Kaplan B 1963 Symbol formation. Wiley, New York

Werner A, Malterud K 2003 Is it hard work behaving as a credible patient: encounters between women with chronic pain and their doctors. Social Science and Medicine 57:1409–1419

Werner A, Steihaug S, Malterud K 2003 Encountering the continuing challenges for women with chronic pain: recovery through recognition. Qualitative Health Research 13:491–509

Wertsch J V, Tulviste P 1996 L S Vygotsky and contemporary developmental psychology. In: Daniels H (ed) An introduction to Vygotsky. Routledge, London, pp 53–74

Wesley A L, Gatchel R J, Garofalo J P, Polatin P B 1999 Toward more accurate use of the Beck depression inventory with chronic back pain patients. Clinical Journal of Pain 15:117–121

Wetherell M, Maybin J 1996 The distributed self: a social constructionist perspective. In: Stevens R (ed) Understanding the self. Sage Publications, London, pp 219–279

Wethington E, Moen P, Glasgow N, Pillemer K 2000 Multiple roles, social integration, and health. In: Pillemer K, Moen P (eds) Social integration in the second half of life. Johns Hopkins University Press, Baltimore, pp 48–71

Whitbeck C 1981 A theory of health. In: Caplan A L, Englehardt H T, McCartney J J (eds) Concepts of health and disease: interdisciplinary perspective. Addison-Wesley, Reading, pp 611–626

White K 2002 An introduction to the sociology of health and illness. Sage Publications, London

White M, Epston D 1990 Narrative means to therapeutic ends. Norton, New York

White P D, Naish V A B 2001 Graded exercise therapy for chronic fatigue syndrome: an audit. Physiotherapy 87: 285–288

Whitehead M 1988 The health divide. Penguin Books, Harmondsworth

Whitehead M 1989 Swimming upstream: trends and prospects in education for health. Research Report no. 5. King's Fund, London

Whittaker C A 1980 A note on developmental trends in the symbolic play of hospitalized profoundly retarded children. Journal of Child Psychology and Psychiatry and Allied Disciplines 21:253–261

Whittaker C A 1984 Cognitive development and aspects of prelinguistic and manual communication in severely and profoundly retarded children. Paper by proxy to the American Academy of Child Psychiatry, Toronto, October

Whittaker C A 1996 Spontaneous proximal communication in children with autism and severe learning disabilities: issues for therapeutic intervention. Paper to International Conference on Therapeutic Interventions in Autism: Perspectives from Research and Practice, April 1–3, 1996, College of St Hild and St Bede, University of Durham, Durham

Whittaker C A 1997 Key issues in the psychological development of the child: implications for physiotherapy practice. In: French S (ed) Physiotherapy: a psychosocial approach, 2nd edn. Butterworth-Heinemann, Oxford, pp 379–395

Whittaker C, Potter C 1999 Inclusive schools need an inclusive national curriculum. In: Swain J, French S (eds) Therapy and learning difficulties: advocacy, participation and partnership. Butterworth-Heinemann, Oxford, pp 131–145

Whittaker C A, Reynolds J 2000 Hand signalling in dyadic proximal communication: social strengths of children with autism who do not speak. Child Language Teaching and Therapy 16:43–57

Whitty P, Jones I 1995 Public health heresy: a challenge to the purchasing orthodoxy. In: Davey B, Gray A, Seale C (eds) Health and disease: a reader, 2nd edn. Open University Press, Buckingham, pp 384–387

Widdershoven G A M 1993 The story of life: hermeneutic perspectives on the relationship between narrative and life history. In: Josselson R, Lieblich A (eds) The narrative study of lives, vol. 1. Sage Publications, Thousand Oaks, pp 1–20

Widdershoven G A M, Smits M-J 1996 Ethics and narratives. In: Josselson R (ed) The narrative study of lives, vol. 4. Ethics and process. Sage Publications, Thousand Oaks, pp 275–287

Wiedenfeld S A, O'Leary A, Bandura A, Brown S, Levine S, Raska K 1990 Impact of perceived self-efficacy in coping with stressors on components of the immune system. Journal of Personality and Social Psychology 59:1082–1094

Wiener C L 1975 The burden of rheumatoid arthritis: tolerating the uncertainty. Social Science and Medicine 9: 97–104

Wikstrom I, Isacsson A, Jacobsson L 2001 Leisure activities in rheumatoid arthritis: change after disease onset and associated factors. British Journal of Occupational Therapy 64:87–92

Wilding P 1982 Professional power and social welfare. Routledge and Kegan Paul, London

Wilensky H L 1964 The professionalization of everyone? American Journal of Sociology 70:137–158

Wilkinson R G 2001 Social status, inequality and health. In: Heller T, Muston R, Sidell M, Lloyd C (eds) Working for health. Sage Publications, London, pp 69–76

Wilkinson S, Kitzinger C 1994 Women and health: feminist perspectives. Taylor and Francis, London

Williams B 1985 Are persons bodies? In: Williams B (ed) Problems of the self. Cambridge University Press, Cambridge, pp 76–81

Williams J I 1986 Physiotherapy is handling. Physiotherapy 72:66–70

Williams J I 1989 Illness behaviour to wellness behaviour: the 'school for bravery' approach. Physiotherapy 75:2–7

Williams A 1997 Pitfalls on the road to ethical approval. Nurse Researcher 5(1):15–22

Williams A C deC 1999 Measures of function and psychology. In: Wall P D, Melzack R (eds) Textbook of pain, 4th edn. Churchill Livingstone, Edinburgh, pp 427–444

Williams B, Barlow J 1998 Falling out with my shadow: lay perceptions of the body in the context of arthritis. In: Nettleton S, Watson J (eds) The body in everyday life. Routledge, London, pp 124–141

Williams D A, Keefe F J 1991 Pain beliefs and the use of cognitive-behavioral coping strategies. Pain 46:185–190

Williams A C deC, Richardson P H 1993 What does the BDI measure in chronic pain? Pain 55:259–266

Williams P L, Webb C 1994 Clinical supervision skills: a Delphi and critical incident technique study. Medical Teacher 16:139–158

Williams A C deC, Richardson P H, Nicholas M K, Pither C E, Harding V R, Ridout K L, Ralphs J A, Richardson I H, Justins D M, Chamberlain J H 1996 Inpatient vs outpatient pain management: results of a randomised controlled trial. Pain 66:13–22

Williams J M G, Watts F N, MacLeod C, Mathews A 1997 Cognitive psychology and emotional disorders, 2nd edn. John Wiley, Chichester

Wilson L 1989 Dilemma of 172 recorded languages. Therapy Weekly 16(20):3

Wilson J 1999 Acknowledging the expertise of patients and their organisations. British Medical Journal 319: 771–774

Wiltse L L, Rocchio P D 1975 Preoperative psychological tests as predictors of success of chemonucleolysis in the treatment of low-back syndrome. Journal of Bone and Joint Surgery American 57:478–483

Wing L, Gould J, Yeats S R, Brierley L M 1977 Symbolic play in severely mentally retarded and in autistic children. Journal of Child Psychology and Psychiatry and Allied Disciplines 18:167–178

Winslade J, Crocket K, Monk G 1996 The therapeutic relationship. In: Monk G, Winslade J, Crocket K, Epston D (eds) Narrative therapy in practice: the archaeology of hope. Jossey-Bass, San Francisco, pp 53–81

Wittink H, Hoskins Michel T 1997 Chronic pain management for physical therapists. Butterworth-Heinemann, Boston

Witz A 1992 Professions and patriarchy. Routledge, London

Wolff M S, Michel T H, Krebs D E, Watts N T 1991 Chronic pain – assessment of orthopedic physical therapists' knowledge and attitudes. Physical Therapy 71:207–214

Woodward R V, Broom D H, Legge D G 1995 Diagnosis in chronic illness: disabling or enabling – the case of chronic fatigue syndrome. Journal of the Royal Society of Medicine 88:325–329

Woolley M 1993 Acquired hearing loss: acquired oppression. In: Swain J, Finkelstein V, French S, Oliver M (eds) Disabling barriers – enabling environments. Sage Publications, London, pp 78–84

Worden J W 1976 Personal death awareness. Prentice-Hall, Englewood Cliffs

Worden J W 1983 Grief counselling and grief therapy. Tavistock Publications, London

Worden J W 1991 Grief counselling and grief therapy, 2nd edn. Springer, New York

World Bank 1994 Averting the old age crisis: policies to protect the old and promote growth. Oxford University Press, New York

World Health Organization 1946 Constitution. World Health Organization, Geneva

World Health Organization 1977 Health for all by the year 2000. World Health Organization, Geneva

World Health Organization 1978 The declaration of Alma Ata. World Health Organization, Geneva

World Health Organization 1985 Health for all in Europe by the year 2000: regional targets. World Health Organization, Copenhagen

World Health Organization 1988 Learning to work together for health. World Health Organization, Geneva

Worthington R C 1989 The chronically ill child and recurring family grief. Journal of Family Practice 29:397–400

Wright R 1969 Hysterectomy: past, present and future (editorial). Obstetrics and Gynecology 33.560–563

Wright C 1973 Personal view. British Medical Journal 4:45

Wright-St Clair V 2001 Caring: the moral motivation for good occupational therapy practice. Australian Occupational Therapy Journal 48:187–199

Wringe C 1991 Education, schooling and the world of work. In: Corson D (ed) Education for work: background to policy and curriculum. Multilingual Matters, Clevedon, pp 33–46

Yandell D 1999 Did Descartes abandon dualism? The nature of the union of mind and body. British Journal for the History of Philosophy 7:199–217

Yardley L 1999 Understanding embodied experience: beyond mind–body dualism in health research. In: Murray M, Chamberlain K (eds) Qualitative health psychology: theories and methods. Sage Publications, London, pp 31–46

Yirmiya N, Shulman C 1995 Seriation, conservation and theory of mind abilities in individuals with autism, mental retardation and normal development. Proceedings of the International Conference on Psychological Perspectives in Autism. Autism Research Unit, Sunderland, pp 105–116

Young J, McNicoll, P 1998 Against all odds: positive life experiences of people with advanced amyotrophic lateral sclerosis. Health and Social Work 23:35–43

Zarb G 1992 On the road to Damascus: first steps towards changing the relations of research production. Disability, Handicap and Society 7:125–138

Zarb G 1995 Modelling the social model of disability. Critical Public Health 6:21–29

Zautra A J, Manne S L 1992 Coping with rheumatoid arthritis: a review of a decade of research. Annals of Behavioral Medicine 14:31–39

Zautra A, Burleson M, Smith C, Blalock S 1995 Arthritis and perceptions of quality of life: an examination of positive and negative affect in rheumatoid arthritis patients. Health Psychology 14:399–408

Zborowski M 1952 Cultural components in responses to pain. Journal of Social Issues 8:16–30

Zborowski M 1969 People in pain. Jossey-Bass, San Francisco

Zigmond A S, Snaith R P 1983 The hospital anxiety and depression scale. Acta Psychiatrica Scandinavica 67: 361–370

Zola I K 1966 Culture and symptoms – an analysis of patients' presenting complaints. American Sociological Review 31:615–630

Zwarenstein M, Reeves S, Barr H, Hammick M, Koppel L, Atkins J 2002 Interprofessional education: effects on professional practice and healthcare outcomes. Cochrane Review. Cochrane Library, 2. Update Software, Oxford

Index

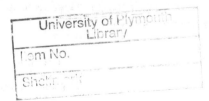